Natural Cures®

Secrets "They" Don't Want You to Know About

New & Updated for 2014

Natural Cures®

Secrets "They" Don't Want
You to Know About

New & Updated for 2014

Kevin Trudeau

Natural Cures® Secrets "They" Don't Want You to Know About Updated & New for 2014

This edition published by Natural Press, LLC
For information, address:

Natural Press, LLC
PO Box 8568
Pueblo, CO 81001

ISBN 13: 978-0-9911782-1-6

Interior design: The Printed Page, Phoenix, AZ

Manufactured in the United States of America

10 9 8 7 6 5 4 3 2 1

First Version

Contents

DISCLAIMER

You must know that everything I say in this book is simply my opinion and that there are many people who vehemently disagree with my conclusions. If you do anything I recommend without the supervision of a licensed medical doctor, it is at your own risk. The publisher, the author, the distributors and bookstores, present this information for educational purposes only. I am not making an attempt to prescribe any medical treatment, since under the laws of the United States only a licensed medical doctor (an MD) can do so. (How sad!)

This book contains only my opinions, thoughts, and conclusions. Again, it is for educational purposes only and you and only you are responsible if you choose to do anything based on what you read.

Kevin Trudeau

Acknowledgments

I would like to acknowledge the many people around the world who helped make this book and this mission possible. I can't name you all, but you know who you are. It's an honor to serve with you on this noble mission to educate the world about the evils of greed and the benefits of using natural methods to prevent and cure disease.

Ironically, I'd also like to thank the Federal Trade Commission and the Food and Drug Administration. Both agencies have inspired me to write this book, much like Goliath inspired David; and like David, with my measly slingshot I vow to help stop the needless suffering that their corruption has caused millions of people around the world.

Read This First

I congratulate you for having the courage to read this book. Your interest tells me that you're either sick and looking for natural cures, or you're worried about getting sick. You may also be concerned about the health and wellbeing of your family and friends. In order to get the most benefit from the information presented here, it's imperative that you read the book from start to finish. Don't jump ahead, or jump around the book looking for an immediate answer to a health related question. This applies to those of you who've seen my infomercial and may want the answer to a specific illness mentioned in the program. All of the information is presented in a specific order for a reason. Please be assured that if you start at the beginning and read the book in its entirety, by the time you reach the end you'll have a better understanding of the cause of your disease and you'll know that there is a natural cure for it. You'll also know what steps to take in order to cure yourself and remain healthy for life without drugs and surgery.

Please note that there are many important concepts discussed within these pages. Because these concepts are an important foundation to everything else that I discuss, in many instances I repeat them. This is done purposely, because in order for you to benefit from this information you must absolutely know, backwards and forwards, the basic foundational principles.

So let's begin the journey, and when you reach the end of this book I promise you, you'll never be the same!

Yours in health,

Kevin Trudeau

Introduction

Bill Gates was interviewed on The Larry King Show and when asked about his incredible wealth and success, he said "Larry, I was at the right place at the right time, and luck has a lot to do with that."

I believe that by reading this book, you are at the right place at the right time, right now. Maybe luck has something to do with it.

Bill continued, "But Larry, there were a lot of people at the same place I was. One difference was I had vision. I saw the potential that was there. And I took massive and immediate action."

Folks, as you read this book, will you see the potential that utilizing this information can have on your own health and wellbeing? Do you have the vision that you can prevent and cure almost all illness and disease with natural methods, without drugs, and without surgery? And will you take massive and immediate action by implementing the recommendations? If you do, you will succeed in your quest for longevity, health, and vitality.

There are natural cures for virtually every disease. The drug companies, the government, and a host of other organizations do not want you to know what these natural cures are. This book will give them to you. Since I first published it, I've received tens of thousands of letters and emails from people all around the world telling me how utilizing the information I've shared has changed their lives for the better. I hope it will have a positive impact on your life as well.

You'll be learning some new and exciting things here. The concepts are logical, easy to understand, and filled with common sense. However, the conclusions go against conventional wisdom. For you to fully grasp this information it's important that you ask yourself now just how "teachable" you are.

There is, in fact, a "teachability index," which will determine how easy learning new concepts will be for you. This teachability index consists of two variables. First, is your willingness to learn. Since you purchased this book, and you're taking the time to read it, on a scale of one to ten, you probably have a pretty high willingness to learn. However, the second variable is your willingness to accept change. If you're a ten on willingness to learn, but a zero on willingness to accept change, ten times zero is zero; therefore, your teachability index is nonexistent.

You must have a high willingness to accept change in order to fully grasp these concepts and benefit from them. I sincerely hope that you have a high teachability index.

As you read, please consider another important component to fully implementing the information in your daily life. Information is only useful when it is used. It can only be used when it's fully internalized; when you don't have to "think about it."

The four stages one goes through when learning any new information are:

1. Unconscious incompetence—this is the stage where you don't know that you don't know.

2. Conscious incompetence—this is the stage where you know you don't know.

3. Conscious competence—this is when you know that you know, but you have to consciously think about it.

4. Unconscious competence—this is when it's second nature; when the information is part of you and you know it as intrinsically as you know your own name; it's fully internalized and automatic.

When you read this book you'll go through the first three stages. When you finish, you'll have to implement the information for a time before reaching level four. When you do, you will quite possibly live a life that's healthy and disease free. You might even be fortunate enough to never get sick again. That may sound ambitious, but it is a real possibility. If you're ready, let the journey begin.

I Should Be Dead By Now

I was driving down the Tri-State Highway outside of Chicago, Illinois, in my brand new Corvette enjoying a beautiful sunny day. Suddenly I felt an enormous ripping pain in my chest. I could barely breathe; the pain was excruciating. I immediately pulled off to the side of the road. My life virtually flashed before my eyes and I thought, "Oh my God I'm having a heart attack and I'm only twenty-one years old!"

Just as quickly as the pain came, it vanished. I was left disoriented, and in a state of shock about what had just happened. I looked down at my new car phone, (yes, in the good old days before cell phones). I picked it up, called my secretary, and said, "I think I just had a heart attack."

Luckily within a few moments I felt fine. I figured that if it was a heart attack, it most likely didn't cause any major damage. But something was obviously wrong.

Over the next week I was examined by three of the top heart specialists in America. Through the use of the most advanced medical diagnostic devices, I learned that I had been born with a deformed heart; a severe mitral valve prolapse that would cause me major problems for the rest of my life. There was no cure.

Skeptical, yet open to new ideas...What did I have to lose?

These top medical minds recommended experimental drugs, or risky surgery, both of which I was told had little promise. My life expectancy was to be very short.

I struggled to come up with an effective plan that could solve my medical dilemma. I was twenty-one years old with my whole life in front of me. I had to do something!

Months earlier I'd attended a lecture wherein I heard about a Harvard medical doctor named Yiwen Y. Tang, founder of the Century Clinic in Reno, Nevada. (Today the clinic is called Sierra Integrative Medical Center.) This MD, who'd been a MASH surgeon during the Korean War, had decided that standard medical procedures—drugs and surgery were not the best way to cure and prevent diseases. Instead, he was using a diagnostic device developed in Germany by Dr. Reinhold Voll called the Dermatron machine. Allegedly, in a matter of minutes, it could diagnose a person's medical problems. When the diagnosis was complete, homeopathic remedies were given to correct the imbalances and reverse and cure the disease.

At the time it sounded like hocus pocus. The words homeostasis, holistic healing, homeopathic remedies, acupuncture meridians, energy frequencies, imbalances, and the like were used in the lecture, replacing the standard vernacular that I knew: germs, bacteria, viruses, drugs, surgery, and genetics. Skeptical, yet open to new ideas, I flew to Reno to meet Dr. Tang. What did I have to lose?

Upon my arrival, the doctor asked me why I was there. Most of his patients were old and had severe medical problems. I, on the other hand, appeared to be healthy, and young, so he was puzzled by my desire for a diagnosis. I wanted to see if this Dermatron machine was legitimate, so I simply said, "I feel great. I just want a basic checkup."

He tested me with his magic machine and within two minutes the probe touched my heart meridian and registered very low energy. Dr. Tang looked at me with concern and said, "Son you have a heart problem." I was shocked by how quickly the diagnosis came. He just as quickly said, "Let me find out where it is."

He touched other meridian points. When he got to the mitral valve, once again, the machine registered very low energy. He looked at me and said matter-of-factly, "You have a mitral valve prolapse."

Needless to say, I was impressed. The medical doctors took days of testing to diagnose my mitral valve prolapse. This "energy machine" diagnosed it within minutes. I looked at Dr. Tang and said, "Yes I know, and I understand it's incurable." His response startled me. "In America it's incurable, but there are natural treatments in other countries that can reverse this problem in a matter of weeks. Unfortunately the FDA has not approved these treatments. So, yes, in America it is incurable."

He went on to explain a procedure of live cell injections that was available in Switzerland, or Mexico, but not accessible via legal treatment in the United States. The procedure would correct the problem by rebuilding the heart, ensuring that it would never return. I couldn't believe my ears. Effective natural treatments that are not approved by the FDA? Impossible!

This happened over twenty years ago. The treatment was inexpensive, all natural, painless, quick, and it *worked*. And to this day, that therapy is still illegal in America.

The most amazing part of this story is, after I received the natural treatment that was forbidden in America, I went back to the medical doctors who originally diagnosed my heart problem and asked to be tested again. My request was met with indignation. I was told that being tested again was a waste of time and money because it was impossible for the condition to change in two months. I demanded that they retest me anyway. The doctors humored me and they were stunned to find that I no longer had a mitral valve prolapse.

I was so excited to share how my problem had been cured. I thought certainly these doctors would want to know about an all natural treatment that could cure the incurable. Imagine my shock when I was told that the treatment could not have cured my disease but, rather, I must have been misdiagnosed in the first place. They tried to tell me that I never actually had the condition.

I couldn't believe my ears. These medical doctors would not accept the facts: I had a severe mitral valve prolapse—the pictures confirmed it; and then I no longer had a mitral valve prolapse—the pictures confirmed that, too.

I began to think of all of the people who would come to these medical doctors only to be told the bold-faced lie that their condition was incurable and could only be treated with drugs and surgery. Knowing that the established medical community would deny the existence of natural cures, and allow millions of people to suffer, and in many cases die, absolutely enraged me.

That event set in motion my lifelong mission of searching for natural remedies that don't include drugs or surgery, and natural treatments that prevent and cure illness and disease. It also exposed me to the organizations, companies, and government agencies that do not want you to know about these cures.

Today I live a full, healthy, and dynamic life. I don't take any drugs and I've had no surgeries. I haven't had a prescription or nonprescription drug in over twenty years. I virtually never get sick. Colds, flu, and all illnesses seem to pass me by. I've had numerous blood tests and other diagnostic tests every few years, just to make sure everything is within the normal range. The medical professionals who've examined and reviewed these results are amazed at the level of health that I enjoy. Am I lucky? Is it just genetics? Or are there some specific things that one can do to have a disease and illness-free life and enjoy vibrant health? Is it possible for you to go week after week, year after year, and never get sick? I strongly believe the answer is yes. This book specifically outlines the following things:

✔ Yes, there are all natural non-drug and nonsurgical cures for most every illness and disease.

✔ Yes, there are organizations, government agencies, companies and entire industries that are spending billions of dollars trying to hide these natural cures from you.

✔ Yes, every single nonprescription and prescription drug has adverse side effects and should virtually never be taken (with exceptions that I'll explain later).

It's important to note that I'm oversimplifying things in this book. That's because I'm not writing it for the medical community, scientists, researchers, or MDs. They're not going to agree with anything I say anyway. I'm writing this in plain English so that you can understand it.

Medical science always presents things as fact when actually it's opinion, based on information they have at the time. Throughout history, medical "facts" have been disproved time and time again.

The medical industry presents itself as the only source of truth when it comes to health, illness, and disease. They use words like "credible scientific evidence," "scientifically tested," and "scientifically proven." But what they're really presenting are theories, and theories change constantly. Here are examples of "medical facts" that have been proven wrong:

✔ Bloodletting was once proven to cure most illnesses. Now it is considered totally ineffective.

✔ Margarine was considered healthier than butter. Now research suggests that the opposite is true.

✔ Eggs were considered bad because of high cholesterol. Now research suggests that they aren't bad at all, they're actually healthy.

✔ Alcohol in all forms was said to be unhealthy and therefore should not be consumed. Then the medical community said that red wine was actually healthy for the heart, but other forms of alcohol were not. Now "medical science" says that all alcohol in moderation has health benefits.

✔ Chocolate and oily foods were touted to be a cause of acne. Now research suggests that they don't contribute to acne.

✔ Coffee was thought to be unhealthy. Now it's been discovered that coffee is a major source of antioxidants as well as a protective against liver cancer.

✔ Coconut oil was believed to be an unhealthy saturated fat. Now science says that coconut oil does not have a negative effect on cholesterol and is in fact good for the heart.

✔ Homosexuality was once classified as a disease.

✔ Medical doctors claimed that baby formula was much better than breast milk for children. Now the exact opposite is shown to be true.

✔ Milk was recommended for coating the stomach and alleviating stomach ulcers. Now it's discouraged and has been found to aggravate ulcers.

✔ Medical science at one time stated that diet had no effect on disease or illness. Now we're told that diet has a huge effect on the prevention and cause of disease.

✔ Medical science once had evidence that removing the tonsils and the appendix improved health and should be done to virtually everyone. Now the medical community has reversed that theory.

✔ Children with asthma were told to stay in enclosed pool areas because the humidity was good for their condition. Now research suggests that the chlorine in the air from pools actually makes asthma worse.

✔ The most obvious example of all is the fact that there are thousands of drugs that have been approved by the FDA because they were scientifically proven to cure, or prevent disease, and they were found to be safe to use. Then, years later, they've been taken off the market because they either did not cure or prevent those diseases, or the side effects were so adverse that they're too dangerous to use.

It saddens me when I see doctors on TV stating things as *fact* when they should be qualifying their comments with such phrases as: "it appears," "based on the current research we have," "it seems that," or "we believe this to be true, however, we also know that as more research and observations are evaluated this may change in the future."

This is not happening. Medical doctors are still looked upon as gods. Whatever they say is taken as absolutely true. No one else can say anything about health, illness, or disease with the credibility of a medical doctor. In my opinion, that's just wrong. Medical doctors are trained to prescribe drugs, or cut out parts of a person's anatomy (surgery). They aren't trained in preventing disease and, most importantly, they have little to no training in, or exposure to treatments other than drugs or surgery.

> They aren't trained in preventing disease...

Another example of medical facts reversed is the diet industry. First, a low-calorie diet was said to be the only way to lose weight. Then experts said, "It's not the calories, but the amount of fat you consume that will determine your weight." Now the rage of the day is "It's not the calories and it's not the fat, it's sugar and the high-glycemic carbohydrates that cause obesity." The fact is, nobody really knows.

A hundred years ago people believed they knew all there was about the cure and prevention of disease. We look back at them and we're amazed at just how little they really knew. We laugh at the thought of something like bloodletting curing a disease. Well, guess what? Fifty years from now people will laugh when they look at some of the archaic and horrible so-called cures that we're using today.

I realize that as more research and data become available, there's an excellent chance that many of the theories and opinions I've included in this book may be modified, improved, or even changed completely. Well, since there are virtually no medical facts, only medical opinions, you'll need to choose the opinion that makes the best sense for you.

How did I come up with my opinions? I've traveled over five million miles to bring you this information. I've been in all fifty states in the U.S. and traveled to countries all over the world. Over the last twenty years I have talked with thousands of healthcare providers. I've listened to tens of thousands of people who've had serious medical conditions cured by natural therapies; many after drugs and surgery had failed them.

I have so much firsthand experience with this that I believe I have the unique perspective necessary to come up with my bold conclusions. The biggest acknowledgment I must give is to the tens of thousands of dedicated healthcare professionals around the world who refuse to use drugs and surgery, yet routinely see their patients cured of diseases and go on to live vibrant healthy lives. These natural healthcare providers see people cured of cancer, diabetes, heart disease, chronic pain, headaches, arthritis, allergies, depression, and the list goes on.

The question is no longer whether diseases can be prevented or cured faster and more effectively without drugs and surgery. The real question is why are healthcare providers, who do not use drugs and surgery, being prosecuted as criminals because they cure people of cancer, AIDS, and hundreds of other chronic diseases? Natural therapies work. Natural therapies can work better than drugs or surgery. Those who are using natural therapies to cure and prevent disease, and have a higher success rate and fewer adverse side effects than drug or surgical treatments, are being prosecuted for breaking the law. The question is, why are inexpensive, all natural, safe, effective treatments being suppressed? Let's find out...

CHAPTER 2

What's Wrong With Healthcare In America?

Standard medical science is failing. More people are getting medical treatment, taking more drugs, having more diagnostic testing, and having more surgeries than ever before in history. Yet more people are getting sick than ever before. Today you have a higher chance of getting cancer than ever before in history, and yet with many types of cancer you would have the same chance of dying as you did in 1950. I would call that a miserable failure.

The average American has over thirty different prescription and nonprescription drugs in their medicine cabinet. Do you think they're healthy? Obviously not. Who are the real winners in the cure and prevention of disease? It's certainly not those people taking multiple prescriptions every day. The winners are the drug companies and the healthcare companies. The drug companies' profits are at an all-time high.

And let's look at the diet industry:

- ✔ More people are on diets than ever before.
- ✔ More people take more diet products than ever before.
- ✔ More people exercise than ever before.

And yet, according to the Centers for Disease Control and Prevention, more than one-third (35.7%) of adults living in America are obese. Not just a bit overweight, but obese.

Who are the winners in the war on obesity? The corporations that sell diet food, diet pills, and other weight loss aids, that's who!

What should (and could) the state of our health and fitness look like? An ideal scenario would be one where you never have to take a single drug and you never get sick. You wake up in the morning feeling great, full of energy and vitality. You go throughout your day with a bounce in your step and a smile on your face. You don't feel stressed, anxious, or depressed. You don't feel tired. You've got no headaches or pain in your body. You aren't overweight, and you don't get colds, or the flu, or other illnesses. You're not ravenous with your appetite. You eat what you want and you're never that hungry. You don't deprive yourself of the foods you enjoy. You go to sleep and get a wonderful full night's rest. Your sexual desires are healthy and strong, and you're capable of both giving and receiving sexual pleasure. Your skin, hair, and nails look healthy and radiant. You have strength and tone in your muscles. Your body is graceful and flexible. You're firm, strong, vibrant, and you feel great! That's the description of a healthy person.

> We're also brainwashed into believing that it's "natural" to take drugs.

Most people have no idea how good their body is designed to feel. We've been brainwashed into believing that it's natural for a human being to get colds and flu, have aches and pains, and other medical problems. You do not have to get sick. Being sick is not "normal," it's abnormal. We're also brainwashed into believing that it's "natural" to take drugs. We're programmed to believe that we "need" drugs in order to be healthy.

Is there a place for surgery and drugs? Sure. Medical science has done a very good job at addressing symptoms. However, the treatment of a symptom has two flaws. First, the treatment itself often causes more problems, which then have to be treated. Second, the cause of the symptom is usually never addressed. When you don't address the cause, you're setting up more problems later on. That said, if you're in an emergency situation like a bad accident, of course drugs and surgery can save your life. However, drugs and surgery have failed at preventing illness and they do not address the cause of illness. If you fall off a ladder and puncture a kidney, of course you want to be rushed to the nearest emergency room and have a trained doctor use drugs and surgery to save your life. But if you want to stay healthy and never have disease, drugs and surgery are not the answer.

So, if trillions of dollars in scientific research has failed to produce ways of preventing and curing illness and disease, and all natural inexpensive prevention methods and cures exist, why aren't we hearing about them? The answer may surprise you.

CHAPTER 3

It's All About the Money

My contention is that there are all natural cures for virtually every ailment. These cures are being hidden from you by the pharmaceutical industry, the Food and Drug Administration, and the Federal Trade Commission, as well as other groups. The question that arises most often when I make this statement is, "Why? What is the motive for such a thing to occur?" The answer is simple: money and power.

All publicly traded corporations have a legal responsibility to increase profits. It's the law. Think about it: The only way companies make increased profits is by producing their product at the lowest possible cost, selling it at the highest possible price, and selling as much as they possibly can. Every decision a company makes is to increase profits.

In business, is everything always about the money? Yes. Throughout the history of big business, planned obsolescence has been standard operating procedure. This is when a product is manufactured in such a way that it will wear out or need to be replaced. The product could have been made to last a long time;

but in order for the company to ensure future profits, it knowingly manufactured an item that was inherently flawed. Thus it planned for the product's obsolescence, all in the name of profit.

Consider the drug industry. Let's say you sell insulin to diabetics. Would you be happy if someone discovered an herb that cured a person's diabetes so that they never needed insulin again? Of course not. You'd be out of business. Healthcare, defined as the treatment, prevention, and diagnosis of disease, is the most profitable industry in the world. As long as people are sick, billions of dollars in profit are made every year. There are enormous amounts of money to be made as long as people stay sick. A healthy person, on the other hand, does not need to buy drugs, doesn't get medical treatment, and is therefore a liability to the corporations involved in healthcare. If every person were healthy and disease-free, the drug companies and virtually the entire healthcare industry would be out of business.

> This money machine does not make its profits by keeping people healthy...

To the drug companies and the corporations involved in healthcare, as long as you're sick, there's money to be made; you're a potentially good customer. There's no financial incentive for the healthcare industry to prevent or cure disease, because the industry is driven to make money.

Let's examine a fictitious (or maybe not so fictitious) scenario. Imagine there's a scientist working in a lab somewhere who makes a breakthrough discovery: a small plant is found in the Amazon that, when brewed into a tea and consumed, eliminates all cancer in the body within one week.

Imagine this researcher proclaiming that he has given this tea to one thousand cancer patients and that every single one of them, within a week and without having undergone surgery, was found to have absolutely no cancer in their body. Eureka! A cure for cancer! An inexpensive, simple plant that you make into a tea and drink. It's all natural, has no side effects, and costs pennies.

Imagine this scientist announcing his discovery to the world. Certainly he'd win a Nobel Prize, right? Certainly the world medical community would be rejoicing. No more cancer!

Unfortunately, you'll never hear this story. Not because it isn't true, but because if a simple herbal tea that cured all cancer was being sold there would be no need for the American Cancer Society. No need for any of the drug companies that manufacture and sell cancer drugs. There would be no need for any cancer research funding. Cancer clinics around the world would close. Hundreds of thousands of people would be put out of work. Entire industries would shut down and billions of dollars in profit would no longer be funneling in to the kingpins who control the cancer industry.

So if such a person made this discovery, what do you think would happen? In some cases these people simply vanish. In others, they're given hundreds of millions of dollars for their research. And in still other cases the federal government raids these researchers' offices, confiscates the data, and jails them for practicing medicine without a license. Is this fantasy or is it the truth? Well, the healthcare industry has a dirty little secret, and I am blowing the whistle on it.

It's all about the money. Hospitals, drug companies, and the entire healthcare industry should really be called the "sick care" industry. This money machine does not make its profits by keeping people healthy, but rather by finding sick people and then selling them their outrageously expensive drugs and medical procedures. And they make over $1.3 trillion annually doing it. I've listened to these people. I've heard CEOs of major pharmaceutical companies say things like, "I don't care how much liver damage this drug causes, get it approved by the FDA. Do it and our stock price goes up threefold."

That is why I am mad as hell, and I am not going to take it anymore. Is it always just about the money? Are natural remedies and cures being suppressed and hidden just because greedy people and corporations want to make more money? Is it true that money makes the world go 'round? Yes. You must understand that the number one motivator in the world is making money. So let's look at who's involved...

CHAPTER 4

Who Are They?

Drugs and surgery are being promoted as the only answer to the prevention and cure of illness and disease. Natural cures are being suppressed and hidden from the public. So who's involved in this cover up?

- ✔ **The Pharmaceutical Companies.** These include not only the companies that sell drugs, but also companies that research and develop drugs. It also includes the suppliers in the healthcare industry who provide things like syringes, gauze, medical tape, tubing, plastic bottles, tongue depressors, etc. The profits this group of companies makes is astronomical.

- ✔ **The Food Companies**. You may ask: how do food companies get involved in healthcare? Well, there's a huge correlation between food and healthcare. Keep in mind many food companies are directly or indirectly involved in the pharmaceutical industry through corporate ownership, affiliated business transactions, or by the officers and directors owning stock in the pharmaceutical companies. Food companies include those that manufacture and sell food, and they also include fast food restaurants and the suppliers of the food industry—the actual growers of the food.

✔ **The Trade Associations.** The number of associations involved in the healthcare industry is enormous. Keep in mind, these associations are not in place to eliminate disease or keep people healthy. When you read their charters you find that they are there to promote the disease in an effort to get additional funding, and to protect their members, which are the drug companies and doctors! You've heard of some of them: American Medical Association, American Heart Association, American Lung Association, or American Cancer Society. There are many more than you probably know of—countless numbers of them. You might not be aware that these associations are incredibly powerful. Remember, these are not organizations with a goal of curing and preventing disease, or protecting the consumer. These associations don't represent sick people, they represent their members: The companies, the corporations, and the people making the money. And the people running these associations, of course, have an interest in keeping their cushy jobs.

✔ **Charities and Foundations.** These organizations sound great, but have you met the people who run them? The officers and directors of most charities and foundations have huge salaries and enormous expense accounts. They usually fly first-class, sometimes on private jets. They stay in the most expensive hotels and eat in the finest restaurants with your donations. Some foundations and charities have been found to spend over 40 percent of all of their donations on "administrative costs." Think about it. If a foundation used the money it received to cure a disease, there'd be no further need for the foundation. Consider this: the Jerry Lewis Telethon has raised over $1 billion for muscular dystrophy, yet more people have muscular dystrophy today than ever before.

✔ **Lobbyists**. This is the hidden, secret group of people in Washington that most of you have no idea even exists. These people make on average between $300,000 to $400,000 a year, plus hundreds of thousands more in perks. Their job is simply to walk up to a congressman or senator and try to persuade them to pass a certain piece of legislation, or vote a certain way. How do they do that? Well, the lobbyist can't walk up to a member of Congress and say, "Please vote a certain way on this bill and I'll give you 200,000 dollars." That would be called a bribe. But what the lobbyist can do is say, "Do you have a son or a daughter, Mr. Congressman? You do? Fantastic. I know your son or daughter has absolutely no experience whatsoever, but we'd like to give your son or daughter a job for $200,000 a year. And the best part is they don't even have to show up for work. Oh, by the way Mr. Congressman, would you please vote a certain way on this particular piece of legislation which helps who I represent?" Lobbyists absolutely bribe members of Congress, although Congress has passed laws that make these bribes legally not bribes, by disguising them as other things. Lobbyists may make huge donations to a congressman's favorite charity or school or hire companies that the congressman is affiliated with. Folks, that's what is happening in Washington. But according to the law it's not called a bribe or payoff, it's technically legal. And who made the law? The congressmen. Hmm, pretty interesting, isn't it? They make a law to make sure that what they do is legal.

✔ **Government Agencies**. Primarily the Food and Drug Administration (FDA) and the Federal Trade Commission (FTC). Isn't it surprising that it's the Food AND Drug Administration? (Why not two separate agencies?) This organization is one of the most powerful organizations in the country. They use Gestapo-like tactics to put natural cures out of business. They act as judge, jury, and executioner. They raid companies, unannounced, to seize products such as herbal remedies, vitamins and minerals, computers, files, research data, and equipment. They conduct these raids with armed agents with guns drawn. They seize harmless products, papers, documents, and computers without provocation, with no customer or consumer complaints, and without warning.

Let's look now at how these organizations make it all about the money.

Legal responsibility to shareholders

Virtually every pharmaceutical company is a publicly traded company, which means that the officers and directors have a legal responsibility to increase shareholder value. That means that the officers and directors of virtually every pharmaceutical company have a legal responsibility to increase profits. The only way they can increase profits is to sell more of what they sell and produce those products at a lower cost. Drug companies, therefore, have one goal: To sell more drugs and produce those drugs as inexpensively as possible. Once a drug is approved and the pharmaceutical company has the patent, it becomes the only company that can sell that drug. Getting a patented drug is an automatic billion dollars in the bank. This is why you will never see a pharmaceutical company promoting a natural cure. Natural cures cannot be patented. You can only make profits if you have a patented drug. There are no large profits in selling a natural cure that can't be patented. When you have a patented product you are the only company that can sell it. There's no competition. But if you're selling a natural product, a hundred other companies could sell the same product! Because of that competition, the prices will come down and the profits are reduced. That is why the drug industry will only promote patented drugs, because that's where the profits are. This is also why the drug companies gave tens of millions of dollars to lobbyists to get the FDA to make a new "law." Listen to this carefully. The FDA has the power to make laws and enforce them. It can make these laws without congressional approval or debate. In order to protect the profits of the drug industry the FDA passed the most incredibly insane law of all time. And here it is: "Only a drug can cure, prevent or treat a disease." Think about the ramifications. The FDA has now guaranteed and protected the profits of the drug companies! Only a patented drug, according to the FDA, can treat, prevent, or cure a disease. First off, we know this is blatantly untrue. The disease scurvy, for example, which is simply a vitamin C deficiency, is treated, prevented, and cured by eating citrus fruit. According to the FDA's law, however, if you were to holdup an orange and say, "This orange is the cure for the disease of scurvy," you would go to jail for selling a "drug" without a license. I'm not kidding. According to the FDA, as soon as you made a disease claim in reference to taking an orange, the orange was no longer an orange, but magically became a "drug" according to the FDA. And since that "drug" has not been patented or approved by the FDA, you are selling a "drug" without a license, which is a criminal offense. This is how the FDA works to protect the profits of the pharmaceutical company and suppress and hide information about natural remedies.

> The pharmaceutical companies give huge cash incentives and information to the doctors…

And just when you think it being all about the money can't get any worse, it does.

Manipulation

You are being duped into buying their drugs. Let's look at how the drug companies accomplish this. Years ago, they basically had to make sure that you were sick and had a problem that a drug could ameliorate. Second, they had to make sure that the doctors prescribed their particular drug. That still goes on. The pharmaceutical companies give huge cash incentives and information to the doctors about the drugs they make to ensure that the doctors, who are in fact legal drug pushers, get their drugs to you via prescription. Remember, the pharmaceutical companies have ensured that you're sick. How do they do that? This is going to blow your mind, but it's sadly true. One of the major reasons there's so much sickness and disease is because of the poisons you are putting in your body. The number one poison you put in your body consists of prescription and nonprescription drugs! That's right. The prescription and nonprescription drugs you're taking to eliminate your symptoms are, in fact, one of the major reasons that you get sick. The pharmaceutical companies know that all drugs have side effects. This is the dirty little secret they don't want you to know. Just as the tobacco industry knew that cigarettes were addictive and could cause lung cancer, yet lied for decades about this fact, the pharmaceutical industry today knows that all drugs have negative side effects and can cause further illness.

Why is the drug industry keeping this information secret? Because it's profitable. Look at the cycle: You start taking a drug to handle a certain symptom. A few months later you develop another medical condition. This new condition, unknown to you, was actually caused by the first drug you were taking. You start taking another drug for this new medical condition. The drug seems to work. Your condition gets better. A few months later, you develop yet another series of medical problems. And you're given still more drugs for the latest conditions… See how profitable this is? The cycle guarantees additional drug sales and profits for the drug companies.

Do you wonder how this is allowed to go on? I'll tell you: Virtually all drug research is funded by the pharmaceutical industry itself, that's how. And in nearly every study, drugs are found to be safe and effective. But of course, that's not true. Think of all of the drugs that were once proven to be safe and effective and approved by the FDA. Then, years later, these same drugs were found to be dangerous. They caused all kinds of severe medical conditions, which then led the FDA to take them off the market. Interestingly enough, they were only taken off the market after the drug companies made millions of dollars in profits.

Advertising

Another way you're being manipulated by it being all about the money is that the pharmaceutical industry is doing something that it hadn't done historically—advertising its drugs directly to the consumer. Close to two-thirds of all advertising in America is for drugs. It's estimated that the drug industry spends well in excess of $10 billion a year on advertising. These ads show beautiful, happy people, and give you the impression that they're taking this wonderful drug and that their lives are so much better. They're actors. Even when well-known figures and famous actors publicly endorse a drug or foundation (usually funded by pharmaceutical companies), ostensibly because they or a close friend or relative has suffered with a particular disease, they're being paid enormous sums to do so. These ads are not truthful.

Collusion

The Food and Drug Administration, the Federal Trade Commission and the pharmaceutical industry have an unholy alliance. The regulating government body should be governing, regulating and protecting consumers from the drug companies' insatiable desire to make profits. But it isn't. They work together to increase profits and power. A law was passed in Congress with virtually no debate which increased the FDA's dependence on large drug companies for its funding. Yes, you read that correctly. The FDA gets funding directly from the drug industry. And guess who owns stock in these drug companies? Would it surprise you that many members of the FDA and FTC own stock in drug companies? Would it surprise you that many members of Congress own stock in drug companies? Would it also surprise you that members of the news media, that are supposed to be impartially presenting news, own stock in drug companies? And the corporations that own television networks, radio networks, newspapers, and magazines all have financial ties to the pharmaceutical industry? That's one of the reasons you hear so much about drugs on the news and read so many positive articles about them in magazines and newspapers. These organizations get financial benefit from the drugs they help to sell.

> The FDA gets funding directly from the drug industry.

Doesn't it surprise you that you almost never hear any positive news about an herbal remedy, a natural remedy, or a homeopathic remedy in mainstream media? Could it be that there's no profit in those remedies? Remember, natural remedies cannot be patented.

The FDA says that there is not, and never will be, a natural remedy that can cure, prevent, or treat a disease. Because if a natural remedy did, then it would have to be classified as a "drug" and once it's classified as a drug it has to go through 800 million dollars' worth of testing that the FDA requires to approve it as a new drug. This cannot be done. Why? Because a natural remedy cannot be patented and there's no company that can spend $800 million to get a natural remedy approved as a new drug because it won't own a patent for that drug and therefore can't make that money back plus tenfold profits. This is why the FDA and drug companies love this system. It prevents any natural remedy from being touted as a cure or preventative of disease when in fact many of them are.

Can you see how the pharmaceutical industry is committed to wiping out non-patentable, all natural cures for disease? It's spending hundreds of millions of dollars to try to get you to believe that drugs are safe and effective and all natural cures are ineffective and dangerous. It's the drugs that are dangerous and cause disease. And the current research shows that drugs do not cure disease either. Natural remedies are generally safe, effective, and have virtually no side effects. Technically, all natural remedies do not cure disease either, because only the body can do that. But these remedies help the body cure itself.

Government Mandates of Drug Use

Another technique that the drug industry uses to make sure sales of drugs continue to increase is to get the federal government to pass laws requiring people to take drugs. There are three methods employed. First, pass a law requiring that children must take a certain drug, such as vaccines. Second, pass a law requiring all federal employees and military personnel to take a certain drug. Third, get the government to pay for drug usage for the poor and elderly through Social Security, Medicare, and Medicaid. When this happens…bam! Billions of dollars in profits.

Censorship of Opposing Ideas

We live in America—the supposed land of free speech. Well, speech is not free. If your speech happens to threaten the profits of big business, you are going to be bound, gagged, ridiculed and persecuted. A plethora of books is written about the drug industry, the FDA, the FTC, and the collusion between the associations, corporations, lobbyists, and certain government regulators and how they work together to suppress natural, inexpensive ways to prevent and cure disease. But they rarely, if ever, get published, because if a publisher puts out a book that's bashing the pharmaceutical industry, or certain government agencies, or big business, the publishing company may be blacklisted and have its other books taken out of distribution, which would cost them millions of dollars in profits.

And it's not just books that are censored. News organizations will block unflattering stories involving these companies, too. Several years ago, a couple of reporters did an exposé on the company now infamous for genetically modifying (and ruining) our food: Monsanto. This story was about the growth hormone rBGH that's used in dairy cows. It revealed that this hormone was making the animals sick and making the milk and dairy products from these cows poisonous. However, the news organization they wrote the story for refused to run it and tried to pay them hush money. Why? Because Monsanto put pressure on the news organization!

Censorship of Advertising

Let's say you're the president of a major television network. The network is owned by another multinational company that owns a drug company, or has a huge interest in one. Your network gets two-thirds, or close to 70 percent, of its advertising revenue directly from the drug industry. Now imagine a guy comes to you and says, "I'd like to advertise my book entitled *How the Drug Companies Are Ripping Off America.*" Would you, as the president of that company, run that ad? Of course not. You'd get fired. Because that ad could have a negative impact on the sales and profits of the drug companies in which the owner of the network has a major equity position. Folks, this is what is happening. *It's all about the money.*

Debunking Natural Remedies

In an actual memorandum, the U.S. federal government states that one of the most effective tools to get people to believe the government's opinion is to put together a well-orchestrated debunking campaign. What this means is there is a coordinated effort between the FDA, the FTC, the healthcare associations, and the entire pharmaceutical industry as well as some major news organizations to produce scare tactic stories about natural alternatives and suppress the truth about the ineffectiveness and dangers of drugs. There's a litany of inexpensive, highly effective natural cures that are being labeled as "snake oil" or simply hidden from the public.

The FDA has led the way in this battle against natural cures. In the 1970s the FDA attempted to make vitamin supplements prescription drugs. They claimed that vitamins were so dangerous they should only be prescribed by doctors. The public was outraged and Congress rejected the idea. In 1993 the FDA tried to classify certain minerals and amino acids as prescription drugs. Again, a public outcry caused Congress to act. The FDA has gone after companies that sell natural remedies via the Internet. It claims these companies are selling "drugs" without a license.

In 2013 an *Associated Press* story claimed that vitamins and food supplements were deemed ineffective. Here's a quote from this story: "The government doesn't recommend routine vitamin supplementation as a way to prevent chronic diseases."

The article later quotes a medical doctor who says, "Most people who buy multivitamins and other supplements are generally healthy." Exactly. So, the doctor, along with the government, recommends that they stop? Sounds ludicrous, but I am not making this up.

There are thousands of studies showing that natural remedies are not only effective, but they can be more effective than a drug counterpart. An example is Vitamin E. In major double-blind studies, Vitamin E was found as effective or more effective as a blood thinner than its drug counterpart. But why aren't we given Vitamin E instead of the drug? The facts are clear: natural remedies could financially devastate the pharmaceutical industry.

Did you know that there are different standards used in what's classified as news and advertising? If information is presented by a politician or government agency, such as the FDA or FTC, news organizations present that information as factual, rarely if ever investigating the claims or seeking an opposing viewpoint. The government has the ability to influence the masses without opposition.

Lawsuits

The industry uses lawsuits to spread negative information about natural remedies. Keep in mind the pharmaceutical industry is the most powerful, profitable business in the world. It can afford to file outrageous, frivolous lawsuits against small independent companies that threaten profits, and drive them right out of business.

Lawsuits are also routinely filed against individual healthcare practitioners who are curing people without drugs or surgery. Not only are civil lawsuits filed against them, but many of these health-care providers are being prosecuted criminally for curing people's diseases. They're being charged with practicing medicine without a license or dispensing drugs without a license.

The bottom line is that there are natural, inexpensive, safe cures for almost every disease. The pharmaceutical industry, the FTC, the FDA and the rest of "them" are suppressing this information. The pharmaceutical industry, the drug industry, the food industry, the associations and government agencies, all have a major financial incentive to keep people sick. There are billions of dollars in profits as long as people stay sick and there are billions of dollars in profits as long as people take more and more drugs. Remember, it's always all about the money!

So if we can't believe our government; if we can't believe what we see on television, or what we hear on the radio, or what we read in newspapers and magazines; if we can't believe what we hear from professors and doctors since they're all paid spokespeople for the pharmaceutical industry, then who *can* we believe when it comes to information about health and the treatment, prevention, and cure of disease? It only makes sense that you can't believe anyone who has a financial interest in selling you something. You can't even believe alternative healthcare practitioners who are trying to sell you vitamins. If a licensed healthcare practitioner tells you the benefits of a vitamin, herb, or mineral and he's encouraging you to buy from him at a profit, maybe he's being sincere and truthful, but the financial incentive may impede your ability to get unbiased information. The officers and directors of vitamin, mineral, herb, and homeopathic companies have financial motivations to sell their products just like the officers and directors of pharmaceutical companies. And as long as someone is selling something, it's all about the money. Always.

> And as long as someone is selling something, it's all about the money.

So again, the question is who can you listen to? The answer: You can listen to ME! You might laugh, but it's true.

People all around the world come up to me and ask, "Where do I go for information about health? Who can I trust? Where can I get information about the prevention or curing of a disease? There's so much conflicting information out there, and I just don't know where to go to find the answers." This is the big problem. With the Internet there is more information available than ever before, but when you go on online everyone is trying to sell you something. So when you're reading an article you don't know if the information is true, or just designed to get you to buy a product. WebMD is a perfect example. This is a publicly traded company where the officers and directors have made millions of dollars in profits.

WebMD, in my opinion, is nothing more than a front for the pharmaceutical industry encouraging you to buy and use drugs and get expensive medical procedures. It tries to make you think it's an unbiased source of information when this is categorically untrue. How can they be unbiased when they accept advertising from drug companies? How can they be unbiased when they're publicly traded? How can they be unbiased when their only motivation is to make money?

What makes me different? The answer is simple. For me, it's not all about the money. It's not that I think making money is bad. Giving a good quality service at a good value is an admirable thing to do. Making a profit and enjoying a beautiful lifestyle is not bad. Making money at the expense of employees, customers and the environment is bad.

Here is how I've solved the problem: I do not take any advertising. I do not sell any natural cure products: I only inform. And that's why you can listen to what I am saying in this book, on my website www.NaturalCuresBook.com, and in my newsletter that you can subscribe to by going to www.NaturalCuresBook.com/newsletter.

People approach me regularly offering me money to endorse their product, to recommend their product, or to talk positively about one product, or bash another, but I'm not interested in that. What I'm interested in is sharing information that helps people. So let's get on with that....

CHAPTER 5

Why Are We Sick?

Over the years, the pharmaceutical industry has come up with different theories about why people get sick. Antibiotics were touted as the cure all. The theory was that all disease was caused by germs, primarily bacteria. This theory has been proven wrong. Stronger and stronger antibiotics continue to be developed, and yet people continue to get sicker, and sicker. More people are getting more diseases than ever before.

The next theory was that viruses were the cause of all illness and disease. Unfortunately, few people know that antibiotics have no effect on viruses. The doctors continually prescribe antibiotics at the drop of a hat. People have been brainwashed into thinking they need antibiotics when they feel sick, so they demand them. Doctors, who are in business to make money, understand that patients are essentially customers and so to keep the customers happy they prescribe the antibiotics. According to the Associated Press it's estimated that about half of the antibiotic prescriptions written each year are unnecessary. Still, people continue to get more sicknesses and diseases.

One current theory is that a large percentage of disease and illness is caused by genetic defects. Of course they tell us the only answer is drugs. A new method of making billions of dollars is to come up with a genetic defect for every problem a person has. "Oh, you're fat because you have a genetic defect, and a drug is being worked on that can solve that genetic defect and make you thin." "Diabetes is nothing more than genetics, so we'll work on a drug that will correct that genetic disposition." Keep in mind that drug companies really do *not* want to cure disease as they claim. If they came up with a cure, they'd be out of business.

> If they came up with a cure, they'd be out of business.

Take herpes for example. Herpes is a virus. Ads on TV regularly say there is no cure for herpes, therefore, in order to suppress the symptoms, take our wonderful drug every day for the rest of your life. Imagine what would happen to the publicly traded company that makes the drug if they announced, "Here is a cure for herpes. Simply take this herb for thirty days and you'll never have a herpetic breakout ever again. By the way, this herb is not patented and it costs only three dollars."

That company would lose billions of dollars in profits. Its stock price would plummet. Therefore, there's no incentive to cure herpes. The incentive is to keep the public brainwashed into believing there is no cure for herpes, and the only solution to the "symptoms" is drugs. Remember, the FDA and the drug companies work hand in hand. If I happen to know a cure for herpes, I can't say so. Because if I *do* I'm now making a medical claim and, according to the FDA, I'm breaking the law. Even if what I'm saying is true, I am still breaking the law. The FDA will then come in with their federal agents with their guns drawn, arrest me, throw me in jail, confiscate any papers I have, and any of the harmless herb, suppress the information and outlaw it because there is no "credible scientific evidence." They will then put out press releases stating that

I'm a charlatan selling snake oil and have no scientific evidence to substantiate my claim. Unfortunately, that's how the system works.

So why do you get sick? Is it germs? Bacteria? Is it viruses? Genetics? Well let's think about it. You don't *catch* cancer. Your body develops cancer. You don't catch diabetes. Your body develops diabetes. You don't catch obesity. Your body becomes obese. You don't catch headaches, fibromyalgia, arthritis, PMS, or impotence. These are conditions that develop within the body. They're not caused by a germ, or a virus. Drugs are not the answer. You don't have a headache because you have an aspirin deficiency. The question is why do human beings have so much illness? Is there a way that we can do some simple things to keep us illness free, and full of life, energy, and vitality? Yes.

Let's go back to the cause of all disease and the reason why we're sick. Based on personal experience, reading thousands of pages of documents, and hearing the firsthand accounts from thousands of people and healthcare practitioners around the world, I've come up with what I believe to be the cause of virtually all sickness and disease in the body. There are two main reasons why you get sick:

1. You "catch" something. This means your body picked up a "germ," generally a virus or bacteria.

2. You "develop" an illness or disease. This means there is some imbalance in the body, something is not working right.

Common diseases in this category include: cancer, diabetes, acid reflux, arthritis, heart disease, etc. In our search for the ultimate cause of all illness and the ultimate cure for all illnesses, we need to ask, "What caused that?" With this in mind, let's start with "catching something."

One may say that the "cause" of catching a germ is pretty evident. You obviously caught the germ from someone else who had it. This is where medical science stops. They claim that drugs must be developed in order to kill those bacteria and viruses. However, they're asking the wrong question. The fact is that we're *all* exposed to bacteria and viruses *daily*. If one person in your home or office has the flu, then every single person has been exposed to the flu virus. Some people succumb to bacteria and viruses and get sick, and others don't. Throughout your life you'll pick up thousands of bacteria and viruses. That's natural. Why, in some cases, does the body not do what it was designed to do, which is fight off the bacteria or virus? The answer: the body is out of balance and the immune system is weak.

When your body is in balance (a state called homeostasis), and your immune system is strong, you don't develop any symptoms of the viruses or bacteria that you pick up.

Now the question becomes, "What is causing the body to be out of balance, and the immune system to be weak?" I'll give you the answer in a moment, but first let's go to the second reason people get sick. Remember, you get sick because you either a) catch something, or b) something develops in the body.

You "catch something" because your body is out of balance and your immune system is weak. You "develop something" either because your body is out of balance, or a "toxin" is getting into your body causing the problem to develop.

If we keep asking the question, "What caused that..." we can then conclude that all your illness comes from one of, or a combination of the following things:

1. You have too many toxins in your body.

2. You have nutritional deficiencies.

3. You are exposed to, and negatively affected by electromagnetic chaos.

4. You have trapped mental and emotional stress.

These are the only four reasons why your immune system could be weak or why genetically weak areas in the body can break down, thus allowing illness and disease to develop. These four things cause the body to be "out of balance." I will address each of these four issues.

Let's start with toxins. What is a toxin? A toxin is a poison. It is a substance that if taken in large doses can cause severe illness or death. In relation to toxins, the question is what is causing toxins to be put into our body? The answer is that we have not been educated to know what these toxins are. And secondly, these toxins are being put in virtually everything we eat without our knowledge.

Now, here is the big one: the most toxic thing you can put in your body, and the number one cause of virtually all illness and disease, is prescription and nonprescription drugs!

In my opinion, one of the main reasons people are sick is because of the number of drugs they take. Why? Because *all* drugs have negative side effects. Let me say it again, all drugs have negative side effects! If you're taking a drug to suppress one symptom, that drug is causing some other problem to start developing in your body.

Even if you stop taking that drug, the wheels have been set in motion, and in a few weeks, or a few months, boom, you have some more symptoms caused by the first drug you took a few months ago. You go to your doctor, and he or she gives you another drug to suppress these new symptoms. This *new* drug has negative side effects, and after you start taking it, again, the wheels will have been set in motion, and *voila*—new symptoms which were in fact caused by the drug you were just taking. You go back to the doctor and get another drug...

Drugs...Cause...Medical...Problems. They do not treat the cause. It's a great business for the drug companies, not so great for you. If they get you taking one drug, they've got you. The likelihood of you taking another drug, and then another, keeps going up and up. The more you take, the sicker you get, simply because drugs are major toxins.

I know some of you are saying, "Drugs can't really be poison, can they?" Oh no? Then how about you take thirty of them right now and see what happens? You'll probably die. If you eat thirty apples are you going to die? Not likely. You may feel full, and you might need to go to the bathroom a lot, but you're probably going to survive an apple overdose.

This relates to nonprescription over-the-counter drugs as well. Let me be very clear. The scary thing is the drug companies and the FDA know it.

A good example of this is Vioxx. Vioxx is a pain medication. It was an outrageously expensive drug that reduced pain no better than an over-the-counter drug. The drug company that sold Vioxx made billions in profits. Whistleblowers now say that both the FDA and the drug manufacturer of Vioxx knew it would cause over 100,000 people to die. Whistleblowers say that the decision was made to let the people die because of the potential profits. In my opinion, this happens all of the time. Over-the-counter drugs are some of the biggest culprits. Many of these drugs were approved by the FDA twenty, thirty, forty years ago. The problem is once a drug is approved by the FDA, whether it's a prescription drug or a nonprescription drug, there is virtually no follow-up research or testing to verify the long-term effectiveness of the drug and the long-term safety. We're seeing now that over-the-counter drugs that have been sold for thirty years are being looked at by some independent organizations and they're being shown to be dangerous and ineffective. They're also being shown to cause illness and disease.

Cholesterol lowering drugs, for example, have an adverse effect on the liver. The liver is the only fat metabolizing organ in the body. The liver is needed for proper body function. When the liver is adversely affected you are prone to diabetes, acid reflux, constipation, colon cancer, heart disease, asthma, arthritis, and dozens of other illnesses and disease.

Do cholesterol-lowering drugs directly cause these illnesses and disease? No one really knows for sure, but it's certainly obvious to anyone with half a brain and a little bit of logic that these absolutely contribute to the development of disease in the body.

> All drugs have negative side effects.

The bottom line is all over-the-counter nonprescription drugs and prescription drugs cause illness and disease. This is the big shocker. The industry that's promoting itself as the group dedicated to the prevention and cure of disease is actually the group causing more sickness and disease. All drugs are chemicals. All drugs have negative side effects. All drugs can cause death. All drugs are poisons. Did you know that more Americans die every year from prescription drugs than from illegal drugs? There are dozens of articles showing how prescription and nonprescription drugs are causing all illness and diseases.

Drugs are toxins. When one has lots of toxins in the body, the body goes out of balance. The immune system is weakened. When this occurs the body cannot fight off the viruses or bacteria that it picks up, thus causing sickness.

"Too many toxins in the body" comes down to this:

1. What goes into the body.
2. What comes out of the body.
3. Exercise.

4. Rest.
5. Thoughts.
6. What you say.

Let's go through this list and address some common misconceptions, and see what you should be doing if you want to eliminate disease. Maybe some of you have a disease or know someone who does. Others may be concerned about getting a disease and want to do the steps necessary to prevent one.

The six areas listed above have a direct relation to toxicity in the body. It's interesting to note that when you are toxic, your body becomes highly acidic. Your body pH should be alkaline. When your body pH is acidic you are susceptible to illness and disease. When your body pH is alkaline, you virtually never get sick. Every single person who has cancer has a pH that is too acidic.

Let me show you how each of the above six areas cause you to become too toxic, thus more acidic, and thus more prone to illness and disease.

What Goes Into the Body

Let's look at what we put into our bodies. We put things into the body in a variety of ways, but mostly through the mouth. Jack LaLane, who was vibrant, healthy and strong well into his nineties before he passed away at ninety-six said it best: "If man made it, don't eat it." What you put into your mouth should be as close as possible to what nature intended. If you go out and eat an apple you may think, "Ah, this is an apple; man didn't make it, so I can eat it." Well, unfortunately there's a problem with that, because many fruits and vegetables today are man-made.

I mentioned Monsanto in an earlier chapter. You've probably heard news in the past couple of years about this huge chemical and agricultural biotechnology company and its genetically modified food. Some say Monsanto is the devil incarnate and I can't say that I disagree. Monsanto supplies a lot of our nation's food, and much of it, including fruits and vegetables, have been genetically modified to become more disease resistant. Remember what I said about the pharmaceutical industry being all about the money? Well, the food industry is all about the money, too.

A food manufacturer, or for that matter a farmer, is in business and has to sell more of his product and produce at the lowest possible cost to make more money. So farmers say, "Hmm, how can I grow the largest yield of apples or carrots, or the most onions on my field? How can I produce them in the shortest period of time, at the lowest cost, so I can sell them at the highest possible profit?"

The answer is mess around with mother nature and change these natural fruits and vegetables with some man-made concoction that came out of a laboratory so that they grow bigger, faster and more resistant to disease. So through genetic modification, your all natural carrot is no longer all natural. It is really a man-made product.

And it gets worse. Because that farmer has to produce more carrots per acre in order to make more profit, he uses chemical fertilizers and pesticides and herbicides. When you eat that "natural" vegetable or piece of fruit, it's loaded with toxic chemicals. It also has less nutritional value than it would have had fifty or sixty years ago.

So, if you're going to eat fruits and vegetables, which I highly encourage you to do, they must be *organically grown*.

Grains such as rice and oats are the same. Buy organic. I don't recommend wheat or wheat flour *at all*, because wheat in this country has been modified so drastically it's not even the same grain it once was. It's "Frankenwheat," full of "man-made" garbage that will make you sick and fat.

In the United States, nearly all of our fruits, vegetables, grains, nuts and seeds are grown with highly poisonous chemical fertilizers, pesticides and herbicides.

The same conditions apply in the meat industry. Like farmers and other food producers, the meat industry needs to create a lot of product cheaply and quickly in order to sell it for as high a profit as possible. To that end, the industry uses hormones to speed an animal's growth (contributing to the record levels of obesity and early puberty in our children), antibiotics to keep an animal healthy in unsanitary and inhumane conditions, and feeds that are unnatural to an animal's diet that not only pump more chemicals into the meat, but also upset animals' systems so that they become out of balance and diseased, and pass those imbalances and diseases along to those who consume the meat. Remember, if it's not organic, *don't eat it.*

> When you eat that "natural" vegetable or piece of fruit, it's loaded with toxic chemicals.

The same holds true with dairy products. Because of the use of drugs, growth hormones, pasteurization and homogenization, dairy products today are a major health concern unless they're organic, not pasteurized, and not homogenized. Pasteurization simply heats the dairy product to a temperature high enough to kill bacteria. The problem is it also kills the living enzymes, making it harder for our bodies to digest. But more importantly, and more dangerous, is homogenization.

Remember the milkman? You may be too young to remember, but milkmen used to deliver bottled milk to our houses. Why couldn't we just buy our milk in the store? Because back then milk spoiled within just a few days. The food industry said, "We're losing money by not selling milk in our stores. It goes bad too quickly." So they came up with a solution—a process called homogenization. When milk was delivered back in the day the cream separated into a layer on top and you had to shake the bottle to blend it. The process of homogenization actually spins the milk at a high rate breaking down the clusters of molecules within it. As a result, not only does the cream not separate, the milk won't spoil quickly. It can last a couple of weeks before going bad.

The problem with homogenized and pasteurized milk, and other dairy products is that with the processing, the clusters of fat molecules are now so small that when we ingest them they get into our blood stream, which they shouldn't, and our bodies set up a defense mechanism that ends up scarring our arteries. The scarring of the arteries causes LDL cholesterol to attach itself to the artery, which leads to a major cause of heart disease, arteriosclerosis. The processed milk's tiny fat molecules are also being assimilated into the lining of the stomach in a way that's incompatible with our bodies. This clogs the system, making it harder to digest food, which in turn contributes to acid reflux, obesity, allergies, and constipation. The bottom line is pasteurized and homogenized dairy products are unnatural.

When you eat fish you're only slightly better off, because many kinds of fish are "farmed," meaning that toxic feed and chemicals are used to make it grow unnaturally fast and to unnaturally large sizes. When you consume this "man-made" fish, you're also taking in the toxins that have been used in its production. Fish in the wild are ostensibly better. However, because of the massive dumping of poisonous chemicals into our lakes, rivers, and oceans, many wild fish have abnormally high levels of toxic chemicals in them as well.

I know this sounds terrible. I know you're probably wondering *what do I do? How do I eat?* The good news is there are some simple, easy solutions, which I'll explain in a later chapter. I'm trying to point out that you are constantly loading your body with toxins, and this is one of the reasons you get sick. When I tell people they're toxic, most have a hard time believing it, but the fact is you're likely to be toxic right now, just by virtue of the environment.

In 2005, an independent study on women's breast milk showed a startling fact. Virtually all of the women tested, across several states, showed detectable levels of rocket fuel in their breast milk. Yes rocket fuel in breast milk. It wasn't until nearly a decade later in 2013 that NASA announced that it's planning to replace the toxic fuel with a more environmentally friendly one.

We're exposed to environmental toxins constantly. For example when a plane flies overhead there's a "chem-trail." The chemical residues fall down from the sky and we breathe them in. They also contaminate water supplies, which we drink.

What other toxins do we put in our bodies through our mouths? If it's in a box, a jar or a can, it's been processed by the food industry. The food industry puts tens of thousands of chemical ingredients into the food and, in many cases they do not have to list those ingredients on the label. How do they get away with that? They do it through lobbyist friends, and by paying off politicians and members of the Food and Drug Administration. And why is that bad? Because, as I've explained, the additives are toxic. And not only are these chemical additives toxic, when they're put into the food, the processing strips away much of the nutritional value. And in some cases, the additives actually block absorption of nutrients as well.

So, not only are you not getting enough nutrients from the food you're eating, but the few nutrients you are getting are not being absorbed. Why are these food additives put in the food anyway? Well it's very interesting. I was at a health spa where I spoke with a gentleman who was a senior executive at a company that was one of the largest producers of canned goods in the world. We were talking about the food additives and, yes, he admitted that there are thousands and thousands of chemical additives put into the food, and many of these additives are not listed on the label at all. I suggested that these food additives were dangerous to a person's health and were one of the reasons why people are so sick today. He assured me that these chemicals were totally safe, and that they were in such small amounts that they would have no effect on one's body.

I asked, "If they're totally safe, then if I were to give you a glass of one of these chemicals, would you drink it?" He stammered and went back and forth a few times. I must have asked him the question ten times without getting an answer. Finally he said no, he wouldn't drink it because it could potentially be a problem. He admitted that the ingredients were, in fact, toxic. But he repeated that because they were in such small amounts, they had no effect at all on the human body.

I then asked him the million dollar question. I said, "If you're putting such a small amount in, and these ingredients have no effect at all on the human body, then they must have no effect at all on the food. So why do you have to put them in the food?" Again, he couldn't answer. After I continued grilling this man, he reluctantly admitted that they in fact have a major effect. They preserve the food and give it taste. Bingo.

Still, I suspected that there was something else these ingredients did that he wasn't telling. So I searched through my network of insiders, and here is what I discovered: The food industry, just like the tobacco industry, is hiding a dirty little secret. The food industry is putting ingredients in the food purposely, because these secret (and in many cases illegal) ingredients make a person hungry, and make them addicted to the food. Think this is crazy? Remember Coca Cola? Coca Cola was colored sweetened water that had cocaine in it. Coca Cola was the name because Coca referred to the coca plant and Cola referred to the cola nut. The cola nut had the caffeine, and the coca or the cocaine got the person physically addicted. The drug was removed back in the 1920s, without much fanfare or media exposure. Scary, huh? There are more scary things...

Many of the ingredients they put in the food make you depressed, which is good for the drug companies, because if you're depressed, you have to go to the drug companies to treat your depression. Interestingly enough, some of the additives that are put in the food to make you depressed are manufactured by the same companies that sell antidepressant drugs. It's a fantastic business model folks. Remember, it's all about the money.

There's another reason chemical additives and the food processing are bad. Food must have nutritional value for it to be used by the body, but food also has a "vibration." It has a "life force energy." When food is chemically or genetically altered, highly processed, or contains chemical additives, the energetic vibration of the food is altered. When the vibration of food is radically altered consuming that food actually causes the body to go out of balance and causes disease to develop. Yes, you're reading this right. From an energetic standpoint eating a genetically altered apple that's been sprayed with pesticides can give you cancer, as well as dozens of other diseases.

Without giving a physics lesson, when you eat something you're getting the energy from that thing. How do we know this is true? Say you take a pot and you put soil in it. You put in ten pounds of soil, and you put in a little tiny seed, and every day you add some water. Then at the end of a year you have a big plant. Well, take the plant out, shake off the soil from the roots and weigh the soil. Guess what? You still have ten pounds of soil. The only thing you added was some water. If you were to measure the water, you may have added about five pounds of water. Theoretically, the plant should weigh no more than five pounds if it grabbed 100 percent of the water. But the plant weighs fifty pounds. Wow! What happened? How did fifty pounds of mass and matter magically appear? It didn't eat the soil, the ten pounds of soil is still there, and there were only five pounds of water added. How did that plant appear out of virtually nothing? This is a very important point. The plant, like all living things, was created out of "energy." Energy is "invisible matter."

> ...the food industry lobbied the politicians to allow certain man-made ingredients to be classified as all natural.

Human beings are the same. If you take a little baby, and you weigh every bit of food that goes in and then subtract all of the excretions that come out via the urine, stool, and sweat through the skin, you would see that whatever goes in comes out. If ten pounds of food and water are put in, guess what? Ten pounds of stuff comes out. But the baby grows from fifteen pounds to fifty pounds to one hundred and fifty pounds. How does that happen? The answer is that we get the energy from food, from sunlight and from air; and that's how matter is manifested—it's the energy. Everything is energy, including us. We actually become the very energy we take in.

So if we go through everything that we put into our mouth, whatever we eat or drink, we have to ask ourselves is that energy good? Is it as nature intended? Or has it been screwed up by some greedy people who don't care if we get sick?

What should we eat and drink? Ideally you want to eat all natural things, fruits and vegetables, and get them organic. Cooking destroys some of the enzymes, so raw is generally better, but there are some vegetables that are better absorbed when cooked, like tomatoes and carrots. Aim for a hefty amount (between one and two pounds) of organic fruits and vegetables a day. That may sound like a lot, but one piece of fruit can be more than one-fourth a pound. One sweet potato can be one-half a pound.

And don't just look at food labels. You have to read the ingredients. Because even if the label says all natural, that's often a lie. Why? Because the food industry lobbied the politicians to allow certain man-made ingredients to be classified as all natural.

If it's in a box or can, don't even eat it. Buy from the organic section of the grocery store, or better still, buy organic directly from farmer's markets. If you're not eating organic, you're running the risk of ingesting a lot of chemicals that are potentially harmful. These secret chemicals in nonorganic foods are specifically designed to do the following things:

Preserve the food. Sometimes chemicals are added so that food will not spoil even after years of just sitting around. We've all heard the story of the thirty-year-old Twinkie that looked and tasted the same as it did the day it was manufactured.

- ✔ **Taste and texture.** Much of today's food is produced in such an unnatural way that is has very little nutritional value and very little taste. Chemicals must be added to make the food taste like it's supposed to taste. A major hamburger chain adds a chemical to its hamburgers to make them taste like a hamburger!

✔ **To make you hungry.** The food industry knows that it must sell MORE food to make more money. If it can add a chemical that makes you hungrier, you'll eat more food and they'll make more money!

✔ **To make you fatter.** Fat people eat more food. Chemicals are being added to our food that actually make us gain weight. The more fat people, the more profits for the food industry. Shockingly, one such chemical is actually put into most "diet food." How sad that unknowing consumers buy a product that has the word "diet" on it in the hopes of losing weight, when actually eating it causes them to gain weight.

✔ **To get the person addicted to the product.** Food manufacturers are knowingly putting chemicals into the food that cause the consumer to become physically addicted to it. We know that drugs, which are simply chemicals, can be incredibly physically and emotionally addictive. Having a person addicted to your product is good for profits.

✔ **To give you disease.** As outrageous as it seems, it appears that insiders know that certain "food additives" cause specific diseases. If you knew that huge numbers of people would be coming down with a certain disease in the next five or ten years, you could invest in drug companies that are producing drugs that will be prescribed for this "new disease." When I talk about the greed of the people involved, most people reading this have no comprehension of just how the love of money has taken control over these people's actions, ethics, and morals.

Obviously, what I'm sharing here are my own conclusions. They are vehemently denied by the food industry and the FDA, but think about the same type of denials for years by the tobacco industry. I believe time will prove me correct.

The other important issue relating to these chemical additives is that when you ingest them, they do not necessarily leave your body. Chemical fertilizers, pesticides, herbicides, hormones, prescription and nonprescription drugs, and food additives such as artificial sweeteners, stay in the body and lodge in the fatty tissues. Since our brain is mostly fat, a large percentage of these chemicals accumulate there over the years. This is believed to be one of the main reasons that there's an increase in depression, stress and anxiety, and an increase in learning disabilities like attention deficit disorder. These additives stress the body. When the body is "stressed" two things occur:

1. The immune system is suppressed, making you more susceptible to disease.

2. It can turn your body from the natural alkaline pH state, in which disease and illness and sickness cannot survive, to an acidic state in which diseases like cancer, arteriosclerosis and diabetes can thrive.

When you put something in your mouth ask yourself: Could this have been made a hundred years ago? If it couldn't, don't eat it. The reason it is being processed the way it is, is because somebody is making lots of money. As I've said repeatedly, it's always about the money.

> ...chemical additives...do not necessarily leave your body.

If you were to read the labels of everything you put in your mouth, you would see the names of various chemicals. All of the chemicals listed are dangerous poisons. If you were to ingest a large amount of any of those chemicals at one time, you would probably die.

Now think about the 15,000 chemicals that are in our food that do *not* even have to be listed on the label. Remember, you get sick because you either catch something or you develop something. Catching something is not a problem because your body is designed to fight off infection and disease. But when your body is loaded with toxins (from all those chemicals you're ingesting) and your immune system is suppressed because of lack of nutrition or energetic frequency imbalances, you become susceptible to viruses and bacteria. You develop diseases because toxins, nutritional deficiencies, or energetic imbalances allow disease to form in the genetically weak areas of your system.

It's important to understand why we become ill in order for us to totally understand how to *cure* ourselves. If you really understand why you become sick, then you will understand the "natural cures" much more easily. As I mentioned earlier, this may sound overwhelming. Just go with the flow. The good news is you don't have to be a health fanatic to cure yourself and live a life of health and vitality.

Now let's talk about what else you put in your mouth, primarily what *you drink*. There are two problems here. The first one is most people don't drink enough water, and the second, is that the water you drink is toxic. All tap water has chemicals added to it, primarily chlorine and fluoride, both of which have been found to be toxic.

Most people are dehydrated. Dehydration causes all kinds of medical problems including pain, stiffness, arthritis, asthma, allergies and other medical issues. Dehydration means the cells don't have enough fluid. It can affect your energy and your sleep, but the major thing that it affects is the ability to remove toxins and waste out of the body and out of the cells.

Cells can live forever in a laboratory as long as the fluid in which the cell is living is continually cleaned and changed. If you take a cell and add fluid to it, the cell excretes waste matter and toxins. As long as you clean the environment and get rid of the waste matter and toxins, the cell never seems to age. That's pretty staggering. And it's why removing the toxins from your system is so important. It's also why putting the least amount of toxins *into* your body is so important too.

The debate is on about the best type of water. We have tap water, purified water, spring water and distilled water.

Tap water is absolutely the worst kind, because virtually all tap water is contaminated. All tap water has chlorine in it, and most has synthesized fluoride in it. Synthesized fluoride is toxic.

Most countries in Europe do not have water fluoridation. However, here in the U.S., through lobbying, fluoride was sold to municipalities and dumped in our water supplies under the disguise of being good for our teeth. It isn't true. Even the Centers For Disease Control (CDC) has acknowledged that drinking fluoridated water doesn't benefit teeth. Fluoride is dangerous, and should not be consumed. It adversely affects our organs, primarily the thyroid gland.

Spring water is better than tap water. But certain agencies and interest groups publish misleading stories about bottled water not being any better than tap water because the bacteria count in bottled water is higher than that in tap water. These stories point out that there are no bacteria in tap water because of the chlorine. The problem is chlorine is a poison that kills living organisms. We, too, are living organisms. When we drink it, we're drinking poison. Yes, we're taking it in small amounts, but it's still a highly poisonous chemical and should not be consumed.

Chlorine has been shown to contribute to heart disease. It damages the arteries. People worry about cholesterol and focus on lowering it when it comes to heart disease, but cholesterol becomes a problem only when it attaches itself to the artery and then clogs it, restricting blood flow. And cholesterol only attaches itself to the artery when the artery is scarred or damaged.

Primarily, there are four things that cause the arteries to become scarred:

1. **Chlorinated water**. Chlorine in the water that you drink, shower and bathe in, or swim in causes scarring of the arteries, which in turn means no matter how much cholesterol you have or don't have, whatever cholesterol is there will attach itself and begin the clogging process.

2. **Hydrogenated oils or trans fats**. As you look at much of the processed food you buy in boxes, if you read the label you'll often see the words "hydrogenated oil" or "partially hydrogenated oil." These are trans fats. Margarine, for example, is a hydrogenated oil. These trans fats scar the arteries. They cause heart disease and arteriosclerosis.

3. **Homogenized dairy products**. People say, "Well I drink low-fat milk or low-fat yogurt." You're being misled. The fat isn't the problem. When dairy products are homogenized it turns them into a lethal man-made product that causes scarring of the arteries. It is not the fat that'll harm you, it's the homogenization process.

4. **Sugar**. In the last few years it's been discovered that sugar causes inflammation, which contributes to artery damage. A study published in the *Journal of The American College of Cardiology* found that consuming foods high in sugar led to a dysfunction in the layer of cells that line the arteries. Repeated sugar consumption reduces the flexibility of the arteries and leads to heart disease.

Okay, now let's get back to water. What kind of water do *I* drink? Never tap water. I have a reverse osmosis unit in my house. I have the water in my entire house filtered. I also have a distiller, which in addition to steam distillation, also gets rid of the energetic memory attached to the water. I *do* drink bottled water and spring water when I travel.

The reason I brought up the issue about arteriosclerosis is that tap water has chlorine in it. One reason there's so much heart disease today is because people not only drink tap water, they also bathe and shower in it, and swim in chlorinated pools. Since our skin is the largest organ in the body, it's believed that we absorb more chlorine and toxins by taking one shower than by drinking five glasses of water.

In a shower, not only is the chlorine being absorbed through the skin, the toxins are also turned into a gas created by the steam. These toxic fumes in your shower are then inhaled. Consider reducing this exposure by finding a good shower filtration system for your home, or better yet, a whole house filtration system.

Unfortunately, it's not just the water you drink and bathe in. Chlorine is used in the processing of many fruits and vegetables. It's also added to the water used in the irrigation of fruits and vegetables. Chlorine is a major problem.

As you can now understand, our water supply is loaded with toxins. These toxins are getting into our bodies by:

- ✔ Drinking the water

- ✔ Eating or drinking anything made with the water

- ✔ Eating any food that was grown with the water

- ✔ Eating any meat, poultry, fish or dairy where the animal drank the water

✔ Showering, bathing, or swimming in the water

Let's talk about other toxins you may put into your body via what you drink. How about carbonated sodas? Don't drink them. Carbonated beverages block calcium absorption. Calcium is one of the most important building blocks of nutrition. And have you read the ingredients in sodas? They're full of chemicals, plus high fructose corn syrup (which is a poison that makes you fat), and diet sodas are even worse. Artificial sweeteners in diets sodas are mostly, if not all, toxic.

What about alcohol? I mostly avoid it. I prefer to drink purified water and not much else, but sometimes a little wine (preferably red, because of its antioxidants) is okay.

Tea can be good and therapeutic. Choose organic blends.

What about juices? Be wary of store bought juice. It's processed. Unfortunately, when juice is processed, bacteria and mold can develop, which contaminates it. So by law the juice has to be pasteurized, which means it has to be heated to 220 degrees for thirty minutes to kill any bacteria so you don't get sick from it. This kills all of the living enzymes and destroys the natural energy of the fruit. The juice is then filtered, and in many cases, sugar (which isn't listed on the label) is added. It's not healthy, it's man-made, and it's tainted with chemicals and toxins. If you want juice, buy organic fruits and vegetables and juice them yourself at home.

> The things you apply to your skin get into your bloodstream as well.

Another way we absorb toxins is by applying them to our skin. Anything we put on the skin is absorbed into the body. This is why certain drugs (like hormones and nicotine patches) are administered through the skin. Those drugs pass through the skin and end up in the bloodstream. The things you apply to your skin get into your bloodstream as well.

Our friends at the FDA have determined that many chemicals are for "external use only." They're poisonous and cannot be taken internally because they can kill you. But remember, what you put on your body winds up in your body. Do you understand the problem here and why we take in so many toxins? We apply lotions, moisturizers, sunscreens, cosmetics, soap, shampoo, etc. Virtually all of these contain ingredients that even the FDA says are so poisonous that they can't be taken internally. Yet, they are deemed safe enough to be used on the skin. Be wary of this. Look at the products you use and consider making changes to natural products where you can.

For example, coconut oil makes an excellent moisturizer. Apple cider vinegar can be used as a skin toner. Baking soda can be used to brush your teeth and for deodorant. Underarm deodorants and antiperspirants contain chemicals that are believed to be a major cause of breast cancer. Remember, if you can't eat it, do not put it on your skin.

We also absorb toxins through the nose, via poisons in the air. Pollution is obviously a problem, but there are many toxins floating around that people are unaware of, or simply don't think about. Air fresheners are among the worst. Talk about misleading advertising. They claim that these products "freshen" the air, when actually they contain toxic chemicals. Would you consider opening the can and drinking the air freshener? Read the label since they even tell you how poisonous the ingredients are. These products eliminate odors by having you spray a poison in the air. This poison kills the receptors in the nose so that you can't smell the offending odor any more. Air fresheners don't eliminate odors; they eliminate your ability to smell them.

Other airborne toxins include: mold, dust, pollens, and the fumes emitted from carpeting, glue, paint, mattresses, laundry detergent, household cleaners etc. Any aroma that you smell means molecules are in the air and you're breathing them in. We're inhaling toxins on a regular basis. It's impossible to eliminate all of them. However, it is possible to reduce the number of toxins you're inhaling by avoiding commercial household products and using nontoxic products, or making your own. Baking soda, vinegar, and lemon can be used for all kinds of household cleaning, including laundry. An air purifier (with a filter, not an air *freshener*) reduces other airborne toxins.

It's important to note that what you inhale has an effect on such things as appetite, digestion, moods, depression, anxiety, irritability, and sleep. Reducing the toxins that you breathe can have a very profound impact on your health and wellbeing.

We also take in toxins **through our eyes.** The primary type of toxins that enter through the eyes are images that cause bad emotions. There are more violent images on television, in the movies, newspapers and magazines, video games, and books than ever before. Repeated exposure to negative, disturbing images causes the body to become acidic. Today, people are being exposed to over one thousand times the amount of negative images than they were just twenty years ago; and over ten thousand times the amount of negative images compared to seventy-five years ago. Be mindful of what you're watching, reading, and listening to. Too much negative stimulation is toxic and can lead to health problems.

Toxins get into our bodies **through the ears**, via anything we put into them, as well as the sounds we hear. Sounds are vibrations and frequencies. Certain vibrations and frequencies engender life. And other vibrations and frequencies can cause degeneration and death.

If we stop and really listen to all of the sounds around us, we find the majority are unnatural man-made frequencies. These frequencies go in through the ears and affect us right down to our cells. If the frequency is not in tune with what our bodies are equipped to tolerate, it can disrupt the natural balance of the body. The simplest proof of this is how certain music, sounds, and frequencies, can cause a plant to either die or thrive. Think of the opera singer who hits a high note and shatters a crystal glass. That is how powerful vibrations, sounds, and frequencies are. Sounds can affect the body in such a powerful way that even the U.S. military uses sound as a weapon that induces physiological and psychological damage.

Much of the noise we hear is beyond our control, but you should consider making changes to stressful sounds where you can. When you drive, you might listen to calm music rather than frenetic music, or the news. Alarm clocks are now using natural sounds, like waves, or rain to wake a person more gently. Earplugs or headphones can provide relief at times from stressful sounds. Just be mindful of negative sounds and noises and do what you can to minimize your exposure to them.

> Too much negative stimulation is toxic and can lead to health problems.

Now I'd like to you to consider a toxic cause of illness that people have only recently begun to be concerned about. That is electromagnetic fields. Medical science claims there is no evidence to prove that electromagnetic energy has an adverse effect on health. Remember, though, that science has also refuted things throughout history that have later proven to be true. Science claimed that there was no evidence that nutrition had an effect on health; or that cigarettes were addictive. Science stated that anyone believing those things were heretics. The same is true now in relation to electromagnetic energy. Think about it. If a satellite in the sky beams down electromagnetic energy twenty-four hours a day, seven days a week, and this energy is invisible, cannot be detected, yet has the ability to pass through almost any material, and contains so much information that a "receiver" converts it into the music of an orchestra or images on a TV screen, isn't it possible that this energy is also passing through our bodies? Is it possible that this unnatural energy could have a negative impact on our health? Here are a few examples of the sources of unnatural electromagnetic energy bombarding our bodies every day:

- ✔ **Satellites**. There are dozens of satellites beaming down unnatural electromagnetic energy twenty-four hours a day, seven days a week.

- ✔ **Radar**. Radar stations for national defense and weather emit harmful electromagnetic energy twenty-four hours a day, seven days a week. It's interesting to note that many people believe that when these radar stations are put on maximum power during times of heightened security, a higher percentage of people feel ill, fatigued, and depressed. There is also the suggestion that those living close to these powerful radar towers have a higher chance of getting cancer.

- ✔ **Cell phone towers.** These towers push out powerful energy waves on a consistent basis.

- ✔ **Cell phones**. When your cell phone is turned on it produces powerful unnatural electromagnetic energy, as well as drawing in all of the cell phone tower energy. If a cell phone is within just a few feet of you, you are being affected.

- ✔ **Wireless internet routers.** Wi-Fi modems use electromagnetic radiation to send their signals to your computer through walls, exposing you to radiation.

✔ **High-tension power lines.** These lines produce powerful amounts of negative energy affecting all living things in a large area around them.

✔ **Electric wiring**. Wiring encompasses our homes, our offices, our cars, any electronic device we carry, and is even buried under sidewalks and streets.

✔ **Computers, televisions and radios.** When these units are turned on, they emit large amounts of negative electromagnetic energy.

✔ **Fluorescent lights.** It is common knowledge that fluorescent lighting is an unnatural light source and can cause headaches, fatigue, and a weakening of the immune system. They also emit large doses of negative electromagnetic energy.

✔ **Microwave ovens**. The "microwaves" can be released from the oven adversely affecting those around it.

Another dynamic relating to electromagnetic energy is ions. There are positive and negative ions. Positively charged ions have an adverse effect on the body. Negatively charged ions have a positive, health-enhancing effect on the body. Running water such as a stream, waterfalls or the crashing waves of an ocean, emit large amounts of life-enhancing negative ions. The wind blowing through trees also emits these wonderful negative ions. This is why most people feel better when they're in these areas.

Conversely, the wind blowing through tall buildings in cities, or an electric dryer, emits harmful positive ions. If you sit in a Laundromat all day, it's common to feel horrible and fatigued. These harmful positive ions also can suppress your immune system.

Electromagnetic chaos can't be avoided altogether, however, you should try, where possible, to minimize your exposure to it. Turn off Wi-Fi modems at night. Minimize microwave usage. Don't hold your cell phone against your head or body (use a headset). And don't sleep with your cell phone turned on and right next to you. Avoid fluorescent lights. Don't leave televisions on around your house unnecessarily. Consider periodic detox days where you don't use any electronics.

What Comes Out of the Body

I've discussed toxins that are going *into* our bodies, but now let's talk about what goes *out* of the body. Our bodies produce toxins. This is fine, as long as the body's ability to eliminate these toxins is operating properly. Even if you put no toxins into your body, it would still create waste material and toxins. All toxins, whether created by the body or put into the body must be eliminated in order for us to be healthy. When toxins are allowed to accumulate they cause the immune system to be suppressed, and the body to become acidic. Accumulated toxins that have not been flushed out, or eliminated create an environment wherein illness and disease can flourish. We basically eliminate toxins through:

- ✔ The nose
- ✔ The mouth
- ✔ The urinary tract
- ✔ The colon
- ✔ The skin

The nose and mouth eliminate toxins primarily through the lungs. Our urinary tract eliminates toxins primarily through the kidneys and liver. The colon eliminates toxins primarily through the liver, the stomach and small intestine. The skin eliminates toxins primarily through perspiration.

Most people have excess accumulated toxins and waste in their bodies. The two main reasons for this are: 1) they're putting too many toxins into the body on a regular basis, and 2) their elimination channels are clogged, and/or sluggish.

When you take in toxins, and your body creates toxins at a faster rate than you're eliminating them, you build up an accumulation. For example, are your nasal and sinus cavities clear and mucus free? Do you breathe fully and deeply from your diaphragm, allowing your lungs to properly do their job? Do you sweat on a regular basis? Do you drink plenty of pure water, which allows the elimination channels to work more efficiently? Do you have bowel movements daily? A few common things that slow the elimination process are:

- ✔ **Antibiotics**. If you've ever taken an antibiotic you have dramatically slowed your elimination potential via the colon. Antibiotics kill all of the friendly bacteria in the intestine and colon. This allows unfriendly yeast, most notably Candida, to proliferate and infest your digestive system. This yeast overgrowth slows digestion, increases gas, bloating and constipation, and itself creates an abnormal number of toxins.

- ✔ **Lotions and creams.** Most people put lotions and creams all over their skin clogging the pores and suppressing the natural elimination process through the skin. This includes sunscreens, cosmetics, deodorants, and antiperspirants.

- ✔ **Lack of body movement**. Have you ever noticed when you take a dog for a walk, they poop? When you move your body as nature intended, you assist the elimination process. Since most people sit all day, their elimination cycles are suppressed. When you eat, food goes through the digestion process and ends up in the colon ready for elimination. The longer it sits in the colon, the more toxic it becomes. If left long enough, these toxins begin to enter the bloodstream. This can turn into a serious condition resulting in death. Your body's elimination system must be working at optimal levels if you want to live without illness and disease.

Exercise

In order to properly eliminate toxins you must exercise. In simplistic terms, there are seven kinds of exercise:

1. *Slow rhythmic movement.* This is mainly walking. The body is designed to walk, for long distances, and for long periods of time. Walking is probably the most important form of exercise you can do. When you go for a walk, not only are you getting the benefits of the slow rhythmic movement, your lymph system and digestive system are working toxins out of your body. The body is moving and energy is flowing through the meridians. Walking also has a profound effect on your state of mind and happiness factor.

2. *Stretching.* Your body consists of muscles, tendons, and ligaments. If you lived in a natural setting, interacting with nature as we are designed, the natural activities you would be doing throughout your day would cause the frequent stretching of your ligaments, muscles, and tendons. Lack of flexibility allows for negative energy and toxins to accumulate in parts of your body.

3. *Resistance exercise.* This includes any form of movement where resistance is put against a muscle, and the muscle is required to push or pull against the resistance. The most common form of resistance training is weight lifting or the use of resistance machines. Weight training can increase the size and strength of muscles, but it can reduce flexibility, thus hindering the flow of energy through the body. Nevertheless, doing any form of exercise is better than doing none at all.

4. *Postures.* Certain exercise regimes involve postures that are held for a period of time. The most commonly known is yoga. There are many forms of yoga. Not all are posture

based. Some yoga techniques are fluid and movement oriented. The benefits of postures are that they seem to help open up the natural energy channels in the body, and stimulate internal organs.

5. *Aerobic exercise*. Aerobic means "with air." Any form of exercise where you're breathing heavily but can still have a conversation is aerobic exercise. Aerobic exercise stimulates blood flow throughout the body, oxygenates the body and speeds the elimination of toxins.

6. *Anaerobic exercise*. Anaerobic means "without air." Any form of exercise where you are breathing so hard you can barely speak is anaerobic. The benefits are, generally, a tremendous stimulation to your entire system because, in effect, you are putting the survival of every cell in your body at risk because of the lack of oxygen. This is helpful in "reprogramming the body" and allowing it to increase the elimination of toxins and stop any cellular activity that's abnormal.

7. *Cellular exercise*. Jumping on a mini-trampoline, also known as a Rebounder, has been shown to stimulate and strengthen every cell in the body. This unique form of exercise dramatically increases the movement through the lymph system, stimulates every cell's elimination of toxins, and increases the strength and vitality of every cell in the body.

The major benefits of exercise include:

✔ **Increased oxygen to the cells**. Most people are deficient in the amount of oxygen they have in their bodies. Viruses and cancer, for example, cannot exist in an oxygen rich environment. An oxygen rich body is an alkaline body. An alkaline body is a body where disease and illness cannot exist.

✔ **Movement of lymph fluid**. The lymphatic system is an important element in the elimination process. Moving the body, as it was intended, increases the movement of lymph fluid, assisting with the elimination of toxins.

✔ **Cell stimulation.** Every cell in the body produces toxic waste. Every cell needs stimulation in order to eliminate its toxic waste and thrive normally. When a cell doesn't eliminate its toxic waste it can behave abnormally, which causes tumors, cancer, or the degeneration of vital organs in the body.

✔ **Opening of energy channels.** Energy flows through channels in the body. When these channels are blocked or congested, energy doesn't flow efficiently causing cell abnormalities and the suppression of the immune system, making the body susceptible to illness.

✔ **Releasing of tension and stress.** Stress is the silent killer. In simplistic terms, stress is holding on to negative energy. When negative energy is held, it can lodge itself into parts of the body.

Rest

Without proper rest, the cells are not given the opportunity to recharge and rejuvenate. Tired cells can't eliminate toxins efficiently. It's also during rest that most healing takes place. Most people don't get enough rest, and the rest they do get is not full and deep.

There are three elements of proper rest:

1. *The time in which you rest.* The most optimum time for the body to rest is when the sun is no longer shining. Ideally, a person would rest and sleep when the sun goes down and arise when the sun comes up. This is the natural cycle. However, most people's life styles do not allow this. Therefore they are resting and sleeping at non-optimal times. Each week a lunar cycle occurs starting at sundown every

Friday, ending at sundown every Saturday. This is absolutely the most ideal time for the body to recharge.

2. *The amount of hours you rest.* Although every person is unique, it appears that most operate better when getting eight hours of sleep. Studies show that people don't function as well if they receive fewer, or more, hours. The majority of people sleep fewer than eight hours, and then try to catch up by occasionally sleeping more. This does not allow optimal rejuvenation of the cells in your body.

3. *Rest and sleep should be deep.* Most people toss and turn at night.

Ideally you would not move for the entire sleep time. When sleep is full and deep, brainwave activity can occur, which stimulates the healing process throughout the body. A person who snores wakes up many times per night and unfortunately never reaches the deepest levels of sleep and so the body is never operating at optimal efficiency.

There's a difference between sleep and rest. The body can rest without going to sleep. Most people never take a "rest" during the day. The common pattern of waking up, working all day nonstop, going to bed late, never getting a full deep eight hours of peaceful sleep, results in a body that slowly begins to break down and never has a chance to heal and recharge. The body is very much like a battery. Like a battery, when the body's energy runs out, it must be recharged. If one did nothing else but get proper rest and sleep, that person's energy levels would skyrocket and they'd experience dramatically less illness and disease.

Thoughts

Thoughts are things. Your body is in fact a powerful electromagnetic transmitter and receiver of energy. Every thought you have can have a powerful impact on the cells in your body. Positive high vibrational thoughts can rid your body of disease. Negative stressful low vibrational thoughts can *give* your body disease.

Science tends not to believe that thoughts can have a profound effect on health. However, it is interesting to point out that medical science can't dispute the "placebo" effect. The placebo effect is when a person is given a "placebo," like a sugar pill, yet their disease is cured. This occurs because the patient thinks that what he or she is taking will cure the disease. This happens in as many as 40 percent of cases. Imagine, up to 40 percent of the time a person with a dreaded disease is cured with his or her own thoughts! Yet, remember our friends at the FDA insist that only a drug can cure disease.

Thoughts can heal, but they can also cause sickness and disease. Stress, which could be defined as negative thoughts, causes the body to become acidic, thus creating an environment for illness and disease. These negative thoughts can be conscious or unconscious. Worrying about money, arguing with relatives, friends, and co-workers, watching scary movies and reading the news, all increase stress levels.

> Thoughts can heal, but they can also cause sickness and disease.

Many negative thoughts are trapped in stressful or traumatic incidences from our past. Several doctors have found that the majority of people with cancer have an incident in their past that caused tremendous grief. Individuals who have heart attacks are found to have suppressed anger. It's interesting to note the correlation between emotions and certain diseases. The good news is this can be reversed.

Author Earl Nightingale discovered what he called "the strangest secret": *You become what you think about.* Positive thoughts and low amounts of stress create an alkaline pH in the body, wherein we don't become ill. Negative thoughts and emotions, and high levels of stress cause the body to become acidic, leading to illness and disease.

What You Say

Words have power. Most people speak words that increase stress and turn the body's pH from alkaline to acidic. Words can change the way we think and feel. Researchers have concluded that speaking the correct form of words and thinking the correct thoughts change a person's DNA.

Of all the things I've talked about in this chapter thus far relating to why we get sick, please do not overlook the power of how you think, and what you say. These two factors dramatically contribute to stress levels. Stress absolutely causes illness and disease. Reducing stress is one of the most powerful natural cures for virtually every disease in the body. This is one of those cures that can't be patented. No one's going to make billions of dollars selling it to you, but simple stress reducing techniques that are effective and inexpensive have been proven to be one of the most powerful natural cures of all time. This is one of the "natural cures" that "they" don't want you to know about.

The conclusion, then, is that we get sick because: We're putting too many toxins in our body and not flushing them out fast enough. We are not putting enough of the necessary nutrients into our body, and the nutrients that *are* going in are not being properly absorbed. We are exposed to, and negatively affected by electromagnetic chaos. And we have trapped mental and emotional stress.

Since all matter consists ultimately of energy, in simplistic terms, the cause of all disease is energetic imbalance.

How To Never Get Sick Again

This chapter will give you the information to help you eliminate any illness or disease and prevent any illness and disease in the future. This information will also allow you to potentially slow down or even reverse the aging process. Keep in mind that this information is my opinion and based on the information currently available.

Right now, you either have some known illness or disease such as cancer, diabetes, etc., or you claim to be healthy. If you claim to be healthy, you probably still experience the occasional aches and pains, fatigue, headaches, indigestion, colds and flu, heartburn, etc. So-called healthy people believe that these occasional conditions are "normal." They are not. A healthy person has little, if any, body odor, no bad breath, no foot odor, their urine and stool don't smell bad, they sleep soundly, they have no skin rashes or dandruff, they're not depressed or stressed and they don't get aches and pains, or colds and flu. Truly healthy people are full of energy and vitality, and never have to take any nonprescription or prescription drug because they never have any symptoms that require medication.

It is hard to find a truly healthy person. Let's examine where you are right now. Most likely, you're full of toxins. You're also probably deficient in necessary nutrients. The energy in your body is not flowing properly. Many of your systems are not operating at optimal levels. You either notice severe symptoms, or you have mild symptoms that you classify as normal.

What can we do to (a) eradicate any and all symptoms you have, thus "curing" the disease or illness and (b) prevent any illness or disease from starting, thus giving you a boost in energy, vitality, and vibrant health?

In general terms, the way to eradicate any illness and disease you may have, prevent illness and disease from occurring in the future, and slow down or potentially reverse the aging process is to do the following:

1. Eliminate the toxins that have built up in your system. You're loaded with toxins. The only question is, how much? You must get these toxins out of your body if you want to cure and prevent illness and disease. Getting the toxins out of your body can immediately increase energy, help you lose weight, eliminate depression and anxiety, and potentially reverse most illnesses and disease. The basic cleanses that you should do are:
    (a) colon cleanse
    (b) liver/gallbladder cleanse
    (c) kidney/bladder cleanse
    (d) heavy metal cleanse
    (e) parasite cleanse
    (f) Candida cleanse
    (g) full-body fat tissue/lymphatic cleanse

A simple Internet search will lead you to options for the aforementioned cleanses.

2. Stop, or at least reduce, the toxins entering your body. It's impossible to totally eliminate toxins from entering your body, but you can dramatically reduce the amount of toxins going in.

3. Make sure your elimination systems are clean and not sluggish, thus allowing the toxins that you do put in your body, and the toxins that develop naturally are getting eliminated quickly and not accumulating.

4. Make sure you're getting proper nutrition in the form of vitamins, minerals, enzymes, cofactors, and life-sustaining "energy," and make sure your system can assimilate these nutrients.

5. Reduce and/or neutralize the electromagnetic energy that is attacking your body's energy field and cells.

6. Reduce stress.

7. Use your mind and words to create a healthy alkaline body pH, and actually change genetically defective DNA structures into healthy DNA structures.

Theoretically, if all of the above were to occur you couldn't get sick. If the cause of all disease is too many toxins, nutritional deficiencies, electromagnetic chaos, and/or stress, then if you did not have toxins in the body, if you did not have nutritional deficiencies, if you did not have exposure to electromagnetic chaos, and if you did not have stress, then you would not have any disease.

I'm going to list many things for you to consider doing that will help you accomplish the recommendations above. Do not be overwhelmed by this list. Don't think that you must do all of these things starting tomorrow if you want to prevent and cure any disease you have. Consider going at an easy pace, and implementing these things slowly and in a way that's comfortable for you. If you do these things, in my opinion, you virtually should never get sick. If you do get sick, the severity and duration of the illness will be short.

> You can help the body heal better and faster, but you can't heal the body.

Remember, the body heals itself. No treatment heals or cures. You can help the body heal better and faster, but you can't heal the body. All of the suggestions in this chapter are designed to help the body heal itself. All of these suggestions are designed to turn your body's pH from acidic, where disease and illness can develop, to the healthy state of alkaline, where disease and illness cannot exist. There is no *one* thing that can turn your body from acidic pH to alkaline pH. It depends upon what's *causing* your body to be acidic and that could be a number of things. But if you do the things in this chapter, your body *can* turn from acidic to alkaline pH. That's one of our ultimate goals and it's one of the simplest ways to determine how healthy you are. If your body's pH is alkaline, it is virtually impossible to get cancer or any other major disease.

Here are what I believe to be the simple all natural, non-drug and nonsurgical ways to prevent and cure every disease.

1. **See a natural healthcare provider on a regular basis.**

   Choose one that doesn't only use drugs or surgery. When you have a car that you love and cherish, you keep it clean on the inside and out. You do not wait for the car to make funny noises or stop running; instead you bring the car in for regular maintenance. This maintenance is designed to prevent major problems from occurring. Your body should be treated in a similar manner. You should be seeing various natural healthcare providers from a variety of disciplines, even when you aren't experiencing symptoms. I believe it's important to be looked at by several people and get multiple opinions. Even though I feel I'm knowledgeable when it comes to the prevention and curing of disease naturally, I also know that getting other perspectives is valuable. Avoid being seen or treated by a doctor who uses drugs and surgery. Choose a licensed healthcare practitioner. Some examples I highly recommend are:

a. Get treated by a bioenergetic synchronization technique practitioner.
Dr. M.T. Morter, Jr., who invented the technique, has trained thousands of people in this treatment. It's painless and takes only a few minutes, and it effectively rebalances the body, reducing or eliminating pain or trauma. It helps the body go from acid to alkaline. For more information, go to www.morterhealth.com.

b. Get a chiropractic adjustment.
If you've never had a chiropractic adjustment, you probably need one. Because of our lifestyle, our spines get misaligned. Realigning the spine allows energy to flow freely throughout the body. I see several different chiropractors, because each has a different style of treatment, and I visit one at least once a month for a tune-up. Even if you have no pain, go get an adjustment. The adjustments are painless and most people feel energized afterwards.

c. See an herbalist.
Seeing a highly-recommended herbalist allows you to be treated effectively, and yet avoid the dangers of drugs. If you've never had a consultation with an herbalist you have no idea what you're missing. When you take

in herbs specifically customized for you, the physical benefits can be enormous.

d. See a homeopathic practitioner.

Homeopathy is a system of treatment in which homeopathic medicines are used to gently bring the body into balance. A good homeopathic doctor does not treat symptoms, but instead, treats the whole person.

e. See a naturopath.

Naturopaths are licensed healthcare practitioners who differ from homeopaths in that they may prescribe *multiple* types of treatment (herbs, supplements, dietary adjustment), yet no prescription drugs or surgery. They use a holistic approach to bring a person to a state of balance, thus allowing the body to cure itself.

2. **Stop taking nonprescription and prescription drugs.**

If you're taking drugs of any kind, do not do this step without consulting your physician. Remember, drugs are poisons. This includes vaccines. Although opinions vary, many experts believe that vaccines are some of the most toxic substances you can put in your body. It is estimated that millions have had to receive medical treatment because of horrible side effects from taking prescription and nonprescription drugs. It's also estimated that tens of millions will develop long-term medical conditions because they took nonprescription and prescription drugs. In my opinion, drugs should only be taken in the most severe cases. This step is so important. You have to know that if you are taking any nonprescription or prescription drugs you absolutely will get sick and develop disease. Let me say that again: If you continue to take nonprescription over-thecounter drugs and/or prescription drugs you absolutely will get sick. Nonprescription drugs and prescription drugs are toxins and they *cause* illness and disease. You must stop taking them if you intend to prevent and cure any disease. You cannot cure your disease if you continue to take nonprescription and prescription drugs. You cannot prevent disease if you continue to take nonprescription and prescription drugs. In my opinion, you should clean out your medicine cabinet and stop giving your money to the criminals who run the drug companies.

3. **Energetic rebalancing.**

Frequency generators have been around for decades. Today there are several machines using frequencies to balance a person's energy, thus eliminating the energetic frequency of the imbalance or disease. When the frequency of the disease you have has been neutralized, the disease goes away. These machines allow the body to cure all diseases. They're fast, painless, and inexpensive, and they are also outlawed by the FDA. Individual practitioners using these machines never publicly claim that they cure anything for fear that the FDA will prosecute them for using an unlicensed medical device and curing people without the legally approved drugs. These machines include the Intero, Vegatest, Dermatron, and others. I've been using this technology for several years, and I have never in that time been sick. When everyone around me got the flu, I never experienced a symptom.

People always want to know what the "natural cure" is for their disease, or what the best way to prevent disease is. If you do the three things I have just mentioned— (1) see several licensed health-care practitioners for individualized treatment; (2) stop taking all nonprescription over-the-counter drugs and prescription drugs (under the supervision of a doctor); and (3) get on an energetic rebalancing program, I believe you will virtually never get sick and you can cure any disease you have, provided you're not past the point of no return. If you *are* past the point of no return and the degeneration or disease is in its most advanced stages, then unfortunately it's too late to implement these cures.

Can energetic rebalancing alone prevent and cure all disease? I believe that it can. I've seen this technology cure people of the most horrific debilitating diseases anyone can imagine. I have seen cancer, diabetes, MS and countless other diseases cured by energetic rebalancing. The thousands of people who are on energetic rebalancing technology virtually never get sick. This is statistically unheard of. However, the FDA, other government agencies, and all of the groups I mentioned previously categorically do not want this technology exposed and they try to debunk it and attack it every chance they can. Why? Because it will cost them billions of dollars in profits if people use this inexpensive technology to prevent and cure their diseases. You can go to the Internet to find various energetic rebalancing treatments. I am on two programs. One is available at www.energeticbalancing.us and www.energeticmatrix.com.

4. **Check your body pH.**

Dr. M.T. Morter (whom I mentioned earlier in the chapter) discovered one of the greatest breakthroughs for health assessment in the last hundred years, yet because this discovery would not increase profits to the pharmaceutical industry it has gone by the wayside without much fanfare. Dr. Morter's discovery should have won him a Nobel Prize. He discovered the powerful truth that when your body's pH is acidic, diseases such as cancer, diabetes, and Multiple Sclerosis can thrive. He also discovered that when a body's pH is alkaline, diseases such as cancer cannot exist. Therefore, one of the most powerful and simplest ways to test your health and/or propensity for disease is to check your body's pH.

The pH testing procedure is something I encourage everyone to do on a regular basis. I check mine monthly. If it's out of the proper range I look at the things I'm doing, or not doing, and I can make simple adjustments to correct the out of balance pH. The reason this is so important is because it takes years to develop most diseases. When you're checking your pH regularly, even if it goes out of balance, as long as you correct it and bring it back into balance, you are never allowing your body the time to develop a disease. In my opinion it's the simplest and easiest way to make sure you never develop any major illnesses.

The above four suggestions are what I call the basic four for the prevention and treatment of all disease. In my opinion, you must do these if you're serious about achieving and maintaining optimal health. However, we know that the causes of all disease are (1) too many toxins in the body, (2) nutritional deficiencies, (3) electromagnetic chaos, and (4) stress. Therefore, we must address each of these with specific recommendations on how to achieve (a) no toxins in the body, (b) no nutritional deficiencies, (c) no electromagnetic chaos, and (d) no stress.

Here are the specific recommendations. Doing these things will turn your body's pH from acid to alkaline and create a state of balance in the body known as *homeostasis*.

A. Clean Out The Toxins That Have Accumulated In Your Body.

It's important to understand that from the time you're born your body is flooded with toxins. These include everything from vaccines, to nonprescription and prescription drugs, the air you breathe, the water you drink as well as shower, bathe and swim in, and all of the chemicals put in your food. They also include all of the toxins from carpeting, paint, non-stick cookware, cosmetics, makeup, soaps, lotions, and sunscreens. For years, your body has been loaded with toxins and these toxins don't fully leave the body. They stay in the fatty tissues; they stay in the organs; they stay in the colon, intestine and throughout your entire body. They are causing you illness and disease. They're suppressing your immune system. If you want to prevent disease you must clean these toxins out.

> If you want to prevent disease you must clean these toxins out.

If the toxins in our bodies are the *cause* of the illnesses and diseases that we're suffering from, then if we clean the toxins out of our bodies, *in most cases*, we'll experience a dramatic reduction, or even a complete elimination, of our symptoms. Simply cleaning toxins out of your body could be the "natural cure" of your disease.

Keep in mind, if you're experiencing symptoms or have a disease, it may have taken years to develop that illness. If you clear out all of the toxins in your system it may take several months after that for the body to heal itself. Do give it some time. This is why, again, I encourage you to be under the care of a licensed healthcare practitioner.

Here are the best ways to clean the toxins out of your system:

1. **Get fifteen colonics in thirty days.**
   Right now as you read this there's an excellent chance that you have several pounds of undigested fecal matter in your colon. This waste matter is suppressing your immune system, potentially causing gas, bloating and constipation, dramatically reducing the assimilation of nutrients, and slowing

your metabolism. Getting a series of fifteen colonics over a thirty-day period is one of the most important first steps in cleansing and detoxifying your body. Most people lose between three and fifteen pounds simply by doing this procedure. The hair, skin, and nails begin to radiate and glow with health. Your energy levels can sky rocket, depression, stress, anxiety and fatigue are usually dramatically reduced or eliminated. Food cravings are reduced or vanish completely.

2. **Do a colon cleanse.**

   If you do the colonics, you won't need a colon cleanse as well. But a clean colon is an important step in ridding your body of accumulated toxins.

3. **Do a liver/gallbladder cleanse.**

   This cleanse generally causes the removal of gallstones that contain accumulated toxins and which people are usually unaware that they have. As a result of their removal, the liver will function more efficiently and when it does, the liver itself removes toxins from the body.

4. **Do a kidney/bladder cleanse.**

   Cleansing the kidney and bladder will help these organs function more efficiently. The kidneys and bladder are filters in the body and when they're sluggish due to toxic build up, it only leans to more toxic accumulation.

5. **Do a heavy metal cleanse.**

   Exposure to heavy metals can create all kinds of problems. Some of these heavy metals can affect the brain. In some cases, heavy metal toxicity leads to Multiple Sclerosis.

6. **Do a parasite cleanse.**

   Parasites, like heavy metals, are a major cause of disease. There are different types of parasites and they affect different parts of the body. Common types are in the intestines and they can prevent the body from absorbing nutrients.

7. **Do a Candida cleanse.**

   If you've ever taken antibiotics any time in your life, you likely have a Candida yeast overgrowth. This overgrowth is most common in the intestine, but it can infiltrate your entire body. This overgrowth can be a cause of virtually every symptom you can imagine: headaches, gas bloating, indigestion, heartburn, nausea, allergies, asthma, fibromyalgia, arthritis, diabetes, constipation, yeast infections, dandruff, acne, bad breath, fatigue, depression, stress, and on and on. Doing a program that eliminates Candida from your body is one of the backbones of good health. The most common side effect of excess Candida is the inability to lose weight. People who eliminate Candida tend to lose weight without trying. Candida also causes food cravings and can make you eat when you're not hungry. When Candida is normalized, a person's appetite can be dramatically reduced.

8. **Do a full-body fat/lymphatic cleanse.**

   The lymph system—the lymph nodes and vessels absorb excess fluid and debris from our bodies. When that system gets congested it leads to problems. Cleansing the lymph system includes dietary changes, dry-brushing, massage and exercise, all of which assist the body in moving fluid through the lymph system. This is necessary, because the lymph system doesn't have a pump the way the circulatory system has the heart.

9. **Drink eight glasses of pure water daily.**

   As I've mentioned previously all tap water is toxic because it contains chlorine. Most tap water also has fluoride, which is one of the most poisonous and disease causing agents you can put in your body. Do not drink or use tap water for any reason except for washing your floor. You need to drink water, though, and the water must be pure. Water is instrumental not only in flushing and nourishing the body, but also in keeping it hydrated and pH balanced. I recommend drinking a minimum of eight large glasses of water daily. Use a water purifier or bottled spring water.

10. **Use a rebounder (mini-trampoline) ten minutes a day.**
    A rebounder is a mini-trampoline. Using this device for just ten minutes a day can provide more cellular benefit than almost any other form of exercise. A rebounder stimulates every cell in the body simultaneously. It strengthens the immune system and it's effective at purging toxins from the cells. It stimulates all major organs and glands, and dramatically strengthens and tones the muscles, tendons, and ligaments. A truly spectacular form of exercise.

11. **Walk one hour a day.**
    The body is designed to walk. Walking outside reduces stress, stimulates the lymphatic system, promotes a lean body, and helps alleviate depression.

12. **Stretch the muscles and tendons.**
    If your body is supple and flexible, energy easily flows and blockages do not occur. When energy flows it's less likely for illness and disease to manifest. I recommend doing yoga, Pilates, martial arts, or any other kind of exercise that leads to stretching on a regular basis. I spend fifteen minutes each morning stretching.

13. **Practice deep breathing.**
    Your lungs need to be used. Most Americans breathe from high up in their chests. If you watch babies breathe naturally, you'll notice that they breathe fully and deeply. Their stomachs and diaphragms expand as well as their chests and backs. Deep breathing everyday stimulates the immune system, increases metabolism, reduces stress, and brings vital oxygen into the body. Most people are oxygen deficient.

Increasing oxygen to the cells can eliminate a multitude of diseases. Cancer, for example, cannot live in an oxygen-rich environment.

14. **Sweat with a regular dry sauna or an infrared sauna (not a wet steam).**

Your body is supposed to sweat. It is a natural way to eliminate toxins. If you don't sweat, toxins build up in the system.

15. **Do oil pulling regularly.**

Oil pulling is when you take a teaspoon or two of oil, generally extra virgin coconut oil, or castor oil, and swish it through the teeth as you would mouthwash. Do this for a few minutes or longer, up to 15 minutes. Coconut oil and castor oil are antibacterial and oil pulling with them will remove bacteria and toxins from parts of your mouth and from between the teeth. Did you know that there's a relationship between oral health and heart health? While the plaque in arteries is not the same as the plaque in between our teeth, there is a link. Bacteria from the mouth can enter the bloodstream through the gums and that same bacteria has been found clumped in artery plaque. Oil pulling removes the toxins and bacteria.

16. **Dry brush massage.**

I mentioned dry-brushing earlier; it assists the lymphatic system. Dry-brushing also exfoliates the skin, and helps rid the body of toxins.

17. **Get a full-body Swedish and/or deep tissue massage on a regular basis.**

The benefits of massage are reflected in your ...

Circulatory System by:
- helping to develop a stronger heart
- improving oxygen supply to cells
- improving the supply of nutrients to cells
- eliminating metabolic wastes

- decreasing blood pressure
- increasing circulation of lymph nodes

Digestive System by:
- relaxing the abdominal and intestinal muscles
- relieving tension
- stimulating activity of liver and kidneys
- eliminating waste material

Muscular System by:
- relaxing or stimulating muscles
- strengthening muscles and connective tissue
- helping to keep muscles flexible and pliable
- relieving soreness, tension, and stiffness

Nervous System by:
- stimulating motor nerve points
- relieving restlessness and insomnia
- promoting a sense of well-being
- relieving pain

Respiratory System by:
- developing respiratory muscles
- draining sluggish lymph nodes

Lymphatic System by:
- cleansing the body of metabolic wastes
- draining sluggish lymph nodes

Integumentary System (the skin) by:
- stimulating blood to better nourish skin
- improving tone and elasticity of skin
- helping to normalize glandular functions

Skeletal System by:
- improving body alignment
- relieving stiff joints
- relieving tired aching feet

There are many kinds of massages. You may like one and not the other. I get at least one massage a week. They're highly therapeutic, and I recommend you get as many as you can as often as you can. Use different massage therapists to experience the full range of treatments.

18. **Do Chi Kung.**

Chi Kung is a series of gentle movements that stimulate strength, energy flow, increased energy, and many other health benefits. I have a friend named Peter Ragnar who lives in Tennessee and is a senior citizen. He has the body and skin of an athlete in his thirties. No one would ever guess this man's age. He practices most of the concepts described in this book. One of the things he does, which he believes is a major cause of his youthful appearance and incredible health, is Chi Kung ten minutes a day. Because the Earth's magnetic energy is so much lower today than it was thousands of years ago, he does the simple movements standing on powerful magnets. This technique is very effective. People who practice Chi Kung usually feel a major increase in physical energy within just a few days. Sleeping is improved and people report an increased sense of peace and wellbeing.

19. **Do Tai Chi.**

Tai Chi is a series of flowing movements designed to center oneself, relieve stress, increase energy flow, increase flexibility and strength, and promote health and wellbeing. I've practiced Tai Chi for over twenty years. There are many different teachers, some better than others, but doing any form of Tai Chi has benefits.

20. **Do a seven to thirty day fast.**

Fasting has numerous benefits, including giving the digestive system a rest so it can heal itself. It also helps rid the body of toxins. Doing a fast can help to reset your eating habits as well. After a fast you are less likely to crave unhealthy food and so you may have an easier time implementing healthy eating habits. Make sure to be under the supervision of a healthcare practitioner if you undertake a fast that's longer than a week.

21. **Get "specialized treatments" as needed.**
Treatments such as reflexology, acupuncture, cranial sacral therapy, reiki, essential oil treatments, and various other holistic, all natural therapies have profound positive effects on health.

Obviously, when a person looks at this list their initial reaction is to be overwhelmed. You may feel there's no way you can do all of these things. That's okay. Start with doing *something*. You'll notice the first thing that I listed was doing fifteen colonics in thirty days. Start with that one. You'll feel more energetic than ever before. Just cleaning the colon, in the vast majority of cases, has been known to cure many diseases.

Each one of the things mentioned above is in fact a "natural cure" that "they" don't want you to know about. They're natural, they're not patentable, nobody's making billions of dollars on them, *and* they expose the fact that the drug industry and the food industry are causing the majority of illness and disease by feeding us chemical poisons. This is a fact that the powers that be don't want you to know, but the fact is indisputable.

B. You Must Stop Putting Toxins into the Body

I just gave you a list of things to do to get toxins *out* of the body. It's important now to reduce the amount of toxins going *into* the body on an ongoing basis. The recommendations that follow will dramatically reduce the amount of toxins you're putting in your body. Keep in mind that all of the recommendations in this chapter have a profound effect on preventing and curing disease, because they're addressing the cause of the symptoms and disease. They also have a profound effect upon changing your body's pH from acidic to alkaline.

Medical science does not want you to know what's causing your disease; they only want to sell you drugs to suppress the symptoms. Imagine a guy who says, "Every time I pour gasoline all over my house and light it with a match it burns to the ground. What's the cure?" You'd laugh at such a ridiculous statement, but that's what people do every day in relation to their own diseases. They don't realize that they're causing the disease with the toxins they put in their bodies.

> ...symptoms didn't develop overnight, and if you stop putting the toxins in, the symptoms are not necessarily going to vanish overnight...

A question that comes up is which of these is more important, or which will have the most profound affect. The answer is every person is different; however, generally speaking, the more powerful techniques are at the top of each list. Sometimes just making one change can eradicate your symptoms. You must keep in mind that your symptoms didn't develop overnight, and if you stop putting the toxins in, the symptoms are not necessarily going to vanish overnight either, although in some cases they do. Generally, it takes weeks or months for the symptoms to slowly diminish unless, as I mentioned, you're at the point of no return.

With that in mind, here is a powerful list of things to do and things *not* to do that will reduce the deadly poisons from going into your body and allow you to prevent and cure illness and disease.

1. **Do not eat any food that's produced or sold by a publicly traded corporation or that is a "brand name" product.**

   This is a tough one. If it comes in any mass produced packaging, then it came from a mass production processing plant. If you have ever been in a mass production food processing facility, you would understand what I'm talking about. Remember that there are over 15,000 chemicals that are routinely put into the food in the processing cycle that do not have to be listed on the label. Even if you read the ingredient list, there's an excellent chance that the food itself has been produced with chemicals and chemicals have been added. So, virtually all food you buy at the supermarket that comes in a package is loaded with chemicals. Mass produced food in packages is categorically unhealthy. If you must buy something in a box, jar, can, or package, buy something that was produced by hand in a small facility and look for the words "100% organic."

2. **Get the metal out of your dental work.**

   It's important for you to know that many people suffer horrible, debilitating symptoms that are *directly caused* by the amalgam (metal) fillings in their dental work. People have seen Multiple Sclerosis symptoms subside after removing these fillings, which generally are 50% mercury. Mercury is a powerful neurotoxin and it can cause neurological problems, mental disorders, chronic illnesses and autoimmune disease. If you currently have metal fillings, see a dentist who can replace them with nontoxic, nonmetal ones.

3. **Stop smoking.**

   This one is patently obvious. Not only should you not smoke, you should not allow anyone to smoke anywhere near you, either. Smoking is a horrible, toxic practice that causes and contributes to countless illnesses. Presumably, if you're interested enough in this book to be reading it, you have the good sense not to smoke. But if you've been unable to quit, you must. Don't use the products made by the pharmaceutical industry. Those, too, are toxins. If you're struggling to quit, consider seeing a hypnotherapist. Many people also find acupuncture helpful.

4. **Don't drink tap water.**
All tap water is loaded with contaminants, toxins, poisons, and known cancer causing agents including fluoride and chlorine. Drinking tap water causes illness and disease.
But you must drink lots of water. However, the water has to be *pure*. Bottled spring water, water filtered using reverse-osmosis, and water purified through steam distillation, are all better options than tap water.

5. **Use a shower filter.**
Your skin absorbs the water from your shower or bath. A hot shower produces steam and that turns many of the chemicals in the water into poisonous gases. These gases are inhaled or absorbed through the skin. A good shower filter removes most of the toxins in the water.

6. **Eat only 100% organic food.**
You want to eat food that has not been grown with chemical fertilizers, pesticides, or herbicides. Organic food has no chemical poison residue, and has higher concentrations of nutrients.

7. **Do not eat in fast food restaurants.**
Fast food is simply some of the most nutritionally deficient and chemically loaded "food" on the planet. If the definition of food was "fuel for the body that also encourages life," fast food could no longer be called food. "Fast, good tasting *poison*," is a more accurate description. Oh, and did I tell you that it's designed to increase your appetite, and make you physically addicted to it. If you eat fifteen meals per week

in a fast food restaurant, you have a 90 percent chance of getting cancer, heart disease, diabetes, acid reflux, obesity, and potentially dozens of other diseases. Avoid it completely.

8. **Never microwave food in plastic containers.**
   I don't use microwaves myself, because I believe it compromises the food by making it energetically toxic to the body, but others disagree. I also believe that being exposed to "microwaves" on a regular basis exposes you to toxins, so I would recommend that you avoid them. But I also understand that may be difficult for many people. If you are going to microwave your food, at least don't use plastic containers when you do it. Use a glass or ceramic, microwave safe dish. When you microwave certain plastics, a chemical called bisphenol A (BPA) can leach out of the plastic and migrate into the food making it toxic.

9. **Eliminate aspartame and monosodium glutamate.**
   Aspartame, aka NutraSweet®, is responsible for many distressing medical problems, ranging from headaches and memory loss, to hyperactivity in children, and seizure disorders. Both monosodium glutamate (MSG) and aspartame can cause harm to the brain and nervous system, and both have been linked to Alzheimer's disease, Lou Gehrig's disease, depression, Multiple Sclerosis, and more. MSG is a major cause of treatable and preventable illnesses such as headaches, asthma, epilepsy, heart irregularities, depression, and attention deficit/hyperactivity disorder.

10. **Do not eat artificial sweeteners (including Splenda).**
    Artificial sweeteners are man-made chemicals. They are poisons and should never be consumed. They cause all kinds of health problems. Instead, use raw organic honey, or coconut sugar, both of which have a lower glycemic index than regular sugar, or use the herb stevia, which comes from a plant.

11. **Do not eat processed sugar.**

There's been a lot written about the dangers of sugar in the past few years. Dr. Robert Lustig, an endocrinologist now famous for his lecture "Sugar: The Bitter Truth," which was written about in the New York Times, has even deemed sugar toxic, and many agree with him. The spike in blood sugar caused by ingesting all types of sugar is apparently worse for the body than previously believed. Sugar causes inflammation. Inflammation is detrimental to the immune system. In addition to leading to obesity and diabetes, new evidence suggests that sugar consumption can also cause damage to the arteries, contributing to heart disease. Minimize your sugar consumption and never eat white sugar. I recommend raw organic honey or coconut sugar in small amounts, or stevia.

12. **Do not drink sodas.**

All sodas are laden with chemical additives and all carbonated soft drinks block calcium absorption. Regular sodas are loaded with sugar. And did you know that Coke contains enough acid it can be used as rust remover? If it does that, what do think it's doing inside your body? *Nothing good*, that's what! Diet sodas have been called the "new crack" because they're so addictive. The artificial sweeteners in diet sodas can actually make you gain weight, because they stimulate the appetite, but they don't satisfy it. Studies have shown that consumption of diet sodas raised blood sugar levels.

13. **Do not eat hydrogenated oil.**

This is classified as a trans fat. Hydrogenated oils are man-made products. They are toxic. More importantly, they attack the artery walls and contribute to heart disease. They also attack the liver, spleen, intestine, kidneys, and gallbladder, causing these internal organs to operate much less efficiently. The bad news is that hydrogenated oil is in virtually every product you buy at the grocery store. The good news is that if you shop at a health food or whole food store, and if you read the labels, you can find many products without hydrogenated oil. This is a good example of how medical science says something is bad, and then later reverses its position. For years heart patients were told to stay away from butter because it was bad for your heart. They were told to use margarine instead. Margarine contains trans fat. Now we hear from the same medical community that margarine is in fact, much worse than butter. Avoid trans fats.

14. **Do not eat homogenized and pasteurized dairy products.**
    All dairy products are not created equal. Raw milk that hasn't been pasteurized or homogenized, that came from a cow that was organically raised, was free-roaming, grass fed and not given antibiotics or growth hormone injections, will affect the body much differently (and better) than pasteurized and homogenized milk coming from a genetically modified cow that has been given antibiotics and growth hormone injections, never been allowed to roam, and has been fed chemically laced growth enhancing feed. Homogenization causes milk and other dairy products to be detrimental to the arteries and thus contribute to heart disease. Standard supermarket varieties of milk and dairy products are unhealthy. Organic raw, unpasteurized, non-homogenized milk, cheese and dairy products are beneficial.

15. **Do not eat high fructose corn syrup.**
    High fructose corn syrup (HFCS) is used primarily for two reasons. First, it is inexpensive. Secondly, it makes you fatter than other sweeteners. The food industry wants you to be fat. Fat people eat more food, thus increasing sales and profits for the food companies. HFCS contributes to

fat deposits in your liver increasing buildup of lipoproteins. It also leads to plaque build-up in your arteries. Consuming it increases the likelihood of diabetes. And, studies have linked mercury with HFCS. As I've mentioned, mercury can cause neurological problems including Multiple Sclerosis. Never eat anything that contains high fructose corn syrup. Nearly *all* processed foods in the grocery store: catsup, relish, barbecue sauce, ice cream, cookies, canned fruit, lunch meats, juices, peanut butter and more contain this poison. If you're currently eating things that contain HFCS and you stop, you'll find that you lose weight. You'll also be at less risk for disease.

16. **Do not use fluoride toothpaste.**

Fluoride is a poison. Its supposed benefits to teeth have been largely overstated. Many studies have challenged the efficacy of fluoride to protect against tooth decay. And yet, it continues to be used as a selling point for toothpaste. Don't buy into that. You do not need fluoride and it is not good for you. Fluoride has been shown to increase absorption of aluminum, which can contribute to Alzheimer's disease. Fluoride has been linked to osteoporosis and bone cancer. You can find non-fluoridated toothpastes online or in a health food store. A paste made with baking soda and coconut oil works well, too.

17. **Do not use nonstick cookware.**

When nonstick cookware is heated to high temperatures it emits toxic fumes that can kill a small bird if it's close enough! These fumes, when inhaled by humans, lead to respiratory disease, weakening of the immune system, cancer, depression, asthma, headaches, and a multitude of other health problems.

18. **Eat only organic, kosher meat and poultry.**

Any meat or poultry that's not organic and kosher is highly toxic. Generally speaking:

o   A conventional animal is injected with growth hormones and antibiotics, meaning that the meat we consume is then loaded with these drugs.

o   A conventional animal is not allowed to roam freely or exercise normally, thus

o   creating a toxic animal that is unnaturally obese and diseased.

o   A conventional animal is fed an unnatural diet of chemicals and feed that it would never eat naturally. Conventional cows, for example, are fed ground up cow parts, pig parts, goat parts, and horse parts. Many of these ground-up animal parts are from diseased animals. Keep in mind that the cow is a vegetarian naturally and is not designed to be eating ground up animals diseased or otherwise.

o   A conventional animal is slaughtered by being shot in the head with a bolt. The animal experiences pain and trauma. Adrenaline, which is poisonous, permeates the animal's tissue. The blood, which is loaded with toxins, also permeates the tissue. The trauma causes the energy field in and around the animal to become highly negative. The animal usually dies in its own urine and feces.

o   A conventional animal is often aged, which means the animal flesh is hung in a dark room and allowed to rot. A green mold covers the rotting animal flesh. This green toxic mold is bacteria that tenderizes the meat, but it also fills the meat with more toxins.

o An organic animal is given no drugs, so its meat is drug free.

o An organic animal is allowed to roam naturally, grow at its normal rate, and is not diseased.

o A grass-fed organic cow eats grass as it would in nature, and the grass has not been laced with chemical fertilizers, herbicides, and pesticides.

o An organic animal that is also kosher is killed in the most humane way possible, by slicing its throat. The animal experiences no pain, is immediately drained of all blood, its internal organs are inspected to make sure the animal is healthy, and the tissue is salted to kill any bacteria.

o Organic kosher meat is not aged.

When I learned all this, I decided to eat only kosher organic meat. For thirty days, every day, I ate some kosher organic meat. I tried to monitor whether I felt any difference. I couldn't detect anything specific or dramatic. I wasn't convinced that it was such a big deal. I decided to throw a barbecue and invited several friends over to my house. I went to the butcher and bought the best, highest quality steaks available, which happened to be conventional, Black Angus aged steaks. I cooked the steaks and served them to my guests. Each one raved about how delicious and tender the steaks were. Some said they were the best they'd ever eaten. I took one bite of mine and immediately felt odd. It was as if I was eating some "bad meat." Everyone else was enjoying theirs. I asked my friend to taste my steak. He loved it. So I took another bite. As I chewed and swallowed my forehead began to sweat, I got pale, and my stomach felt nauseated. I quickly excused myself, went to the bathroom and threw up. This happened because I had eaten only clean meat for so long my body immediately rejected the toxins. The bottom line is, chicken, duck, lamb, beef, and goat are all okay as long as they're organic and kosher. It may be a challenge to find kosher organic meats in some areas, but if you can it's worth it. If you *can't,* there are places online where you can order it and have it delivered via FedEx.

19. **Do not eat farm raised fish.**
Farm raised fish are given antibiotics and often treated with pesticides to combat sea lice. They're highly toxic, fattier than wild fish, and eating them can create inflammation in the body due to their higher ratio of Omega 6 to Omega 3s. A recent study in New York found that farm raised salmon was contaminated with PCBs. PCBs are toxins which have been implicated in causing a variety of diseases including cancer.

20. **Do not eat pork.**
Pork products are laced with disease and viruses. Nearly all pork in the U.S. comes from concentrated animal feeding operations or CAFOs. These toxic breeding grounds for pathogens are inhumane environments where the pigs are cramped on concrete and steel grates. Because there's so much bacteria in these horrible environments, the pigs are treated with large doses of antibiotics. Pigs digest whatever they eat quickly, within a few hours. Cows, for example, take up to twenty-four hours to digest their food. Because the pigs digest food quickly, more of the toxins remain in their system to be stored in their fatty tissues. We consume that tissue and it puts us at risk for illness. Another problem with pork is that pigs have virtually no sweat glands, so they don't release any toxins through perspiration like

other mammals. When you eat pork, you're eating all of the toxins the pig has.

21. **Do not eat shellfish.**

More people are allergic to shellfish than any other food. More people get sick from eating shellfish than any other food. More people die from eating shellfish than any other food. Any fish that does not have scales and fins should be avoided. This includes clams, mussels, shrimp, lobster, crab, squid, eel, catfish, shark, etc. The fish must have scales and fins. Catfish, for example, has fins but no scales. It is interesting that this is one of the kosher dietary laws. Today, we know that fish with scales and fins do not absorb the toxins in the water as readily as fish without both scales and fins. I grew up in the Boston area. I loved my shellfish more than any other seafood. Occasionally, a type of algae in the water called the "red tide" would infest the local shores. When this happened, warnings went out telling people not to eat any shellfish, because doing so could cause sickness or even death. However, you could eat the haddock, mackerel, or flounder. Fish that had scales and fins did not absorb the poisons into its edible flesh; however, shellfish or any fish that did not have both scales and fins would absorb the toxins and could kill you. Avoid all seafood that doesn't have scales and fins.

22. **If you can't eat it, don't put it on your skin.**

Whatever you put on the skin, which is our largest organ, gets absorbed and ends up in the body. Many of the products we put on our skin from antiperspirants, moisturizing lotions, cosmetics, insect repellents, sunscreens, and perfumes are so toxic that if you put them in your mouth they would poison you. I know for many of you it would be unrealistic to exclusively use products that were safe enough to eat. Remember, I said that if you can't do something 100 percent, do the best you can. You can eliminate many toxic products by replacing them with natural products. Extra virgin coconut oil (food grade, not the kind they sell in the drug store) is the best moisturizer you can use. It's emollient, antibacterial, and healthy for the skin. And it's sold in many grocery stores these days. It can also be used to remove makeup and cleanse the face and body. Spread it on and use a warm washcloth to wipe it off. Coconut oil can also be used to condition the hair. Put on before you shower and then wash out. Apple cider vinegar works as a toner for acne prone skin. It can also be used to cleanse the scalp and hair. If you can't eliminate all of the toxic products at least *reduce* the number of them that you put on your skin.

23. **Get an air purifier.**

I recommend an air purifier for your home, work space, and most importantly, your bedroom. Since you're breathing all night long, it would be a good idea to be breathing the cleanest, purest air you can. Your work space is the second most important. There are hundreds of types of air filters and air purifiers on the market. The best ones are so good they can even eliminate the black mold that's causing illness in many homes today. If you have an air purifier, use it regularly and change the filter as directed. If you don't have one, do some research and look for one that's highly rated and powerful enough to eliminate airborne mold.

24. **Use only nontoxic, organic cleaning supplies.**

Cleaning products used in the home have proven to be a leading cause of cancer in children. Toxic cleaning products suppress the immune system and cause disease. This occurs by inhaling the fumes, or through contact with the skin. Buy organic products or make your own with vinegar, baking soda, and lemon. White vinegar cleans glass, chrome, and tile. You can dilute it with water and you can add lemon juice if the smell bothers you. But when you clean with vinegar the smell goes away after a few minutes. Baking soda can clean ovens, sinks, and tubs. Baking soda *and* vinegar, together, create a powerful cleanser. Pour vinegar into a spray bottle; sprinkle baking soda onto a surface and spray it with the vinegar. It will bubble up and effectively clean and disinfect many surfaces in your home.

25. Do not drink canned or bottled juice.

All store-bought canned or bottled juice has been pasteurized making it toxic to the body. The filtering and processing used in juice manufacturing only increases and concentrates the amount of toxic chemicals. Drink only fresh juice made with organic ingredients.

26. Avoid most sunscreens.

They contain toxic chemicals. Oxybenzone, octinoxate and 4-MBC, which are in many sunscreens, are considered harmful and dangerous. Would you eat anything with names like that? If you can't eat it, don't put it on your skin. I don't believe in using *any* sunscreens, personally, but if you're at high risk for skin cancer or you live where the sun is particularly strong, it's understandable that you'd want some protection. My advice is to wear a hat and/or cover your body with light clothing in lieu of sunscreen. But if you absolutely need it, then at least look at the ingredients and avoid the poisons I noted.

27. Take whole food supplements, rather than vitamins.

There are many grades of individual vitamins. Unfortunately, most companies use the cheapest grades available. These inexpensive "vitamins" in many cases are chemically produced and are not natural. It's true that you are likely deficient in vitamins and minerals. The best way to correct this deficiency is by juicing. The second best way is to take *whole food supplements*. These are different from traditional, big-brand-name vitamin and mineral pills. Whole food supplements take organically produced vegetables and fruits and concentrate them into a convenient tablet. When you take a whole food supplement you're getting vitamins and minerals in a proportion that nature intended. You're also getting the enzymes and cofactors present in nature, which includes benefits that science hasn't even discovered yet.

28. **Do not use antiperspirants or deodorants.**
Antiperspirants and deodorants contain toxins, most notably aluminum. These poisons are being put on the skin close to the lymph nodes. Anything absorbed into the skin from the armpit gets drawn into the lymph system and travels to the breasts. I believe one of the major causes of breast cancer in women is the use of these poisonous products. A healthy person should not have an offensive odor if he or she bathes daily. The odor is caused by bacteria, and bathing should take care of that. If that's not enough, consider wiping your underarm with vinegar, preferably apple cider vinegar. Yes, you will smell it at first, but the vinegar odor will dissipate. Vinegar kills bacteria. You can also use baking soda, either like a powder, or wet it and make a thin paste. Some people use coconut oil, which also kills bacteria. Himalayan pink sea salt now comes in bars and can be used for bathing and deodorant. Remember, if you can't eat it, don't put it on your skin. If you *must* use deodorant, look for all natural products that don't contain chemicals.

29. **Do not eat processed flour.**
White processed flour is similar to white sugar in that consuming it raises the blood sugar level. Processed flour comes

from grain that's been chemically treated in the growing process. It's also stripped of its natural fiber and nutrients, and chemically bleached to make it white. White flour mixed with water makes paste. You use it to make papier-mâché. It turns hard as a rock. And that's what happens when you eat it. It is an unnatural product that the body has difficulty digesting. It has little nutritional value, no life energy, spikes your insulin, and causes constipation. Avoid breads, cakes, cookies, pasta and anything else made with white flour. I don't recommend whole wheat flour either, because the wheat supply has been modified and it's no longer a natural product. In place of breads and pasta, eat real grains: oatmeal, brown rice, and quinoa.

30. **Eat nothing that says "fat-free" on the label.**
Food companies want you to buy their products. Whatever the hot button is at the time will determine what their marketing people decide goes on the label. "Fat free" does not mean "healthy." Most fat free products mask the loss of taste (due to removing the fat) by loading them with sugar and chemicals. These things are toxic and detrimental to your health.

31. **Eat nothing that says "sugar-free" on the label.**
If it says sugar free on the label there's a good chance the product is laced with artificial sweeteners. Don't buy it. Obviously, there are many foods that naturally don't contain sugar and I'm not talking about those. I'm talking about processed snacks in the grocery. Avoid them. They're not going to help you lose weight. Eating real, unprocessed food will help you lose weight.

32. **Eat nothing that says "low carbs" or "net carbs" on the label.**
The term "net carbs" is a big scam. Manufacturers load these products with chemicals and artificial sweeteners that they

claim have negligible results on insulin levels, so they don't count these real carbohydrates in the net carb number. It's nonsense. A product that says it has two net carbs could have as many as forty grams of real carbohydrates. Do not buy these products, as you know that the manufacturers are simply trying to take advantage of a fad to sell you their products. Learn about glycemic index and try to eat foods with a lower glycemic index. You don't need to count carbs. If you're not eating processed flour, and instead eating whole grains, and if you're eliminating sugar and processed foods, you don't need to worry about "net carbs."

33. **Do not eat "food bars."**

Food bars are man-made products that are filled with chemicals to provide good taste. They're highly processed and should be avoided. There *are* a few all-raw, organic food bars and these are okay. Be sure to read the ingredient list.

34. **Do not eat diet or protein shakes.**

Like food bars, these are produced by companies whose goal is to make them taste great using the cheapest ingredients possible. They often have chemical additives and/or sugar. Make your own shakes at home with a blender using real ingredients. Smoothies are a great way to get your fruits and vegetables. You can use nuts, nut butters, and seeds to increase the protein content. Chia seeds are a good source of protein and blend well.

35. **Stay away from hot tubs, steam rooms, and chlorine swimming pools.**

Swimming pools and hot tubs are filled with water that's loaded with chlorine. Chlorine is a poisonous chemical. People think swimming in a pool, or relaxing in a hot tub is healthy. The exact opposite is true. They suppress your immune system, dry your skin, and load your body with high levels of chlorine, which can scar your arteries and lead to heart disease. The steam pouring into the steam room is from regular tap water that's loaded with contaminants. A steam room is, in fact, a poisonous gas chamber. Swimming is excellent in the ocean or in a lake. If you have a pool or hot tub, inquire about a filtration system where no chlorine or chemicals are used. The system I use employs ozone and oxygen to purify the water. No chlorine or chemicals are put into my pool or hot tub. If you can't drink the water, don't swim in it. Some people may say you can't drink lake water or ocean water, and that's true. But those waters are living, vitalized natural waters. Chlorinated swimming pools are something not found in nature.

36. **Don't use air fresheners.**

Don't spray anything in the air. Avoid solid air fresheners and the plug-in variety. All they do is put toxic chemicals in the air. It's insane. In my bathrooms I do have a can of organic citrus oil, which is nontoxic and can be purchased at most health food stores. Read the labels. Use 100 percent organic essential oils or air purification systems (filters) to eliminate offensive odors.

37. **Eliminate fluorescent lighting.**

Fluorescent lighting is irritating to the body. It makes you tired and weakens the immune system. Get rid of all florescent lighting and replace it with full spectrum lighting. Full spectrum lighting is similar to natural sunlight, and can have health benefits, most notably increased energy and alleviation of depression.

38. **Reduce air conditioning.**

Generally, air conditioning is not healthy. It makes the air unnatural. And poorly maintained units can contribute to airborne bacteria and fungi. In some climates, it's impossible to live without air conditioning. I get that. But use it less and you'll see a decrease in the amount of colds and flu you get. Where possible, use ceiling fans instead.

39. **Avoid dry cleaning.**

The chemicals in dry cleaning are toxic poisons. Allowing them to come in contact with your skin increases risk of disease. The chemicals have been linked to cancer, liver and nervous system damage, infertility, and hormonal disturbances. Hand wash delicate clothes when possible, or have them laundered and pressed rather than dry cleaned. For garments where that's not feasible, look for dry cleaners that specify that they do not use toxic chemicals.

40. **Buy a vacuum cleaner with a HEPA filter.**

Using a vacuum with a HEPA filter will help reduce the toxins in your home. When you walk into your house from the outside, you track inside environmental toxins and all kinds of allergens. Using a vacuum with a good filter can help people with asthma and allergies. The filter traps fine particles, which benefits everyone, even non-allergy sufferers.

Implementing the recommendations above will reduce the number of toxins going into your body and can also cure disease. These are in fact "natural cures." I've seen people with diabetes stop eating in fast food restaurants and in three weeks they no longer had diabetes. I've seen people who suffer from migraine headaches and constipation problems stop eating pasteurized and homogenized dairy products and the migraines stopped and they became regular. I've seen people with horrible skin rashes and acne use a shower filter and find that their symptoms disappeared, their skin become smooth and beautiful again. Don't be misled into thinking that things as simple as these are not cures. These things are causing your illnesses, and eliminating them can cure you.

C. You must address your nutritional deficiencies.

Many, if not all, diseases are caused at least in part by nutritional deficiencies.

By now, hopefully you understand that you have nutritional deficiencies and you also understand *why* you have them. The reason you're deficient in nutrients is because the food is grown and processed in such a way that its nutritional value is stripped from it before it even reaches you. And because we have so many toxins in our body, we have difficulty absorbing what little nutrition we *are* getting from our food. Many, if not all, diseases are caused at least in part by nutritional deficiencies. If you want to prevent and cure disease you must mitigate your nutritional deficiencies. So let me give you a list of dos and don'ts designed to help your body retain nutrients. For many of you this will be the miraculous all natural cure that you've been looking for.

1. **Eat more fresh organic fruits and vegetables.**
   You don't have to be a vegetarian to be healthy. However, the healthiest people eat a lot of fresh, organic fruits and vegetables. If you were to do just one thing to improve your level of nutrition, I would tell you to eat four pieces of fresh fruit per day and two big raw salads full of vegetables. If you changed nothing else in your diet and just added those two things, many medical conditions would disappear.

2. **Buy a juice machine and use it.**
   Our current food supply is dramatically depleted of vital vitamins and minerals. Organic produce has up to ten times more vitamins and minerals than nonorganic, and it has none of the poisonous residues from the chemical fertilizers, pesticides, and fungicides. Even so, because the soil is

so depleted, organic produce still has less nutritional value than the same produce had fifty years ago. Therefore, it's difficult to get enough of the necessary vitamins, minerals, and enzymes just by eating food. And remember, because of all of the toxins you've ingested, your ability to absorb these nutrients is reduced. Even if you ate nothing but raw, uncooked organic fruits, vegetables, nuts, and seeds, your body would still have nutritional deficiencies. The best way to correct this is to make fresh juice using organic fruits and vegetables. Drinking three to four glasses of fresh juice gives your body a good dose of living enzymes, as well as many vitamins and minerals in their natural state as nature intended.

3. **Eat raw organic nuts and seeds.**
   Raw means uncooked. Stay away from roasted and salted nuts and seeds. Ideally, buy them in the shell; they retain more nutrients. There's tremendous life force in nuts and seeds. They're great to snack on throughout the day. One caveat: They're dense in calories and high in fat. So try to keep your snacking to between one to three ounces a day.

4. **Get natural sunlight.**
   Go for a walk in the sun. Your body benefits from sunlight. Do not use sunglasses. The sun enters through the eyes and stimulates energy in the entire body. Let some of your skin be exposed to the sun, because sunlight on the skin helps the body produce much needed Vitamin D. This natural source of Vitamin D dramatically reduces the risk of developing several kinds of cancer. Remember, it's the sun that creates growth in plants. The solar energy from sun can be alkalizing to the body; it reduces depression and strengthens the immune system.

5. **Eat an organic apple a day.**

    It's true, an apple a day keeps the doctor away! This is a "natural cure" for dozens of diseases. It is in fact a superfood.

6. **Take all natural Vitamin E.**

    One of the most important vitamins you are deficient in, in my opinion, is Vitamin E. Taking Vitamin E can prevent a number of conditions including heart disease as well as eliminate varicose veins, improve sexual performance, reduce or alleviate depression,and a whole host of other disorders.

7. **Take liquid colloidal minerals daily.**

    You are deficient in minerals. Nutritional deficiencies lead to disease. Correcting these deficiencies cures disease. Colloidal minerals provide structure to tissues in your body. They also support an adequate acid-base balance in your body. They support the many processes of enzymes as well.

8. **Drink the "magic juices."**

    There are several fruits that have miraculous healing properties in the body. These are: noni, goji, mangosteen, acai berry and aloe vera. Aloe vera is technically a succulent plant, but I'm including it in this group. Some of these fruits are from other parts of the world and so they're difficult to buy fresh. While I generally discourage one from buying bottled juice, most of these must be purchased bottled. Unfortunately, they're pasteurized, because the government requires that. Pasteurization is not ideal, however the positive outweighs the negative in this case. I highly encourage you to buy and drink these juices. They provide super nutrition and they help cleanse and detoxify the body as well.

9. **Take a whole food supplement daily.**

    Whole food supplements are not synthetic vitamins and minerals. They are "concentrated real food." They contain nutrients, living enzymes, and life force energy in the proportion that nature intended. Whole food supplements include chlorella, blue-green algae, spirulina, royal jelly, and other types of concentrated whole herbs, plants, dehydrated juices, and/or sprouts. Remember, your body is deficient in vitamins, minerals and enzymes. There's no way you can get all of the nutrients you need just by eating food. You would have to eat ten to twenty times the amount of food you're eating now, and it would all have to be organic for you to meet your minimum nutritional needs. Since nutritional deficiencies cause disease, it's essential that you take a supplement with the proper amount of vitamins, minerals, and enzymes to help your body to operate at its best, and prevent diseases from developing.

10. **Eat raw organic honey, bee propolis, royal jelly, and bee pollen.**

    Raw organic bee products and honey are super nutritious foods. Royal jelly, for example, is an excellent health tonic that has been found to reduce tumors. It benefits the immune system and improves a number of conditions including asthma, allergies, insomnia, and high cholesterol. It also helps combat menopausal symptoms, stomach ulcers, liver disease, pancreatitis, kidney disease and bone fractures. Bee pollen boosts the immune system, treats allergies and can prevent the onset of asthma. It also aids digestion. Take bee products with meals for the best absorption.

11. **Get an oxygen water cooler.**

    For a variety of reasons, your body is deficient in oxygen. Bringing the level of oxygen to where it should be alkalizes the body and creates an environment where disease cannot exist. One of the best ways to get more oxygen into the body is through water. Do not buy oxygenated water at the store. The oxygen dissipates rapidly and by the time you buy it, any oxygen that was added is likely gone. I have water coolers in my home and office that add the oxygen when the water is dispensed. Most people feel an immediate rush of energy and increased vitality.

12. **Take digestive enzymes.**

One of the main causes of indigestion, heartburn, gas, bloating, and constipation is a lack of digestive enzymes in the stomach and intestine. Because of antibiotics, other prescription and nonprescription drugs, chlorinated and fluoridated water, most people don't have enough digestive enzymes in their system, which slows the metabolism and blocks the absorption of nutrients. It's essential to take digestive enzymes for a period of time until your body is cleansed and rejuvenated, and can produce the correct amount on its own. Taking digestive enzymes can eliminate acid reflux, heartburn, indigestion, gas, bloating, and constipation. The majority of people who begin taking digestive enzymes lose between five and ten pounds in the first thirty days.

13. **Eat probiotic foods.**

Probiotic foods contain microorganisms that are similar to the microorganisms found in the human digestive system. They benefit the immune system. Organic yogurt with live cultures is a good source of probiotics. Fermented foods like miso, sauerkraut, tempeh, and kimchi are also good sources.

14. **Use Himalayan pink sea salt.**

Regular table salt is poison. Sea salt is infinitely better for you. Himalayan pink sea salt contains the full spectrum of minerals and trace elements. Replacing your white nutrient stripped salt with Himalayan pink sea salt will help balance your body's pH and also improve circulation. Regular table salt is considered unhealthy and can exacerbate high blood pressure. This sea salt, used in moderation (too much of *any* form of sodium is not good), can help normalize blood pressure.

15. **Eat organic dark chocolate.**

    Dark chocolate has a lot of antioxidants. Antioxidants help rid the body of free radicals that cause oxidative damage to the cells. This slows the aging process, and also protects against some forms of cancer. Dark chocolate benefits the heart by lowering blood pressure. It benefits the brain by increasing blood flow, which helps cognitive function. Don't over indulge, because it's also high in fat and calories, but an ounce a day will benefit your health without weight gain. Be sure that the kind of dark chocolate you're eating is 70 percent cacao, or higher to receive the benefits.

16. **Take an omega-3 supplement.**

    Omega-3s (essential fatty acids) help lower triglycerides and blood pressure. They also help treat arthritis and depression. They're primarily available in fish oil capsules, (purchase a brand that assures *no mercury*), but they're also available as flaxseed oil capsules. They reduce inflammation throughout the body, which assists in disease prevention.

17. **Eat snacks.**

    Don't go hungry. What I mean by *eat snacks* is eat in between meals if you're hungry. However, my definition of snack and your definition of snack are probably two different things. My definition of "snack" is: organic apples, pears, or other organic fruit, organic raw nuts and seeds, organic raw celery, carrots, cucumbers or other vegetables, or freshly made juices, organic chicken salad, tuna salad, or other organic beef or poultry... you get the idea. I mean healthy snacks, not junk food or sweets. And my point is, you don't need to go hungry to be healthy.

As I've said repeatedly, you are nutritionally deficient. Virtually *every* disease has been linked to nutritional deficiencies and research is conclusive that when nutritional deficiencies are addressed many diseases vanish. Adding appropriate snacks is one way to bolster your level of nutrition. Food is medicine. So be sure that you're eating the healthiest foods possible. Can eating some raw organic honey cure a disease? Can eating an organic apple cure a disease? Can drinking some goji juice or mangosteen juice cure a disease? The answer: Absolutely. You bet it can.

D. Neutralize electromagnetic chaos

As you now know, electromagnetic chaos can cause your body to develop disease. We can't eliminate electromagnetic chaos, but we can reduce our exposure to it. Reducing, eliminating, or neutralizing these powerful negative frequencies can and does result in the "curing" of symptoms and disease. I've seen men with erectile dysfunction and prostate cancer cured by simply discontinuing the use of laptop computers. Why? Because in their case the powerful wireless devices in the laptops were causing their disease. I've seen people with migraines, fatigue, and depression be cured just by wearing an electromagnetic chaos eliminator because their symptoms were caused by sitting in front of a computer screen all day long at work. Cell phones do cause cancer. Laptop computers do cause cancer. High-definition TVs do cause cancer. As a matter of fact, all of these things not only cause cancer, but they also suppress the body's immune system and make us susceptible to all kinds of diseases. The manufacturers of these devices deny these allegations, of course, because there's too much money to be lost. Remember, it's always all about the money. But there are scientists and researchers who assert that these devices cause disease. So let me give you some recommendations for managing electromagnetic chaos.

1. **Use crystals to neutralize electromagnetic chaos.**

   As I mentioned, we're being bombarded by electromagnetic energy from hundreds of sources, including satellites, high-tension power lines, computers, cell phones, global positioning systems in our cars, wireless telephones, remote controls, high-definition TVs, etc. We can't eliminate the electromagnetic energy around us. We can only do things to neutralize the negative effects. Crystals help neutralize these negative energies. Some can be put in your home or office near your computer and minimize the negative energy in the space around you; others can be carried in your purse or pocket, or worn as a pendant. When I say *crystals*, I'm speaking of naturally formed crystals of quartz, amethyst, etc., not the kind on a chandelier. You can find them online and also in stores that specialize in gem stones and new age material. They are inexpensive and work brilliantly.

2. **Use electronic and wireless devices less.**

   It appears that some of the most negative effects of electromagnetic energy come from wireless devices such as cell phones, laptops, as well as high-definition TVs. I know it's impossible to eliminate the use of these devices; however, you should at least be aware of their powerful adverse effects and limit their use as best as you can.

3. **Reduce TV time.**

   Televisions produce unhealthy electromagnetic energy. High-definition televisions have an *especially* powerful negative electromagnetic energy. The images on TV are largely stress invoking. This doesn't mean you can never watch it, but if you're watching TV every night, seven days a week and you're watching things that are violent or otherwise stressful, that's not conducive to healing or maintaining good health.

4. **Get a magnetic mattress pad.**

    The Earth, at one time, had a magnetic level (called gauss) of 4.0. Today the Earth's gauss is .04. Sleeping on a mattress pad filled with magnets stimulates energy flowing through the body as nature intended. It has been said to alleviate pain, slow the aging process, increase energy, and help alkalize the body.

5. **Use magnetic finger and toe rings.**

    These are inexpensive and easy to use. Simply wear a specially designed magnetic ring on the small finger of each hand, and if you want even more benefit, wear the toe brace on each foot. These are worn while you sleep. The health benefits seem to be almost unbelievable. This device appears to radically slow the aging process. People report looking and feeling younger as time goes on.

6. **Stay away from electric tumble dryers.**

    These devices produce massive amounts of positive ions. Positive ions suppress the immune system, make you fatigued, and can cause depression and anxiety. Do this experiment: Go to a Laundromat and sit in front of the tumble dryers in operation, and notice how you feel after just thirty minutes. Then notice how you feel for the rest of the day. Compare this to taking a walk on the beach or being near running water, or an area with lots of trees. These conditions produce life-enhancing negative ions. The comparison in how you feel can be dramatic. The clothes that come out of the tumble dryer are also charged with these ions that have a negative effect on your emotions and physiology. You will actually feel better if you wear clothes that have been line dried in fresh air.

7. **Add living plants to your home.**
   Real living plants add oxygen to the air, balance the energy in the space, produce life-enhancing negative ions, and are incredibly beneficial to the health of human beings. Fill your house with living plants and flowers. You will feel the difference and benefit from the moment you do it.

8. **Wear white.**
   Colors affect energy. The closer you get to white, the more positive energy you bring into your energetic field. This may not be practical in everyday situations; however, having some white or light colored clothing as your general around-the-house attire can make you feel much better.

9. **Use feng shui in your home and office.**
   This ancient method of arranging things allows energy to flow better, reducing stress, increasing prosperity, and generating vibrant health.

As simple as some of these things seem, they *can* be the "natural cure" you're looking for. I know there are a lot of recommendations and it's unlikely that you'll do every single one. Do as many as you can. With the majority of people one thing is not the cause of their illnesses, it's a combination of things. And often one thing is not going to be the cure. You need to do a variety of things to change your health. You must change your lifestyle. If you're not well, the lifestyle you were experiencing (the way you took care of yourself) created the conditions for sickness to develop. So adopt a number of these positive changes to improve the quality of your lifestyle and the quality of your health will improve as well.

E. You must reduce stress.

Stress is the silent killer. Mental and emotional stress affects every cell in the body. The mind can turn the body's pH from acidic to alkaline in a matter of minutes. Stress can adversely affect your body's genetic makeup. The mind can positively or negatively affect DNA. If you want to prevent disease, be happy, eliminate depression and fatigue, and cure illness, you must reduce stress in your body. It is impossible to "eliminate *all* stress," but you can certainly *reduce* stress. Can eliminating stress cure a disease? The surprising answer is *yes*. Healthcare practitioners around the world have proven repeatedly that by simply reducing stress, diseases are cured. The "placebo affect" has shown that up to 40 percent of people cure themselves with nothing more than their thoughts. That comes directly from the pharmaceutical industry's own literature and it's *a natural cure they don't want you to know about.*

> Stress can adversely affect your body's genetic makeup

So let me give you a list of what *I* think are the most powerful ways to reduce stress. I recommend doing as many of these things as you can. And I urge you to begin doing them as soon and as often as you can.

1. **Listen to de-stressing CDs.**
   One of the best ways to eliminate stress is to regularly listen to CDs specifically designed for that purpose. You can find them online. You need headphones when you use this specially created music (and in some cases words) because the frequencies are designed in such a way that they go into one ear or the other and at carefully selected time intervals. These CDs stimulate the brain to release healing hormones, and dramatically release tension that's been trapped in the body. Your pH levels can be radically changed in a matter of minutes with these powerful tools.

2. **Meditate.**

   There are many forms of meditation to choose from. You can practice the technique you prefer if you have one. Or if you're new to meditation, start by taking some time, perhaps once a day, to sit in silence for several minutes. Start off with 15 minutes and try to build up to 30 minutes or even an hour if you can. Close your eyes and be still. Sit or lie in a comfortable position and do nothing but focus on your breath. As thoughts come up, let them go and bring your attention back to your breath. If you prefer, you can focus on a word like "peace," but try to quiet your mind and allow yourself to be still in silence. Doing this regularly has healing benefits. It's good for the brain, and over time, it can improve your overall health and wellbeing.

3. **Laugh.**

   Laughing is one of the most powerfully beneficial and healing things you can do. Children laugh, on average, 10,000 times per week. Adults laugh, on average, five times per week. Laughing stimulates the immune system, reduces depression and alkalizes the body. In the book *The Anatomy of an Illness*, we hear the amazing story of a cancer patient who, given six months to live, used laughter to eliminate his cancer. The popular documentary *The Secret* showed a woman who watched funny movies and laughed each day to eradicate her breast cancer quickly and without radiation or chemotherapy. Laugh daily, as often as you can, even if you have nothing to laugh about. You'll feel better and your body will be healthier.

4. **Smile.**

   The physical act of smiling strengthens the immune system and releases endorphins from the brain, making you feel better. The act of smiling also changes your energetic field, as evidenced by Kirlian photography. Make it a habit to notice if you're smiling or not. Smile for no reason and do it often.

5. **Get and give hugs.**

Human contact is essential in order to thrive. Babies who are given all of the nutrition they need, but receive no physical contact grow less, cry more, and come down with more illnesses than babies who are cuddled regularly. Our immune systems are strengthened when we physically hug another human being. Ask yourself how many hugs you gave and got yesterday. You should be hugging every day as often as possible. It's a gratifying way to experience increased health.

6. **Speak powerful words.**

Words create. What you say is what you get. Most people get hung by their own tongue. When you say something you energetically put the wheels in motion that will manifest it into reality. Speak positively and use words as a tool to make what you desire come to pass. Say things like: I am healthy, I am happy, I am excited about life. Or say whatever is it that you want to occur. Say it as if it's true, and in the present tense, not: I *want* to be healthy. Instead affirm: I *am* healthy. It doesn't matter if you are not actually healthy in the moment. You are using the right words to make it so. Speaking in these affirmative ways impresses your subconscious mind powerfully. If you say I *want* something, rather than I *am* or I *have*, your subconscious will obediently agree with what you say and you will remain *wanting* that thing.

7. **Don't use a cell phone and drive at the same time.**

Holding a cell phone and driving is illegal in many states, as it should be, since it selfishly endangers others. But I discourage hands-free cell phone use as well. Driving is stressful enough. When you're talking on a cell phone and driving simultaneously, the physical and psychological stress can be even greater. If you're trying to reduce stress in order to bring your body into balance, driving and talking on the phone is not going to help. When driving, consider listening to soothing music to help counter the stress. Just make sure it's not so soothing that it puts you to sleep.

8. **Sleep eight hours.**

Ideally, get a full eight hours of solid, deep, restful sleep every night. This is easier said than done, but do what you can to get there. Power down your electronics at least an hour before bed. Don't have them on in your bedroom, especially if they emit any light. Even a small amount of light can affect sleep quality. Use earplugs if noise keeps you awake. If your mattress isn't comfortable replace it. Set the temperature where it's not too hot or too cold. Use comfortable sleepwear. Avoid caffeine within several hours of going to bed and avoid eating too close to bedtime. If drinking causes you to go to the bathroom several times a night, consider drinking your fluids earlier in the day and stop ingesting them a couple of hours before bed so you can sleep through the night.

9. **Rest from Friday sundown to Saturday sundown.**

Each week the moon cycles are in position to promote healing and rejuvenation in the body. Resting during this time promotes the optimal rejuvenation of your cells. "Rest" doesn't mean lying in your bed, necessarily, but if you're that tired, it's fine. Rest means no work, or stressful obligations. Have family time, or consider silent time with yourself to read, write in a journal, think your own thoughts, plan your next week... Whatever, just so long as you give your body some time to wind down. You can't be your best if you never take the time to replenish your energy. Scheduling the time to do that can really help you find balance in your life.

10. **Go to bed at approximately 10:00 p.m. and arise at approximately 6:00 a.m.**

    In Ayurvedic medicine it is believed that there are cycles that are the most conducive for certain activities. Going to bed at 10:00 p.m. and rising at 6:00 a.m. appears to allow the body to rest the deepest, rejuvenate the most, and gives one the most energy throughout the day. Hormones that heal the body are released only between 10:00 p.m. and 2:00 a.m., and they're only released when the body is in deep sleep.

11. **Take an afternoon fifteen minute break.**

    Most people wake up to an alarm, rush to work, stress, worry and work all day, rush to get home, eat a meal, and sit in front of the television. Then they go to bed and prepare to repeat the process again the next day. A fifteen minute relaxation break, ideally using special music or relaxation CDs, allows the body a mini-rest to decompress, and rejuvenate sufficiently to get you through the rest of the day with better energy and clarity.

12. **Get rolfing.**

    Rolfing is a type of deep-tissue massage technique that releases the fasciae (connective tissues between the muscle and the bone) and dramatically improves posture and balance, and integrates the entire body. Rolfing is generally done once per week for fifteen weeks. Each session is like a deep-tissue massage and takes approximately an hour and a half. You can find trained Rolfing practitioners in your area. I highly recommend this.

13. **Don't read the newspaper.**

    Most of us get our news online so this applies to online reading as well. You can't bombard your mind with negative thoughts and expect your body's pH to remain alkaline. The newspaper is filled with negativity, which causes anxiety. The news is almost always misleading, slanted, or in some cases, completely untrue. So more often than not, it's not the best use of your energy to focus on it. Yes, we live in the real world and we want to know what's going on, but it's problematic to dwell on and react to a negative story. The emotions become involved and stress levels go up. When you feel yourself getting anxious, realize that your pH is becoming more acidic. Our goal is to keep your pH level alkaline.

14. **Avoid watching the news.**
Watching the news on television fills your mind with negative images that can have a profound effect on wellbeing. I've done my own study and found that one's pH level can go from a healthy alkaline state, to the cancer-prone acidic state after just thirty minutes of watching a stressful news broadcast. If you want to stay up on current events glance at the major headlines, or briefly listen to the radio news and then move on with your day. If there's something you *really* need to know, someone will surely tell you. Don't dwell on stressful stories when you're trying to heal yourself, or stay well.

15. **Have sex regularly.**
There are many benefits to sexual activity, including strengthening the immune system, reducing stress, lowering blood pressure, and improving sleep quality. There have even been studies suggesting that having sex a few times a week can make both men and women look several years younger. This study also said that the benefits came with having sex with a consistent partner. (I'm not telling you to go out and have a bunch of one night stands.) Casual sex would actually be detrimental and not lead to stress reduction.

16. **Commit reckless acts of kindness.**
Each day make it a goal, then ultimately a habit to be kind to everyone you meet. The act of showing kindness stimulates

the body's immune system and gives one a greater sense of peace. It causes stress when you interact with hostility or mean-spiritedness toward another. If you're annoyed, in the moment, you may think you feel better by snapping at someone or being rude, but the body says otherwise by becoming stressed. (Remember those pH levels?) We're all connected and what goes around comes around. So send out kindness and you can relax, knowing that that's what you have coming back to you.

17. **Listen to nice music.**

Certain kinds of music have been shown to kill plants and to suppress the immune system in humans. Certain music also has been shown to make the body acidic. Baroque classical music seems to promote health and vitality in plants, and it seems to encourage the same in humans. You can sense which types of music are healing and relaxing for you. It's different for everyone, but the point is to recognize what makes you feel good and peaceful, rather than anxious, because the music that puts you at ease is going to benefit your health.

18. **Get out of debt.**

Financial pressure causes an increase in stress, which can lead to disease. There are several organizations that can assist you in managing, reducing, and eliminating debt. Consider Debtors Anonymous if you think you have a chronic problem. When you free yourself from financial worry you're more likely to be relaxed, happier and healthier.

19. **Drive less.**

Driving causes a lot of stress. If you're driving a lot in your life, see if you can make any changes. Car pool? Public transportation? Even making a switch a couple of times a week can make a difference if you commute regularly. If you take a bus or train, you can rest on the way, or catch up on reading so you don't have to be in constant stress mode the entire trip. If you live in a city, but you drive everywhere, consider walking, riding a bike, or taking a bus now and then for a break from driving. It'll be better for you *and* for the environment.

20. **Be thankful.**

Thoughts are things. Thoughts are powerful. When you wake up in the morning, take a moment to be thankful for the day. Before you eat a meal, take a moment and be thankful for the food. Before you go to bed, reflect and be thankful for the people and experiences you have. Living a life of gratitude creates happiness and peace, reduces stress, and promotes general health.

21. **Get an inversion table.**

Machines are available online and in fitness equipment stores that allow you to tilt your body into an inverted position or hang completely upside down. This process is believed to decompress the spine, relieve back pain, increase blood and oxygen to the brain, reduce stress and potentially slow the aging process. I own one of these machines myself and use it a few times a week. It only takes three minutes and you feel absolutely fantastic.

22. **Use foot orthotics.**

Good foot orthotics can promote general health and can eliminate foot, joint, and back pain. If you walk a lot, have an injury that makes walking painful, or you have arthritis or diabetes, this is worth looking into. Some prescribers/sellers are better than others. Be sure to work with a company or doctor who specializes in orthotics and get recommendations.

23. **Get a range of motion machine.**

How would you like to get the benefits of thirty minutes of aerobics, forty-five minutes of stretching, and forty-five minutes of strength training in just four minutes? There's a machine called the "range of motion machine" which does just that. It's expensive, but highly recommended.

24. **Be lighthearted.**

There are tens of thousands of people around the world who live past the age of one hundred. Research conducted on these centenarians has found that one of the major common denominators is that they take life lightly. They strive to be happy. It's a good reminder. Hold grudges less. Smile more. Don't stress over things unnecessarily. Remember, stress is one of the things that contribute to an acidic pH, which creates an environment conducive to disease.

25. **Stay away from psychiatrists.**

Psychiatrists almost always prescribe drugs to their patients. These drugs are some of the most dangerous pharmaceuticals available today. Did you know that many of the violent acts committed in schools in the past several years were perpetrated by someone who had either taken, or was currently taking a psychiatric drug? The research has become so compelling that there are warnings that certain psychiatric drugs actually increase the propensity to commit suicide. Avoid psychiatrists and the drugs they prescribe.

26. **Do not use an alarm clock.**

Or if you do, don't use one that shocks you awake with a loud, harsh noise. Most people wake to the sound of a loud alarm clock. This shocks the system and starts the body off in a stress mode for the day. It's important, and better for you, to awaken slowly and gently. There are alarm clocks that wake you with gentle tones or natural sounds like ocean waves that start off low in volume and slowly get louder. There are also clocks that wake you with a light that gradually increases in brightness. This little change in the way you awaken can have profound effects on your emotions and your body's pH.

27. **Use aromatherapy.**

Smells have a powerful effect on the body. Certain smells evoke chemical reactions. They can be soothing and healing. Essential oils have many health benefits in addition to wonderfully pleasant aromas. Seek out an aromatherapy expert to help you choose the essential oils and aromas specifically for you.

28. **Use Thought Field Therapy or the Emotional Freedom Technique (tapping).**

Phobias, stress, compulsions, and other dysfunctional problems can be treated by using a technique that involves tapping meridian points on the body with one's fingers. Thought Field Therapy was developed by Roger Callahan. His book is called *Tapping the Power Within*. The Emotional Freedom Technique, developed by Gary Craig, is a similar modality. Both approaches are derived from acupuncture and help a person release energy blockages.

29. **Get a pet.**

Research indicates that having a pet leads to a longer life and less disease. Pets give unconditional love and allow us a nonjudgmental being to give love to. The process of being loved and giving love strengthens our immune system, reduces stress, and has a variety of emotional and physical benefits.

30. **Write down goals.**

Write down what you want. Something magical occurs when you physically write down the things you want in life. This is one of the most powerful secrets used by the super wealthy. Just as I advised you how to speak your powerful thoughts earlier (*I am* healthy, rather than *I want to be* healthy), write powerful words. You might even write then with gratitude as if they're already true. For example: "Thank you for my healing," as if it's already accomplished.

31. **Plant a garden.**

Being in the physical universe, working with living things and creating things with our hands is incredibly beneficial. Working in a garden provides an outdoor environment, exercise, stress reduction, and many more mental, emotional, and physical benefits. It's awe-inspiring to start with a tiny seed or a small plant and watch it flourish into something amazing. Gardening will connect you with how wonderful and creative the universe is.

32. **Cook.**

When we create something with our hands we benefit emotionally and physically. When you cook food from scratch you take a much needed mental break, and you can create great tasting, incredibly healthy meals. I personally cook almost every day.

33. **Don't eat late.**

It is best to stop eating at 7:00 p.m. You'll sleep better, wake more refreshed, and find it easier to manage your weight.

34. **Dance and sing.**

Dancing and singing are great ways to release stress in the body. They are fun, and have a positive impact on our emotions and our physiology. Sing in the shower, or the car, if you're shy. Dance while you brush your teeth. However you do it, let dancing and singing be an expression of the joy within you. The more you express joy, the more you'll create within your life.

35. **Find your life's purpose.**

I put this last, although it's the most important. The reason it's last is because it is probably the hardest. Most people go throughout life without ever finding their true life's purpose. I can tell you from experience how stressful life can be when you are going day after day feeling like you're not doing what you were put on Earth to do. I experienced that myself early in my career when my focus was solely on making money at all costs. Today, my stress levels are at the lowest they've ever been, yet the amount of stressors in my life are the highest. Why? Because I've found my life's purpose, and that is to expose corporate and government corruption, and help people cure themselves of disease without drugs and surgery. My life is no longer about making money. Instead, I'm motivated to get true, honest healing information to people around the world, and to stop the insatiable greed going on primarily in the pharmaceutical companies and healthcare industry all around the globe.

Finding your life purpose, I believe, can help you be happier and healthier than ever before. It is hard to do, but I encourage you to consider where you are, and what your purpose is. Maybe your purpose is to help others achieve their purpose. Maybe your purpose in life is to make your own home and family happy and healthy. Maybe it's to help support me in my quest of educating people around the world on natural healing methods. I gratefully ask that you support me by reading the monthly newsletter (which can be ordered at www.NaturalCuresBook.com/newsletter) and writing me with your success stories at mystory@NaturalCuresSuccess.com. Stay connected so you can keep up with new articles. They'll be helpful to you in many areas of your life. I'd also love for you to direct positive energy and thoughts toward me and my mission. I am thanking you in advance for your support, and I hope the information in this book will be the miracle you've been looking for.

There you have my basic list of things to do and things to avoid that can bring your body back to a state of balance, eliminating disease and illness. It would be silly for anyone to believe that a person could do *all* of these things *all of the time*. Ideally, do as many as you can as often as you can. Doing even a little bit is better than none at all. For example, you may not be able to eliminate something 100 percent. At least cut back or reduce, or try eliminating it for a day or two. The more you do these things, and the more often you do them, the healthier and younger you will feel.

What you have in this chapter is what I believe to be the method to cure the incurable; the secrets to a long healthy disease-free life, full of energy and vitality, and in my opinion, the fountain of youth. These are some of the cures *they don't want you to know about.* Since I strongly believe that the cause of all disease is too many toxins in the body, nutritional deficiencies, exposure to electromagnetic chaos, and stress, the way to prevent and cure every disease is simply eliminate toxins in the body, eliminate nutritional deficiencies, eliminate or reduce exposure to electromagnetic chaos, and eliminate or reduce stress. The suggestions are simple, yet powerful and effective. I encourage you to start implementing some of these things immediately. I believe that you'll start feeling better remarkably quickly. I get letters and emails every week with people telling me of their success as they've been implementing the recommendations

> These techniques are powerful because they address the "cause" of all disease and illness.

in this chapter. These techniques are powerful because they address the "cause" of all disease and illness.

Now, I want to specifically address a very important issue facing not only America, but people all over the world. That issue is... LOSING WEIGHT! Let's learn the truth about why you're fat and how to lose weight once and for all, and keep it off forever.

CHAPTER 7

Why People Are Fat

If you want to get rich, write a book on how to lose weight. Americans are obsessed with losing weight. Yet Americans are among the fattest people in the world. Statistics vary, but at the moment, according to the Centers for Disease Control and Prevention, over 35 percent of Americans are *obese,* and nearly 70 percent are overweight. Still, we're doing more to lose weight, than ever. There are more diet books available than ever before. More people are on diets than ever before. More people drink diet sodas, eat diet, prepackaged food, and take diet pills than ever before. More people exercise than ever before. But the fact is, with all of the effort we've put into losing weight, as a nation, we're still *fatter* than ever before. Why is this?

Although rates of obesity have risen in other countries, the United States has had the distinction of being the *fattest country in the entire world* until recently, in 2013, when Mexico surpassed us to claim that honor.

First, we'll focus on the fundamentals so you can understand *why* you're overweight and how you've been lied to.

The United States government, through various agencies, has had a standard party line on the obesity epidemic. As I mentioned earlier in the book, "experts" state things as *fact* when, in reality, their statements are opinions, not facts. What the federal agencies say concerning obesity has constantly changed over time. Years ago the standard party line was the four basic food groups: **meat, dairy, grains, plus fruits and vegetables**. No one really questioned where those four basic food groups came from. I remember a food group poster in school back in the sixties. When I looked at it closely, I noticed that on the bottom it said that it was sponsored by the American Dairy Association. No wonder dairy products had their own food group. Isn't it surprising that the dairy association, whose only objective is to increase the consumption of dairy products (and thus profits), would strategically put a poster in school designed to brainwash kids into believing that in order to be healthy they had to eat dairy products at every meal? It's *always* been "*all about the money.*"

> ...we'll focus on the fundamentals so you can understand why you're overweight and how you've been lied to.

The party line for obesity has always been, "If you want to lose weight you must eat fewer calories and exercise more." However, there are "experts" who claim to have "scientific proof" that calories are not the issue at all; it's *fat* that you must consume less of to lose weight. Then there are still *other* experts who have just as much scientific evidence to prove that fat is not the issue after all; the real culprit is carbohydrates. And yet *another* group of experts claim that "food combining" is the secret to losing weight. Then there's a long line of still more experts, each holding a stack of research espousing their so-called "fact" about losing weight: the glycemic index, insulin secretion, hormonal imbalances, genetics... the list goes on and on.

As I said in the beginning of the book, no one really knows anything when it comes to medicine, health, disease, illness, sickness, or obesity. We all look at studies, general observations, personal experiences, other people's anecdotes, and we come up with conclusions that make the most sense to us. However, why one person is fat and another skinny, no one really knows. Everyone is just presenting a theory, including me. I'm going to present my theory as to why you're fat, and I'm going to explain a system that will allow you to lose weight easier than ever before and keep it off once and for all. I could, as everyone else does, present my information as the absolute gospel truth, and though I believe that it *is*, it would be arrogant to say so. As I've done before, I'll preface my theory by saying that "it is based on the information I have at the time. As more information becomes available my theory may be altered, or improved." With that said, let's look at something we all know is true.

Everyone reading this knows someone who does not exercise; who eats huge amounts of food, including the so-called fattening foods like pizza, pasta, ice cream, cookies, and cakes—you name it, they eat it. We all know someone like this who, nonetheless, is as skinny as a rail and never gains a pound.

When I was growing up my own brother could eat anything he wanted, in any amount, at any time of the day, and he **Never Gained Any Weight.** If I'd eaten the same amount and did exactly the same things he did in terms of exercise, I would have blown up to 300 pounds.

Some people's bodies seem genetically designed to be thin, while other's bodies seem genetically destined to be fat. At least that's how it appears. However, I was looking through history books about Nazi concentration camps in World War II and noticed that the people behind the barbed wire were *all* skinny. There were no fat people there. I wondered if some of those people were genetically predisposed to be thin and others predisposed to be fat. I wondered if those who made it out of the concentration camps and went back to their normal routines, remained thin and other people, because of their genetic predisposition, got fatter. The point is it doesn't make a difference what your genetic predisposition is; if you're not eating any food for a long period of time, you're going to get skinny. But that doesn't answer the question about why a person in America is more likely to be fat than a person in another country.

Based on personal experience, thousands of scientific papers, and interviews with thousands of people in nearly every state in over a fifteen-year period, I've come up with some interesting conclusions about why people, Americans in particular, are fat.

1. **Most fat people have a low metabolism.**
   This means that you can eat some food and even if you eat a small amount your body won't burn it off very quickly. Instead, it turns into fat. If you had a high metabolism you could eat large amounts of food and it wouldn't turn to fat in your body. So, the number one reason a person is fat is because of a low metabolism.

   Why is this so specific to America, (and Mexico, apparently) as opposed to other countries? I will explain. But first, what exactly is metabolism? In simple terms, there are certain organs and glands in the body that regulate how your body burns food for fuel and how it converts food into fat. These include the thyroid, pancreas, liver, stomach, small and large intestines, and colon. When you have a slow metabolism, there's a good chance that some of these organs and glands are not working at optimal levels. Always remember, if you find a problem where the body is not operating as it is supposed to, you have to ask the question, "What caused that not to operate properly?" You must always look for the cause first.

There are many causes for low metabolism, including yo-yo dieting. If you've repeatedly lost and gained weight I can tell you that your metabolism is all screwed up.

So, let's look at each one of these reasons, and find out what caused the malfunction.

o **Most Fat People Have an Under-active Thyroid.**
   If you have an under-active thyroid (called a hypoactive thyroid), your body's ability to convert food to energy is slow, and the likelihood that the food you eat will turn into fat is greater than usual. What is the number one cause of a hypoactive thyroid? There's no consensus. But it appears that one contributing factor is the fluoride in the water that you drink. Fluoride is not added to drinking water in most other countries. This is *one* of the reasons Americans have such a high propensity for an under-active thyroid, a low metabolism, and being overweight. Bear in mind it's just *one* contributing factor. There's no one thing that causes obesity; it's a number of things

o **Most Fat People Have a Pancreas that Does Not Work Properly.**
   The pancreas secretes insulin. Fat people appear to have a pancreas that secretes insulin at a faster rate than thin people. A fat person's pancreas also secretes more insulin than that of a thin person. What causes the pancreas to secrete more insulin at a faster rate? The answer: No one really knows. But based on the information we have, it appears to be caused by some of the chemical additives contained in the food served in America. Many of these food additives are not put in food in other countries. It also appears that the large amounts of refined sugar cause this pancreatic problem as well. America's food has more

processed sugar and high fructose corn syrup than food in other countries.

o **Most Fat People Have a Clogged and Sluggish Liver.** The liver is a detoxifying organ. When it's clogged, your metabolism slows down. What causes the liver to clog up? The number one reason your liver is not operating properly is the nonprescription and prescription drugs you've taken throughout your life. Most notably, if you take cholesterol reducing drugs, your liver is definitely clogged. Chlorine and fluoride in the water is another cause of a clogged liver. Chemical additives in processed food, fast food and animal fats clog the liver. Refined sugar, high fructose corn syrup and white flour clog the liver. Artificial sweeteners, monosodium glutamate, and preservatives clog the liver. The bottom line is the pharmaceutical companies clog your liver and the publicly traded food industry clogs your liver.

o **Most Fat People Have A Sluggish Digestive System** Overweight people seem to have a problem producing digestive enzymes. If you're not producing enough digestive enzymes your food doesn't get converted into energy and there's a higher chance it will be stored as fat. What's the reason for not producing enough digestive enzymes? It appears to be the chemical additives that are in the American food supply. The small and large intestines of overweight people are generally not as healthy as those of thin people. What is the cause of this? Candida yeast overgrowth. Why would someone have a yeast overgrowth? Antibiotics. Antibiotics kill all of the friendly bacteria in the intestines, which allow Candida (the unfriendly bacteria) to proliferate in the digestive system. This slows digestion and elimination.

So, if we were to ask *what is the number one reason for a slow metabolism*, the answer would be: "What you put in your body." The poisons you put in your body affect your metabolism. These toxins include: nonprescription and prescription drugs, chemical pesticides used in the process of growing food, artificial food additives, and the chemicals added to our water, primarily chlorine and fluoride.

There's another reason your metabolism is low. It has to do with exercise. The more muscle you have, the higher your metabolism. Americans, by and large, tend not to have a lot of muscle in their bodies. This means that calories aren't burned as effectively as they could be. The second most important issue in relation to exercise is sitting too much and walking too little. The human body is designed to walk. A study of thin Europeans, Africans, Chinese, and South Americans showed that the common denominator amongst the lean subjects in the study was the amount of walking they did daily. People who walk a lot every day tend to be thin. People who walk less than a tenth of a mile per day tend to be overweight.

2. **The majority of people who are overweight eat when they're not hungry.**
   This is caused by two factors: (a) emotional eating, or (b) physiological food cravings. Emotional eating is triggered by stress or stressful situations. Physiological food cravings are generally caused by the toxins you put in your body, or Candida yeast overgrowth.

3. **Most fat people have a large appetite.**
   If you're overweight you probably find yourself hungry a lot of the time. The hunger is generally caused by the body's inability to assimilate nutrients due to lack of digestive enzymes and Candida yeast overgrowth. Another reason you're hungry is that certain food additives increase hunger.

4. **Most fat people have hormonal imbalances.**

   If you're overweight, statistics show there's a high likelihood that your body is secreting too much of certain hormones and not enough of others. This imbalance is generally caused by excess toxins in the body and by a sedentary lifestyle.

5. **Most fat people eat larger portions than thin people.**

   This is caused by a combination of things: larger appetite, inability to assimilate nutrients, physiological cravings, stress, emotional issues, and the increase in the size of portions packaged and sold by the food industry. In Europe, for example, candy bars and snack food come in packages that are smaller than American-sized portions. Restaurants in Europe serve portions 30 to 40 percent smaller than their American counterparts.

6. **Fat people consume more "diet food."**

   Here is a major mind blower. Most diet food actually makes you fatter. Diet products, i.e. those labeled: "diet," "low-fat," "sugar-free," "low-calorie," "light," "low-carb," "lean," etc., are filled with either artificial sweeteners, high levels of sugar (added to low-fat foods), or chemical additives that make you fatter, not thinner. This is the dirty little secret the food industry does not want you to know. These additives can increase your appetite and make you physically addicted to the food, causing you to gain weight.

7. **Most fat people's bodies are highly toxic.**

   Toxins lodge primarily in the colon and fat cells throughout the body. When the body is high in toxins it retains water and increases its fat stores in an effort to dilute the poisons.

8. **Most fat people eat before they go to bed.**

   When you sleep, your metabolism slows considerably. When you eat late at night, food doesn't get a chance to burn off and it converts to fat easier.

9. **Most fat people are affected by the growth hormone put in meat and dairy products.**

   Our meat and dairy supply is loaded with growth hormones. These hormones are given to the animals to speed their growth in order to increase production and profits. When you consume nonorganic meat and dairy you're also consuming growth hormones. This contributes to obesity, and it's also one of the reasons children today are maturing earlier and earlier.

10. **Most fat people see themselves as fat.**

   Remember Earl Nightingale's discovery, "The Strangest Secret"? After years of research he discovered that *people become what they think about.* Fat people constantly think about their weight, thus creating the undesired result.

The dirty little secret the food industry doesn't want you to know.

Here I am blowing the whistle on what I believe to be one of the greatest, most devious lies in American history. The food industry consists of publicly traded corporations. These companies have one objective: To increase profits. The only way a food company can increase profits is to produce their products at the lowest possible cost and sell them at the highest possible price, and sell as much of them as they can.

The people running the food companies, the officers and directors, do not care about the health and wellbeing of the American public. They care only about the profits. You may have a hard time understanding or believing just how greedy these people can be. Did you know that there are a number of billionaires in prisons around the world? Why? Because the more money they make, the more money they need to make. For many of these people it becomes an addiction. Some of the officers and directors of food companies are so consumed with making more money they'll do anything, and knowingly hurt anybody, including you, just to make more money. It's sad, but true.

When the executives of food companies think only about how to increase profits, and they need to come up with ways to make their product (food) cheaper, those ways include genetic engineering the food and spraying chemical poisons on it, so that the crops won't be damaged by disease or bugs. The soil is loaded with chemicals to make the plants grow faster, the animals are pumped full of growth hormone to make them grow faster. These companies will do anything to get their products produced less expensively. They also want to sell these products at the highest possible price, and they want to sell massive amounts of them. So here's what happens. In making their products faster and cheaper, they become highly toxic. If you've ever been in a mass production facility you would be appalled at how food is "made."

These food companies must also be sure that you continue to buy and eat more food. They have laboratories where thousands of chemical additives are researched and tested. These laboratories are in secret locations with tighter security than the CIA headquarters. The objective is to make the food physically addictive, to make it increase your appetite, and to make it cause you to gain weight. Two common additives that appear to do this include the artificial sweetener aspartame and the sweetener high fructose corn syrup. Like the tobacco industry, the executives of the food industry vehemently deny these allegations. Remember, the tobacco industry denied knowingly making cigarettes physically addictive.

The fact is the American food supply will make you fat no matter what you do. This is why when thin people from other countries come to America, they seem to gain weight even though it appears that they're not eating any differently than they had previously.

When first lady Michelle Obama began encouraging people to exercise more and eat healthier food, some politicians actually railed against this. Some even suggested that Obama was endangering people and blaming an increase in pedestrian deaths on her campaign to get people to walk more. How likely do you think it is that some of those same politicians had financial ties to the food industry? The food industry is so profit driven it does not want people to eat less and get fit! The food industry wants you fat and eating more and more food every year.

This is the reason diet products in the form of pills, powders, food bars, and prepackaged diet foods will never work. The good news is that knowing the truth allows you to take simple steps to lose weight faster and easier than ever before. This knowledge also allows you to eat the foods you enjoy, never deprive yourself, and stay thin for life.

CHAPTER 8

How to Lose Weight Effortlessly and Keep It Off

I struggled with my weight for much of my life. I was a fat kid. I tried every diet, every weight loss pill, and I even hired a personal trainer, exercising as much as five hours a day. Whatever I lost, I put right back on. While I was losing weight I was hungry, tired, and grumpy. I never understood what the problem was, until I went overseas and found the answer. While living abroad I ate everything I wanted, and yet I began to lose weight without even trying. This led me to the discovery of the reasons why Americans are so overweight, and it showed me an easy, workable solution.

Though this isn't a explicitly a weight loss book (for more weight loss suggestions, listen to my book on CD, *Weight Loss Secrets "They" Don't Want You to Know About* which you can find at www. NaturalCuresBook.com if you don't already have it), I *am* going to give you a list of simple steps that will help you lose weight and keep it off once and for all. Many readers have implemented the recommendations that follow with great success. You may have heard some of their stories in my infomercial. I can assure you that following these steps will turn your body into a fat-burning furnace and bring your weight to its ideal place. These steps have tremendous health benefits as well.

1. **Drink a glass of water immediately upon arising.**

   This starts the body's metabolism and cleansing. Ideally, the water should be distilled, no tap water, and it should be room temperature or slightly warm, not cold. For an added boost, squeeze some lemon into the water. Warm water aids digestion. And the lemon stimulates the liver and aids in detoxification. And for even *more* of a boost, add a dash of cayenne pepper. The hot pepper detoxifies, boosts blood flow, and helps with weight loss.

2. **Drink eight glasses of distilled water each day.**

   People think drinking water will make them bloated. The exact opposite is true. If you're overweight you need to flush the toxins from your fat cells. Water, and lots of it, is absolutely needed to lose weight.

3. **Eat a big breakfast.**

   Many overweight people eat a small breakfast, or none at all, and then eat large amounts later in the day. This is not a good approach for weight loss or weight maintenance. You'll lose more weight if you make breakfast a large meal and dinner a lighter meal. Your breakfast should consist of as much as you want of the following items (everything should be organic): apples, pears, berries, kiwis, pineapples, grapefruit, plums, peaches, prunes, figs, raw butter (raw means not pasteurized or homogenized), raw milk, plain yogurt (this means no sugar or added fruit), wild smoked salmon, beef in any form as long as it's organic, chicken in any form as long as it's organic, lamb in any form as long as it's organic, tuna, sardines, eggs, tomatoes, peppers, salsa, celery, carrots, any green leafy vegetables, potatoes (preferably sweet potatoes) in limited amounts, coffee in limited amounts made with pure water (not tap water) with raw milk or cream and raw honey (in small amounts) or stevia as a sweetener, and organic tea (no pesticides). Notice what is *not* on this list? Anything made with flour or wheat. Bagels, toast, donuts, etc. Limit refined carbohydrates.

4. **Eat organic grapefruit all day.**
   Remember the grapefruit diet? Well, it turns out that there actually *is* an enzyme in grapefruit that burns fat. Eating grapefruits all day, as many and as often as you desire, will speed the fat burning process.

5. **Eat organic apples all day.**
   The old saying is true: An apple a day keeps the doctor away. Apples are loaded with fiber and nutrients; they normalize the blood sugar and decrease appetite. You should eat at least one organic apple every day.

6. **Eat a huge salad at lunch and dinner.**
   Use a few cups of fresh organic leafy greens as the base of your meal. Leafy greens include romaine, spinach, kale, arugula, Swiss chard, and others. Iceberg lettuce does not count. If you do make it your base, you can add other organic vegetables and some lean protein and even a grain, like brown rice or quinoa. For dressing, use olive oil and lemon and lime, or organic vinegar. If you really want to speed the weight loss process, use organic apple cider vinegar. Add some organic Himalayan pink sea salt, fresh ground pepper, or some garlic for taste. Do not use processed salad dressings from the supermarket. They will contain chemicals and often sugar or high fructose corn syrup as well. If you *don't* make salad the meal, at least eat a huge salad *along with* your meal. I don't care if your lunch is a cheeseburger

and french fries (as long as it's organic), eat a huge salad first and you'll be amazed by how you lose weight.

7. **Eat only organic meat, poultry, and fish.**
One of the reasons you are overweight is because of the growth hormones put in meat and poultry. If you want to lose weight, eat as much meat and poultry as you like as long as it is organic, grass fed, ideally kosher, and most importantly, has not been given growth hormones. The fish you eat should not be farm raised.

8. **Eat hot peppers.**
Anything spicy or hot will increase your metabolism and make you burn fat quicker. Imagine for breakfast having some scrambled eggs, some lamb chops, and some chopped peppers. Smother the eggs with some organic hot salsa and you will simply lose weight faster.

9. **Use organic apple cider vinegar.**
Take a couple of teaspoons of organic apple cider vinegar in a cup of distilled water before meals and you'll be amazed at how your clothes will become bigger in no time. This vinegar suppresses the appetite and also lowers blood sugar levels. It promotes the secretion of hydrochloric acid in the stomach, which promotes good digestion and better assimilation of nutrients. I don't recommend daily use because the acid can be harmful to tooth enamel and high levels can lead to reduced bone density. But using it a couple of times a week is beneficial and will aid weight loss without harmful effects.

10. **Consume organic extra virgin coconut oil.**
Specifically, replace the cooking oil you've been using with coconut oil. (Olive oil is fine, but stop using soybean oil, corn oil, lard or processed butter.) Coconut oil erroneously

got a bad reputation years ago when it was believed that because it's a saturated fat, it clogged the arteries. It's not true. Coconut oil has no cholesterol and it does not affect the body in the same way that saturated animal fat does. The other great thing about coconut oil is that it gives the metabolism a boost, so it aids in weight loss. Don't go crazy with it, because it's still high in calories. But if you use coconut oil in place of other oil, it will help you lose weight. It tastes good enough that you can also use it in place of butter on vegetables, or baked potatoes.

11. **Consume probiotics.**

Probiotic foods are fermented foods. Rich in enzymes, they help the body's digestive system by breaking down sugars. They also help us absorb more nutrients from our food. They promote good bacteria in the intestines and minimize bad bacteria (like Candida). They assist with weight loss by destroying bile salts in the intestines, which reduce the absorption of fat calories. Some probiotic foods you should add to your diet are: plain organic yogurt, kimchi, miso, sauerkraut, pickles and tempeh.

12. **Do not eat after six p.m.**

This takes some getting used to, so do the best you can. If you follow it, you'll be amazed at how much easier it is to lose weight when you stop eating at this hour. I know it's not easy, but the good news is you can eat *well* during the day, and if you stop eating by 6:00 p.m., you'll still lose weight.

13. **Limit dairy products.**

If you are going to consume milk, cheese, butter, or any dairy products, eat only organic ones that have not been pasteurized or homogenized. The dairy products should be labeled "organic and raw." It may be hard to find raw dairy products in some parts of the country. The next best option is organic, not homogenized, but that has been pasteurized. Your last option is organic that has been both pasteurized and homogenized. Ideally, if you want to lose weight, reduce dairy regardless of what you're getting. Avoid milk, cream, cheese and ice cream. Plain yogurt (preferably Greek) is good and does aid weight loss, because the live cultures assist the digestive system. Definitely do not consume any dairy products that are not organic because they will have growth hormones in them which will slow your weight loss.

14. **No white sugar, white flour, or white rice.**
    White sugar is addictive and makes you fat. Use unprocessed sweeteners in small amounts, preferably raw, organic honey, organic coconut sugar, or stevia extract. White flour, as I've mentioned previously, when mixed with water, makes paste. It does the same thing in your body. Eating white flour clogs up your digestive system and slows your metabolism, which keeps you from losing weight. Use organic whole grain flours that have not been processed or stripped of the fiber, or even better, eat whole grains in place of flour-based products. Oatmeal, quinoa and brown rice are good choices. Avoid white rice. White rice is stripped of its fiber and it spikes blood sugar levels, which leads to inflammation.

15. **No wheat.**
    The wheat produced in this country is genetically modified to the point wherein it isn't the same grain it was originally. This "Frankenwheat" is addictive and it irritates the digestive system. This is not exclusive to people who are gluten sensitive. No one should eat wheat. Removing wheat from you diet is one of the best things you can do to lose weight. This means eliminating most bread. This means eliminating pasta. I know that's hard, and will take some getting used to, but replace it with other grains like oatmeal, brown rice and quinoa and you will get used to it.

16. **No diet sodas or diet food.**

    Diet sodas actually make you fat. They're loaded with chemicals that reek havoc on your metabolism. I did an experiment with people who drank diet soft drinks on a regular basis. For two weeks they replaced their diet soda with regular soda. Amazingly, though they were ingesting more calories from the sugar-sweetened soda, no one gained any weight. Even more shocking was that 80 percent of the people actually lost weight. This is *not* an invitation to go drink a bunch of regular soda—I don't advocate that (all sodas are bad for you), but I want you to see how you're being duped as a consumer. Diet sodas are promoted so heavily, because they're cheaper to make than regular sodas, and because the product is so physically addictive it's been called the "new crack." There is simply no benefit to drinking diet soda. It's the same scam with diet *foods*. Don't eat them. They're not healthy and they're full of chemicals that will actually make it more difficult for you to lose weight. Eat real, wholesome food.

17. **No aspartame or ANY artificial sweeteners.**

    Aspartame, which goes by the name NutraSweet®, will make you fat. All other artificial sweeteners, including saccharin, Splenda®, or anything else, should be avoided. These are toxins. I encourage you to *release* toxins, not store them up in your body. Aspartame triggers food cravings (for sugar and carbohydrates), which obviously works *against* weight loss efforts. And it's addictive. If you use it, you'll tend to use it a lot. Don't even start. Stevia is okay, depending on the brand. Don't buy the kind sold in major grocery stores masquerading as stevia. Truvia is *not* stevia, despite the claims. Look at the ingredients. If it lists a lot of chemicals, avoid it. There are good brands of liquid stevia available online containing just stevia extract, vegetable glycerin, and a small amount of alcohol.

18. **No monosodium glutamate.**

Monosodium glutamate (MSG) is an excitotoxin, which means it over stimulates the cells until it kills them. It makes you fat; it can cause all kinds of medical problems (including fibromyalgia), and it can affect your mood making you depressed. It can also be physically addictive. Unfortunately, the food industry has lobbied Congress to pass laws allowing monosodium glutamate to be added to food while not being listed on the label. There are dozens of words such as spices, natural flavoring, hydrolyzed vegetable protein, etc., that are in fact MSG in disguise. This is why I recommend buying organic, where everything in the ingredient list is something you recognize and can pronounce. Also, MSG is in virtually all fast food, including things you would never imagine, like pizza. This is why people in other countries seem to be able to eat all kinds of food without gaining weight. It's not just the food, but the ingredients used in American food processing that keeps us fat.

19. **No high fructose corn syrup.**

This sweetener, like many of the items on this list, makes you fat and it's physically addictive. I know a woman who lost 15 pounds by doing nothing other than removing high fructose corn syrup from her diet. This corn-derived poison has been linked to obesity, hypertension, and diabetes among other problems. Never ever consume it. In fact, just stop buying *any* processed foods, because it is in nearly all of them. Read the labels on the food you buy. You'll be shocked by how ubiquitous high fructose corn syrup is. But once you realize this, and you see how it's added to so many products, you'll be empowered to make better choices and cook your own food.

20. **No fast food or chain restaurants.**

Any chain or franchise restaurant that sells fast food produces it in such a way that it will make you fat. You can actually eat French fries and cheeseburgers and lose weight, provided that the ingredients you use are organic. It's virtually impossible to eat food in a chain or franchise restaurant where the food has *not* been processed to last for years, which means it is full of preservatives. In addition to that there are chemicals added to make the food taste great, get you physically addicted to it, increase your appetite and make you fatter. Remember, these are businesses whose main objective is to make a profit. If the food tastes amazing, gets you physically addicted, increases your appetite, and makes you fat, the restaurant is guaranteed success. They're like drug dealers getting their customers hooked and continually coming back for more. This is the sad truth of what's happening in our food industry today.

21. **Take digestive enzymes.**

There's an excellent chance your body is not producing enough digestive enzymes if you're gaining weight, feeling bloated, and have gas, indigestion, and/or constipation. Go to your health food store and inquire, or do an online search. Try a few kinds to see which one works best for you.

22. **Get fifteen colonics in thirty days.**

This process will clean your colon, making it easier for your body to assimilate nutrients. This reduces hunger, it reduces cravings, and increases metabolism. Colonics also allow your body to digest food faster so that it will not turn to fat.

23. **Do a colon cleanse.**

If you do the fifteen colonics, you won't need a colon cleanse, but if you *don't* do the colonics, you should do one. If you're significantly overweight, your digestive system is more than likely sluggish. You should be moving your bowels *at least* once daily, preferably more. Cleansing the colon will help with weight loss, dramatically increase your metabolism, and benefit your body by eliminating toxins. There are many colon-cleansing programs available. Inquire at your local health food store for recommendations, or research them online.

24. **Do a Candida cleanse.**

If you're overweight, you most certainly have a Candida yeast overgrowth, probably throughout your entire body. Losing weight will be difficult and slow and keeping it off nearly impossible as long as this condition persists. If you wipe out the excess Candida, losing weight will be much easier and keeping it off will be easier, too. There is plenty of information about Candida cleanses online.

25. **Do a liver cleanse.**

If you are overweight your liver is most definitely clogged and needs attention. The liver is one of our most important detox organs. Cleansing the liver will assist it in detoxifying the body's waste, which in turn will help the digestive system process food more efficiently so that you can lose weight more easily. There are many liver cleanses on the market. Research them and see what works best for you. In the meantime, you can help begin the liver cleansing process by eating lots of fresh leafy greens, omitting sugar and food high in animal fats, and drinking distilled water with lemon or with lemon and cayenne pepper first thing every morning.

26. **Fast**

This is intimidating to most people, and it can be difficult, but the benefits are so fantastic I urge you to do it. It will change your body and your life. A twenty-one day organic juice fast will completely detoxify your body, flush out your fat cells, and reset your body's weight set point. It will also leave you thinner, revitalized and feeling like a new (improved) person. Ideally, you should have a juicer and juice the organic fruits and vegetables yourself, emphasizing leafy greens as the base for most of your juices. Organic juice fasting lets the digestive system heal itself by cleansing it and giving it a rest. The first few days are challenging, but it becomes easier and you will soon feel energized. Not only will you shed weight, but some people experience increased wellbeing, more clarity in their thoughts, and an improvement in emotional health. One caveat: a fast that's longer than a few days should be done under the supervision of a professional healthcare provider.

27. **Use infrared saunas.**

Infrared saunas increase metabolism, dramatically reduce toxins, speed weight loss, and burn fat. Ideally they're used on a daily basis, but I realize this is impractical for most people. Do the best you can. Spas and gyms are slowly catching on about the benefits of infrared saunas over traditional saunas, so they're getting easier to find in most big cities.

28. **Add muscle.**

Muscle burns fat. When you add muscle through exercise you're increasing your body's metabolism. Weight training is probably the method you're most familiar with. It's not the method I prefer, but it's better than not adding muscle. The reason it's not my preference is because I believe that it builds muscle in a way that blocks energy rather than allowing it to flow through your body. Blocked energy is not ideal. In my opinion, the best way to add muscle without blocking energy is to do exercises that add muscle, while also stretching the body and keeping it limber. Consider yoga, Pilates, ballet, swimming, or martial arts.

29. **Walk for at least one hour, nonstop, per day.**

    The body is designed to walk. Research shows that slow, rhythmic movement exercise, like walking, resets the body's weight set point and creates a leaner physique. A one-hour walk every day will change your body dramatically in as little as one month.

30. **Rebound.**

    Using a rebounder, or mini-trampoline, stimulates and strengthens every cell in the body simultaneously. Gently jumping up and down on a rebounder for just ten minutes a day stimulates the lymphatic system and increases your metabolism. It is very effective for weight loss and enhances overall health.

31. **Practice deep breathing.**

    Oxygen breaks down and burns fat. Most people do not breathe deeply enough to stimulate their metabolism and fat burning capabilities. Fat is made up of oxygen, hydrogen and carbon. When the oxygen we breathe reaches fat molecules it breaks them down into carbon dioxide and water. The blood then picks up the carbon dioxide and returns it to the lungs and we exhale it. So the more oxygen you use, the more fat you'll burn. Breathe deeply, using your diaphragm. While breathing *alone* won't transform your body (sorry, you still have to exercise!), deep breathing will help tremendously. Try doing it when you wake up, before you go to bed and even occasionally while you're working or waiting in line somewhere. Take in a deep breath, hold it a moment and exhale slowly, then repeat. Do this at least five times and build up to ten times or more. Consider deep breathing while you do your daily activities; it will increase the benefits.

32. **Wear magnetic finger rings.**

Special magnetic rings worn on the little finger of each hand while you sleep can have amazing results. Magnetic rings help speed the metabolism. They also assist with fluid retention.

33. **Cheat once in a while.**

You want ice cream, cookies, cakes, chocolate, French fries, pizza, potato chips? Don't completely deprive yourself. It's better to eat a little something without guilt than not eat it and feel bad about it. Not eating food and being stressed about it can make you fat, because after a while, you'll rebel and binge to the point where your eating will be out of control. Allow yourself a little bit of whatever it is you're craving. If you follow my recommendations, the boost you'll get from how wonderful your weight loss looks will help you change your eating habits. When you start omitting processed foods, you'll stop craving them, because the chemicals that keep you addicted will be out of your system. Ideally, if you *are* going to cheat and want cookies, cakes, ice cream, potato chips, etc., don't buy these products from the supermarket. Go to a health food store and buy the natural or organic counterpart. The advantage is that if you choose wisely, you can enjoy these treats without all of the processing and chemicals that make and keep you fat.

34. **Reduce or eliminate the "uncontrollable" urge to eat when you're not hungry.**

If you're an emotional eater and have uncontrollable urges and compulsions to eat when you're not hungry you may benefit from hypnosis. Look for a licensed hypnotherapist. You may also benefit from a process called "tapping." Look into the Emotional Freedom Technique (EFT) or Thought Field Therapy (TRT). Both employ tapping and can be used to eliminate compulsions. I recommend the book *Tapping The Healer Within: How to Instantly Conquer Fears, Anxieties, and Emotional Distress* by Roger Callahan.

It's amazing that little things can make a difference. When looking at this list, a good way to attack it is to pick one thing on the list and do that for a few days. Then, look for another thing on the list and while still doing the first thing, add the second. Do that until you feel comfortable adding something else. These techniques absolutely work and they will not only help you lose weight, but they'll benefit your health overall.

CHAPTER 9

How to Read Food Labels

Hopefully by now you're convinced that there most definitely *are* toxic chemicals in the majority of the food you purchase in major supermarkets, or eat in most fast food restaurants. Our food supply is different than it was seventy-five, fifty, or even as recently as twenty-five years ago. Many of you eat the same brands and products today that you ate twenty or thirty years ago, without realizing that the product is no longer the same; it's been modified. Today that same product could contain a hundred times the number of chemical toxins that it contained twenty-five or fifty years ago. In an effort to produce food more cheaply, make it last longer, make you physically addicted to it, increase your appetite, and make you fat, food manufacturers process and load their products with chemicals that add toxins and destroy the living enzymes. This wipes out much of the food's nutritional value.

The bottom line is that today it's nearly impossible to go to a supermarket or fast food restaurant and buy anything to eat or drink that's *not* full of chemicals, reduced in nutritional value, or energetically altered. Ideally, you would never eat in fast food restaurants, and never buy anything mass-produced by large food manufacturers. You'd buy *only* organic fruits, vegetables, nuts, seeds, grains, meats, eggs, and dairy products and make everything in your house from scratch. But, realistically, most of us can't do that, at least not all of the time. So is it a lost cause, or is there something you can do to eat food that has fewer toxins, more nutrition, and that hasn't been energetically altered? The answer is yes. It may not be perfect, but it'll be infinitely better than what you're doing now.

> Our food supply is different than it was seventy-five, fifty, or even as recently as twenty-five years ago.

When you go food shopping, **avoid major supermarkets**. When you shop for food, consider, instead, going to a farmer's market. Buy organic fruits, vegetables, nuts, grains, herbs and spices from small independent growers whom you can meet and talk with, so you can feel confident that what you're buying is actually good for you. In some areas there are "food co-ops" wherein members organize and make the decisions about what food is sold and where it comes from. I recommend these, because they're generally run by people with a sincere interest in bringing good quality food to their communities. If you live in a house with a yard, consider planting fruit trees, or a vegetable garden. Even if you live in an apartment, you can grow some vegetables (like tomatoes, mushrooms, carrots and radishes) in pots indoors, or on a terrace, or rooftop.

The most convenient way to shop for high quality food is go to a whole food or natural health food store where they sell organic products. When you go to these stores, you have a better chance of finding things that aren't loaded with toxins, or energetically altered, the way the products in regular supermarkets are. Keep in mind, though, that not everything they sell in these natural or whole food stores is good for you. Remember, it's always all about the money. In some cases, these stores are also publicly traded companies that have to make a profit, so you have to read the labels. The key to reading labels is not to read the front of the package. This is where the company does its advertising, and where the marketing department has spent millions of dollars researching what will make you think it is healthy so you'll buy it. Take the box, package or jar, (no cans—avoid canned food, because can linings have the toxin Bisphenol A in them) and look for the *ingredients list*. I'm going to give you the most important words you should look for and avoid. When you see these, do not buy that product. Just say *no*, and put it back.

1. **Anything You Can't Pronounce**

   If you can't pronounce the word, it's a chemical. They can call it anything they want. They can say that it comes from a plant, or that it's all natural. But it's not true. Keep in mind food manufacturers lobby Congress to get legislation passed that allows these food manufactures to call chemicals "all natural ingredients." Bottom line: if you can't pronounce it, don't buy it.

2. **Monosodium Glutamate**

   Never buy anything with monosodium glutamate (MSG) in it. MSG is an excitotoxin, which means it damages nerve cells. It's dangerous; it makes you fat, increases your appetite, and causes all types of physical and medical problems.

3. **Sugar**

   The sugar used in processed food is refined, which means they've taken natural sugarcane and turned it into a drug. It's added to food for its sweetness, but also for its chemically addictive qualities. It is also laced with the chemicals used in growing sugarcane. Avoid it entirely.

4. **High Fructose Corn Syrup**

   This corn derived, toxic sweetener is highly addictive, and makes you fat. It can lead to plaque buildup and narrowing of the arteries. It also contributes to fat deposits in your liver.

5. **Aspartame**

   This sweetener is an excitotoxin, which, like MSG, can damage nerve cells. It makes you fat, it makes you hungry, it makes you depressed, and it leads to all types of medical conditions including PMS, chronic fatigue syndrome, fibromyalgia, and migraines.

6. **Dextrose**

   This is a chemically made sweetener. It's a simple carbohydrate, a source of "empty calories" and consuming it can lead to weight gain.

7. **Sucralose-Splenda®**

   This chemical sweetener is poisonous and makes you fat. It was produced so that the food industry could capitalize on the low-carbohydrate craze. Now, products can have "no- carbohydrates" or "low-carbohydrates" and still taste sweet. The problem is that it's artificial, and these man-made sweeteners do in fact increase your appetite, make you depressed, cause all types of symptoms (including migraine headaches, PMS, depression, fibromyalgia, and allergies), and most importantly, make you fat.

8. **Artificial Color**

   Stay away from food dyes. They're chemical poisons. Many of the food dyes in American products are acknowledged to be toxic and banned elsewhere in the world. Some of the dyes can cause a list of health problems including tumors, chromosomal damage, hyperactivity, insomnia, aggression and violent behavior, eczema, hives, asthma and others. Anything that has food dye in it is processed, so avoid it.

9. **Natural and Artificial Flavors**

   If it says "natural" or "artificial flavors" on the label, know that this is where lobbyists have done a magnificent job of allowing the food industry to deceive the public. "Natural flavor" is not natural at all and is no better, nor much different from "artificial flavor." Much of the food in today's high-tech processing is so altered that it loses most of its flavor. Consequently, food manufacturers must add chemicals (natural and/or artificial flavors) to make the food taste like it's supposed to. If you were to ask the food companies to individually list the ingredients in "natural" and/or "artificial" flavors, they would refuse. My insiders tell me that if they did reveal that list, the ingredients for both natural and artificial flavors would contain hundreds of chemicals. While a single chemical may not have major immediate negative effects, when you combine two, three, or four of these chemicals, just like in chemistry class, new chemicals are formed. What these new chemicals do is dangerous for the body. Avoid anything with natural and/or artificial flavors on the label.

10. **Spices**

    Be wary when a label says "spices" without specifying what those spices are. More than likely they are *not* merely spices, they also contain chemicals. *Real* spices are great, but if the spices in the product were in fact *real*, they would be able to name them. "Spices" fall under a category similar to natural flavors.

11. **Hydrogenated Oil or Partially Hydrogenated Oil**

    If it's hydrogenated or partially hydrogenated, don't buy it. It's a trans fat. Trans fats cause heart disease, make you fat, and can lead to a whole host of other medical conditions.

12. **Palm Oil**

    A deadly oil that's cheap to manufacture, and causes all types of physical problems. In its oxidized state, which is how it would appear in most foods, palm oil can threaten physiological and biochemical functions of the body. The dangers include toxicity to the heart, kidney, liver and lungs.

13. **Enriched Bleached Wheat Flour and Enriched Bleached White Flour**

    Wheat production and processing in this country has unfortunately ruined it to the point wherein I don't recommend that you eat *any* product made from wheat or wheat flour. No bread, pasta, bagels, muffins, biscuits or cereals—*nothing* made of wheat will do your body any good. I know this is difficult to hear, but it's true. Sadly, wheat is now a toxin. Today's wheat is simply not the same product it was years ago. It was changed in order to make it stronger, and to make it grow better and faster. Wheat now contains sodium azide, which is a known toxin. It also contains new proteins that aren't found in the original version of wheat. Our bodies don't have the enzymes to break down these proteins and so they are impossible to digest. You've probably heard a lot about *gluten intolerance* over the past few years. Gluten is a protein composite that many people can't digest, hence the proliferation of "gluten free" products. But what you may not know is that *no one can properly digest gluten*. Though you may not experience the symptoms of the gluten intolerant, virtually all of us experience systemic inflammation from eating wheat. On top of that, wheat products contain a morphine-like compound that makes them highly addictive.

14. **Soy Protein Isolate**

    This is a common toxic ingredient in protein shakes and protein bars. Stay away from it. You will never see organic soy protein isolate. The reason is that hexane, which is a petroleum solvent similar to gasoline, is often used to process soy protein isolate. The residues of chemicals like hexane remain in the food, but they're never listed on the label.

There you have the main things to stay away from. A good rule of thumb, however, is to read the labels. You may find things not included on this list that you should avoid. If the ingredients you see are not things that you could have in your own kitchen, or if the food is something you couldn't make yourself, stay away from it; it's dangerous.

Now I'd like to point out in greater detail just how different the food from a regular supermarket is compared to its equivalent purchased at a local health food store. Keep in mind that these products may seem nearly identical, but the differences are these: The food from the health food store will have fewer ingredients, the ingredients will be (mostly) organic, and there will be fewer chemicals in the food or no chemicals at all. The food hasn't been stripped of its nutritional value, and it hasn't been energetically destroyed.

> Keep in mind that most food producers want you to crave their food so you'll eat more of it.

The food from the health food store also tastes better because it's made with whole food ingredients. When you eat it you don't get constipation, bloating, or gas. Most people eat less because the nutrients are greater and more easily assimilated so you don't crave as much. Keep in mind that most food producers want you to crave their food so you'll eat more of it. That's how they increase their profits. Bottom line is the food from the health food store, generally, will have more nutrition, will have nothing energetically destroyed, will taste better, and have virtually no toxins in it. So let's go through a few products and note the differences on the labels.

A. Pancake Syrup

Health Food Store
    Product name: Organic maple syrup
    Ingredients: 100 percent raw, unprocessed, unfiltered maple syrup
Supermarket
    Product name: Aunt Jemima Original Syrup
    Ingredients: Corn syrup, high fructose corn syrup, water, cellulose gum, caramel color, salt, sodium benzoate, ascorbic acid, artificial flavors, natural flavors, sodium hexametaphosphate

B. Potato Chips

Health Food Store
    Product name: Potato chips
    Ingredients: Organic potatoes, organic sunflower oil, sea salt
Supermarket
    Product name: Pringles Potato Chips
    Ingredients: Dried potatoes, corn oil, cottonseed oil, sunflower oil, yellow corn meal, wheat starch, maltodextrin, salt, dextrose, whey, buttermilk, dried tomato, dried garlic, partially hydrogenated soybean oil, monosodium glutamate, corn syrup solids, dried onion, sodium casonate, multicacid, spices, annatto extract, modified corn starch, natural flavors, artificial flavors, disodium inosinate, disodium guanylate

C. Mayonnaise

Health Food Store
    Product name: Organic mayonnaise
    Ingredients: Expeller pressed soybean oil, organic whole eggs, water, organic egg yolks, organic honey, organic white vinegar, sea salt, organic dry mustard, organic lemon juice concentrate
Supermarket
    Product name: Miracle Whip Mayonnaise
    Ingredients: Water, soybean oil, vinegar, high fructose corn syrup, eggs, sugar, modified food starch, salt, mustard flower, artificial color, potassium sorbate, paprika, spices, natural flavors, dried garlic

D. Salad Dressing

Health Food Store

Product name: Salad dressing

Ingredients: Water, expeller pressed canola oil, balsamic vinegar, vine-ripened dried tomatoes, sea salt, garlic, oregano, basil, parsley, black pepper

Supermarket

Product name: Kraft Fat Free Salad Dressing

Ingredients: Water, tomato paste, high fructose corn syrup, vinegar, corn syrup, water, chopped pickles, modified food starch, salt, maltodextrin, soybean oil, egg yolks, xanthan gum, artificial color, mustard flower, potassium sorbate, calcium disodium, EDTA, phosphoric acid, dried onions, guar gum, spices, Vitamin E acetate, lemon juice concentrate, yellow dye #6, natural flavors, oleoresin turmeric, red dye #40, artificial flavors, blue dye #1

E. Granola

Health Food Store

Product name: Granola

Ingredients: Organic rolled oats, organic honey, organic safflower oil, organic sunflower seeds, organic whole wheat flour, organic spiced almonds, organic nonfat dry milk, organic sesame seeds, organic raisins

Supermarket

Product name: Kellogg's Granola

Ingredients: Whole oats, cold grain wheat, brown sugar, corn syrup, raisins, rice, sugar, almonds, partially hydrogenated cottonseed oil, glycerin, modified corn starch, salt, cinnamon, nonfat dry milk, high fructose corn syrup, polyglycerol esters of mono- and diglycerides, malt flavoring, alpha-tocopherol acetate, niacinamide, zinc oxide, sodium ascorbate, ascorbic acid, reduced iron, guar gum, BHT, cryodypyridoxine hydrochloride, riboflavin, Vitamin A palmitate, folic acid, thiamin hydrochloride, Vitamin D, Vitamin B

I hope the pattern here is obvious. The supermarket brand name options clearly contain many chemical ingredients that do not appear in the ingredients list of the equivalent health food store options. If you have the choice to eat something with ingredients you're familiar with, or something with a list of chemicals added to it, I hope you'll go with the ingredients you're familiar with because that product is going to be better for you.

I could do a hundred of these comparisons. There are huge and important differences between what's available in standard supermarkets and what's available in health food or whole food type stores. Keep in mind though, you must read the ingredients yourself. Just because it's in a health food store does not guarantee that it's good. Read the labels and follow my guidelines on what to avoid. When you purchase wisely, you'll be buying products that:

- ✔ Have few or no toxins
- ✔ Have more nutrition than their supermarket equivalent
- ✔ Taste better
- ✔ Make you feel better
- ✔ Will not give you gas, bloating, headaches, constipation, etc.
- ✔ Will not make you hungrier
- ✔ Will not make you fat
- ✔ Will not get you physically addicted
- ✔ And you'll be supporting small, independent, and in many cases local people who are trying to produce products that taste great and are good for you

When you go to your local supermarket and buy name brand products and/or products from major publicly traded food corporations, you're supporting the multinational companies that are hurting local growers and independent farmers, and causing massive amounts of illness and disease not only in America, but in countries around the world. It is my opinion that these large multinational corporations like Monsanto are exploiting and taking advantage of people through their clever use of advertising, and knowingly giving us food filled with chemicals that increase our appetite, get us physically addicted, and make us fat, all in the name of profit. Remember, I'm not being fanatical in advising you to eat more raw fruits, vegetables, nuts, and seeds. I'm recommending that you take small steps and go at a pace that's right for you.

Many of you may feel unwilling to drastically change your eating habits. For example, some of you love snack food and can't imagine giving up treats. That's fine. Go to the health food store and try different kinds of snacks to munch on. Many of them are incredibly delicious. As I write this, I'm thinking about some sweet snacks I recently purchased at my health food store. The first one has four ingredients and no chemicals: Pure raw carob, coconut, pure cane crystals, pure maple syrup. All of the ingredients are organic, raw, and real living food. They taste amazing. Another has these ingredients: Raw organic sunflower seeds, raw organic raisins, raw organic bananas, raw organic maple syrup, and fennel. This snack is sweet and tastes fantastic. Another one is an incredible almond brittle made with raw almonds, pure vanilla beans and crystals of pure cane. It's simple, real, and all natural. And here's the great part: Last night, to see how I would feel, I ate a huge bag of this almond brittle in one sitting. I didn't feel bloated, didn't get a sugar rush, my mood didn't go up or down—I felt absolutely fine and I slept like a baby. If I had done the same thing with some almond or peanut brittle made by a large, publicly traded corporation, I would have felt horrible, bloated, gassy and would have tossed and turned all night.

Just remember that name brand products and large multinational publicly traded corporations are investing tens of millions of dollars in research to find out what the hot buttons are to get you to buy their products. Don't believe their slick ads, and don't believe what's written on the front of the package. Read the ingredients. But do remember as you read them that *in addition* to the chemicals listed there, some of the toxins that were used to process the food may *not,* in fact, be listed. Yes, many toxins that are in the food *do not have to be listed on the ingredients*.

Here is an excerpt from the most recent guidelines of the FDA:

"Is it necessary to declare ingredients in "trace", i.e., incidental amounts? Can sulfites be considered incidental additives?

Answer: FDA does not define "trace amounts"; however, there are some exemptions for declaring ingredients present in "incidental" amounts in a finished food. If an ingredient is present at an incidental level and has no functional or technical effect in the finished product, then it need not be declared on the label."

There you have it. *"If an ingredient is present at an incidental level and has no functional or technical effect in the finished product, then it need not be declared on the label."* Do you see why this does not serve the public well? Who determines whether something has a "functional effect?" If the chemical has no functional effect, then why can't they omit it? And if they're going to include it, how can they know for sure that it will have no adverse effect on the people who consume it? The answer is *they can't know that for sure.* Monsanto is famous for getting away with this kind of thing. They put out harmful chemicals, like saccharine, for instance. Then they declare it "safe" with the FDA's approval, when it's anything *but* safe. It causes cancer; and only after whistle blowers prove the danger, do they make any change to what they're doing.

It's estimated that over 95 percent of all food products have as many as 300 added chemicals that are not listed on the label. This happens because companies have persuaded the FDA that the chemical "has no functional or technical effect on the product." This is the sad truth. This is power of the food industry. And this is why, if you want to eliminate and prevent sickness and disease, you need to stop buying food made by major corporations.

Restaurants

I'm often questioned about eating in restaurants. There are vast differences in the kinds of restaurants you may patronize. I'm not talking about the food. I'm talking about the kind of restaurant. Most restaurants have the following problems:

1. In order to make a profit they have to buy the cheapest food available. Restaurants get their food primarily from large, bulk food suppliers that supply hundreds of restaurants in a given area.

2. Much of the food you eat in any restaurant hasn't been cooked at the restaurant; rather, it's simply been finished off or heated up. This gets worse with restaurants that are vast in number, like fast food places or franchises.

3. Most restaurants use microwave ovens to reheat the food right before serving.

4. Most restaurants, like large food manufacturers, use frying oil all day and in some cases for days on end. The problem with this is once you heat the oil for frying it goes rancid quickly. All of the food that comes out of the rancid oil is carcinogenic.

Recently, I went to a nice restaurant and was about to order, but before doing so, I had some questions. I love fresh guacamole and often make it at home with fresh, raw, organic ingredients. It's absolutely delicious. Guacamole was on the menu so I asked if it was made fresh. The waiter told me that yes, it was. I inquired further. "So you actually take avocados and mash them up in the kitchen, or does it come in a prepackaged mix?" And he said, "Oh, well we do get a mix, but we add water and make it fresh every day."

His idea of fresh and my idea of fresh were completely different. This guacamole was *not* made in the back with fresh avocados, tomatoes, lime juice, onions, etc. Instead, it came as a powdered mix to which water was added. When I asked what the ingredients of the mix were, of course he didn't know. I persuaded him to go and find the package and bring me the ingredient list. There were over three dozen ingredients on the label, including monosodium glutamate.

I asked if the *salad* was fresh. He thought for a moment and said, "No. It actually comes in bags that have been prepackaged." The problem with this, of course, is that in order to retain freshness the "fresh salad" has to be sprayed with chemicals. I asked if the *chicken* was fresh, or did *it* come prepackaged, too. Not surprisingly, it came prepackaged and frozen. Virtually all of the sauces, all of the mixes, and all of the flavoring agents used came in boxes, cans, or packages. This is the unfortunate problem with a lot of restaurant food.

> Even making some simple modifications to your diet could have a dramatic impact.

So, what can you do? Basically, you can be a fanatic and not eat in any restaurant unless it's an all natural, totally organic one, or you can simply eat really well at home and stay away from chains, franchises, and fast food as best you can. When you go to a good quality restaurant, simply ask if you may tour the kitchen and see some of the food being prepared. Most managers welcome this. It'll give you a chance to meet the manager and/or the owner and inquire about how the different dishes are made. Then you can see which dish or dishes include the highest quality and the freshest ingredients. I ask a few questions and make some intelligent choices. Bear in mind, when it comes to eating out, you have to care, but not so much that it makes you crazy. Do what you feel comfortable with, and don't be stressed out about your decisions.

I have a close friend who's not only a vegetarian, but also only eats raw food. She's not stressed out or fanatical about it, that's just what she eats. We went to a restaurant and I ordered some salmon sushi. I knew the salmon was caught in the wild, and the brown rice was made with pure ingredients. I liked the cucumber and onion salad they made as well. The fresh ginger and wasabi were also delicious and made fresh at the restaurant. Although the restaurant does not use organic ingredients, it's a matter of degree. My meal could be classified as relatively healthy. Far from ideal, but also far from something you'd find in a fast food restaurant. At least there were no hydrogenated oils, monosodium glutamate, aspartame or massive amounts of chemicals. My friend, being a vegetarian and a raw foodist, had limited options, but her attitude about what she wanted was the key. She inquired about her choices and made her selections. We had lovely conversation, and her food was secondary in nature to our discussions. She wasn't stressed or uptight. She wasn't judgmental or pushing her ideas and values upon me. Maybe someday I'll eat raw food exclusively too. For right now, I love my organic lamb, chicken, beef and various kinds of cooked food. The point is, knowing all this information doesn't mean you have to do it *all* in order to receive benefits. Do a little or a lot, based on what you feel good about. Even making some simple modifications to your diet could have a dramatic impact.

CHAPTER 10

Still Not Convinced?

This book is filled with some very basic premises from which our conclusions are derived. The most basic is that there *are* natural, non-drug, and nonsurgical ways to prevent and cure virtually every disease. The FDA, the FTC, and the pharmaceutical industry work diligently to prevent you from learning about this information. The news media, including newspapers, magazines, television, and radio, are biased toward the pharmaceutical industry and present half-truths and outright lies in relation to healthcare. If you're still not persuaded that this is true consider these thought provoking ideas:

1. Still not convinced "it's all about the money"? Then consider this:

✔ The *Associated Press* has reported *"drug companies are seeing that cancer can be lucrative."* The article goes on to say how drug companies will be making billions of dollars in profits by selling cancer fighting drugs, even though they *do not work.* The article exposes the fact that curing cancer would be devastating to companies. Companies make money as long as people have cancer and they remain convinced that they need to take drugs. The article also exposes the fact that no research is being done by these drug companies on natural remedies for the treatment of cancer or on the *prevention* of cancer. The big money for these companies is making sure that more people get cancer and more people are brainwashed into buying their overpriced, ineffective and dangerous drugs.

✔ *USA Today* reported that biotech stock prices soared after cancer drug good news. The article pointed out the fact that publicly traded drug companies have only one goal: To increase profits, which means selling more drugs. The article never mentioned if the drugs were effective at preventing or curing cancer. It talked about how much money the companies would make by selling the drugs.

✔ Dozens of companies have been found guilty of failing to recall dangerous products. Several years ago Graco children's products agreed to pay a record $4 million penalty for hiding negative information about problems with their car seats, highchairs, strollers, and other products that resulted in hundreds of injuries and at least six deaths. This is an outrage. The corporate officers and directors should be held accountable for the murder of six people. These individuals made the decision to let people suffer and die so that they could make more money. This goes on all of the time in business. For every company that's caught there are hundreds of other violations that are not exposed. It's always *all about the money*.

✔ I was offered $50 million to recommend certain products when I wrote the first edition of the *Natural Cures* book. The individuals who made this offer even came up with a sophisticated plan of wiring money to numbered Swiss bank accounts. I can assure you that these types of bribes and payoffs are happening regularly in the news media, on television, radio, newspapers, and magazines. I've been offered positive stories on major news stations and in magazines and newspapers *if* I spend huge amounts of money in advertising. This type of corruption is rampant.

✔ Corporations do not want to provide good quality products. They want to get your money. One way to do this is to manufacture products that are of low quality and are guaranteed to break. This way, manufacturers can sell you outrageously priced extended service plans. Consider this when you buy an electronic device such as a computer. Sixty percent of all electronics break down in the first year. The profit made by retailers and the manufacturers in repairing and/or selling new equipment is astronomical. This is done purposely. Where's the Federal Trade Commission? The FTC is not protecting the consumers; it's protecting the profits of the large publicly traded corporations. Similarly, drug companies do not want to cure and prevent disease. They do not care about your health. They do not care about finding out why people are sick or discovering the best ways to prevent sickness and cure illness. Drug companies only want to develop and *sell* patented drugs. This is evidenced by the fact that the majority of their money is not spent on verifying that their drugs are effective and/or safe. The majority of their money is spent on marketing to convince you that you need drugs and that you must buy drugs.

✔ Newspapers, magazines, television, and radio commonly bad mouth all natural products, while at the same time run ads for products that they are *not* bashing. This is done purposely. It occurs blatantly on web sites. It's important to note that there are almost never reports done on companies or products that are the sponsors of those TV stations, radio stations, newspapers, magazines, or web sites. Consider that when companies provide advertising revenue to a "news organization" you never see them run negative stories about those products or companies. Why? Because they don't want to bite the hand that feeds them. But this is an inherent limitation and one that does a disservice to the public. If a company wants to avoid bad press, they can simply payoff the news outlets with advertising money.

✔ Health food and vitamin companies are being gobbled up by the pharmaceutical industry either owned directly or indirectly by them. This is so the drug companies can control all natural vitamins and minerals. When the pharmaceutical companies control this industry, they will either raise the prices dramatically and begin charging much more for all natural herbs, vitamins, and minerals, or they will simply take them off the market,therefore making it impossible for you to have natural options to drugs. This is being done systematically so that the pharmaceutical industry can control and monopolize healthcare. This should be a violation of antitrust laws. The politicians do nothing. The FTC, the agency entrusted with protecting consumers against antitrust violations and monopolies such as this, does nothing. This is corruption at the highest levels of government.

✔ Many "newsletters" or books promote certain supplements. Most people do not know that the owners of these newsletters or books are the same people who actually sell the supplements. This is misleading and fraudulent, but very profitable for the big corporations. Magazines and newspapers commonly run positive articles on products if those companies commit to large advertising contracts. What this means is that you can't believe much of what you read in magazines and newspapers, because you don't know if the article is really a payoff for the prodigious amount of advertising the publisher receives.

2. Still not convinced that the FTC and FDA, as well as maybe TV, radio, and news organizations, are suppressing and censoring information? Then consider this:

✔ The natural supplement ephedra was banned, but the pharmaceutical version, ephedrine, was not banned. The natural version was taken off the market, but the dangerous chemically produced synthetic version is still allowed to be sold. This shows how the FDA protects the pharmaceutical industry.

✔ Drug advertising is everywhere. You see drug ads on TV, hear them on radio, and read them in newspapers and in magazines. Drug companies sponsor sporting events and fill our mailboxes with direct mail campaigns promoting their drugs. These drug ads in many cases have been deemed misleading and/or false, yet the FTC has taken no action against any pharmaceutical company for producing false and misleading ads even though these promotional materials are encouraging people under false pretenses to use these dangerous and ineffective drugs. There has never been a drug ad rejected by a television or radio station, newspaper, or magazine. However television stations, newspapers, magazines, and radio stations will routinely reject advertising for all natural herbal products, homeopathic products, vitamins, minerals, or books that are critical of the pharmaceutical industry.

✔ The most obvious example that the government, as well as the news organizations are suppressing and censoring information is the Monsanto exposé that was squashed by Fox. This is the story where two journalists did a report exposing the growth hormone that Monsanto manufactures and how it was being injected into dairy cows, potentially causing illness and disease and tainting the milk with poisons that harm humans as well. This true story was squashed by Fox. Why? To protect the profits of Monsanto.

3. Still not convinced that the media is biased, deceiving, and lying to you about many topics? Then consider this:

✔ Have you ever read a bad article written about a news organization's sponsors? You'd be hard pressed to recall one of those. It just doesn't happen. This is a blatant example of how the media is biased and succumbs to the whims and pressures of its sponsors. The news media is the mouthpiece of the large corporations that buy the advertising. The *majority* of advertising is from the pharmaceutical industry and the food industry; therefore, it is virtually impossible to hear the truth about how the food being produced by large publicly traded corporations is in fact giving us disease and making us fat, and how the drugs are ineffective and giving us disease.

✔ Many news articles are written by individuals who are on the payroll of the companies profiled in those articles. An example a few years back was an article with the headline: "Despite Known Hazards, Many Potentially Dangerous Dietary Supplements Continue to be Used." This article was written by a doctor who was on the payroll of a drug company. The story wasn't "news." It wasn't true, nor was it unbiased journalism. It was a debunking campaign by the pharmaceutical industry to turn people away from safe and effective natural remedies, and instead, to continue to brainwash people into believing drugs are the only answer for illness and disease. This continues to happen.

✔ Pharmaceutical companies set up and pay for web sites by the hundreds debunking natural remedies. Usually, a small group of people actually runs and maintains hundreds of web sites, so an individual consumer thinks that there are multiple independent organizations around the world saying how bad natural remedies are and how good drugs are. This is propaganda in its most flagrant form.

✔ The four basic food group model promoted for years was actually invented by, promoted by, and funded by the dairy association. The food pyramid today was put into effect by our government after massive lobbying by the food industry. The four basic food groups and the food pyramid have nothing to do with health and nutrition, but are designed to brainwash people into eating a certain way for the benefit of the food industry.

✔ The media hides the truth about the dangers of nonprescription and prescription drugs. There are very few articles written about how lethal over-the-counter nonprescription and prescription drugs really are. However, the number of articles that have been written broadcasting the dangers of natural supplements such as herbs, vitamins and minerals is staggering. The fact is drugs, both over-the-counter nonprescription and prescription ones, are infinitely more dangerous than any vitamin, mineral or herb. There are virtually no reported cases of anyone dying from taking a natural supplement in its proper dose. However, there are hundreds of thousands of documented deaths that have occurred by taking an over-the-counter nonprescription or prescription drug in its proper dosage.

✔ Whistleblowers now report that all forms of media, including radio, TV, newspapers, and magazines, are in fact owned by the sponsors. There are secret meetings with the sponsors who dictate the content of all programming and topics covered or not covered in the media outlets.

4. Still not convinced that right now your body is loaded with toxins causing you all types of illness, disease, depression, stress, and anxiety? Then consider this:

✔ All injections from Botox, collagen, insulin and vaccines are loaded with poisonous toxins. Many of these are animal based and are filled with deadly pathogens and chemicals.

✔ There are so many toxins in our environment and food that even people who live in the most remote parts of the world have been found to have toxins in their fat cells. And this is the case even though the toxins do not exist in their local environment. This is a toxic world, and no one is immune. You are filled with toxins right now.

✔ A study showed that traces of industrial strength fire retardant have turned up in wild and farm-raised salmon around the world. Farm-raised salmon has been found to have troubling levels of PCBs, a known cancer causing agent. When you eat this food the toxins go inside *you*.

✔ The newspaper *The Daily Mail* reported, "Ready to eat salad linked with birth defects… Cancer hazard is in packed salad." The article goes on to expose how premixed ready to eat salad is washed with chlorine. The chlorine is bad enough, but it combines with chemicals naturally present in lettuce to create chlorine byproducts, which can be even more hazardous to your health.

✔ The government has found traces of rocket fuel chemical in milk, green leaf lettuce, and drinking water. The government also acknowledges that these chemicals adversely affect the thyroid, which potentially can make you fat and lead to dozens of other diseases.

✔ *Reuters* reported that air pollution is so bad that it is adversely affecting lung function in teenagers.

✔ *The Daily News* newspaper reported that certain cookies are having hydrogenated oil removed since there is overwhelming evidence that these trans fats cause obesity, clogging of the arteries, heart disease, strokes, and death. This is significant because you have been eating massive amounts of trans fats for the last thirty years, which is one of the major reasons sickness and disease are at an all-time high.

✔ *Reuters* reported that mercury is being released from coal fired power plants and is one of the contributing causes of an increase in autism and other health disorders. It is also believed that whether you live near a power plant or not, you are still affected since once mercury is in the atmosphere it circulates around the globe.

✔ It has been reported that the feed used in U.S. cattle production may be routinely tainted with poisons and disease. The rules and regulations relating to feed are not being complied with. Cattle producers are more interested in making money than safety. They routinely break the law by not complying with safety standards. This means the beef that we're eating is loaded with toxins, poisons, and disease-causing chemicals.

✔ *USA Today* reported the air pollution from other countries drifts into the United States. We breathe in more toxins today than ever before in history. These toxins stay in our body and cause disease.

✔ William Campbell, M.D., stated, "Your daily shower could be killing you softly with the same toxins used to kill lab rats and [used] in chemical weapons." The toxic substances in most municipal water systems have been used in the past to kill laboratory animals and as a weapon of war. It may be more dangerous to shower in municipal water than to drink it.

✔ Genetically modified food is rampant in our food supply. It does not have to be labeled as genetically altered. Now, food manufacturers in a quest to make more money, are changing the nature of things by genetically manufacturing animals and fish. Though genetically modified salmon hasn't been approved by the U.S. yet, just recently in Canada the American company AquaBounty received the green light to manufacture modified fish eggs. Eating genetically modified food means we are ingesting more poisons and toxins.

5. Still not convinced that politicians and various government agencies are corrupt, out of control, and operating un-policed? Then consider this:

✔ The government has changed the definitions of some of the most basic things we know. Example: There was a reported list of the healthiest states in America. Health, in this particular survey, was defined as the number of hospital beds per 1,000 people, and the percentage of children who got all of their recommended vaccinations. They were defining healthiest states as those where people were getting the greatest number of drugs and the most surgery. How insane. The definition for "spices" now includes thousands of deadly chemicals. Roast beef doesn't have to be real roast beef anymore, it can be a man-made product and still be called "roast beef."

✔ Did you know that if you have a child who's been diagnosed with cancer, not giving that child chemotherapy and other drugs can be a criminal offense?

✔ Political insiders are now blowing the whistle on how politics works. Report after report show that politicians have little interest in what's best for the country, the communities, or individual citizens. Every politician has simple objectives:

(a) to get re-elected, (b) to increase their political power and influence, and (c) to increase their personal wealth.

✔ In the last several decades there have been dozens of politicians' "suicides" and accidental deaths; however, none reported as "murders." Doesn't it make you think or at least suspect foul play and corruption?

6. Still not convinced that the FDA is working with big business and major drug companies allowing them to deceive the public and flood the public marketplace with dangerous products? Then consider this:

✔ Cigarettes are obviously bad; however, they are the only product in America where the ingredients do not have to be listed. How can this be? Well, consider that the FDA is in charge and that the politicians who receive huge amounts of donations and lobbying by the tobacco industry tell the FDA what to do.

✔ Federal law prohibits the FDA from using experts with financial conflicts of interest, but the FDA has waived the restriction close to 1,000 times since 1998. Although the FDA does not reveal when financial conflicts exist, since 1992 it has kept the details of any conflict secret so it is not possible to determine the amount of money or the drug companies involved. Two articles ran in *Reuters News* and *USA Today* reporting that 54 percent of the experts the FDA asked for advice on which medicines should be approved for sale have a direct financial interest in the drugs or topics they are evaluating. These financial conflicts of interest typically include stock ownership, consulting fees, or research grants. The *USA Today* article stated, "These pharmaceutical experts, about 300 on eighteen different advisory committees, make decisions that affect the health of millions of Americans and billions of dollars in drug sales. With few exceptions, the FDA follows the committee's advice." The scary part is these people who are making these decisions have a direct financial interest and they benefit based on the decisions they make. The article concluded that at 92 percent of the meetings, at least one member had a financial conflict of interest. At 55 percent of the meetings, half or more of the FDA advisors had conflicts of interest. Conflicts were most frequent at the fifty-seven meetings where broader issues were discussed; 92 percent of those members had conflicts. At the 102 meetings dealing with the fate of a specific drug, 33 percent of the experts had a direct financial interest.

✔ The pharmaceutical industry has more influence with the FDA than the public realizes. In an edition of the prestigious medical journal *Lancet*, editor Richard Horton claimed that the FDA has become a servant to the drug industry. An example: Even though there are multiple deaths caused by certain drugs, the FDA does not recall them from the market, but suggests adding a warning. The *Los Angeles Times* reported that the FDA has withheld safety information from labels that physicians say would call into question the use of the drugs. In the last twenty years, over a million people were killed by drugs that were approved, but never should have been. Before 1990, 60 percent of drugs submitted to the FDA were approved. Today over 80 percent are approved. The *Los Angeles Times* reported that seven killer drugs that were approved by the FDA, and yet were so deadly that they had to be withdrawn, generated over $5 billion for the pharmaceutical industry before the recall. Most shocking is that the FDA knowingly puts children at risk. According to the *LA Times* article, the agency never warned doctors not to administer a drug to infants or other children, even though eight youngsters who were given this drug in clinical studies died. Pediatricians prescribed it widely for infants afflicted with gastric reflux, a common digestive disorder. Patients and their doctors had no way of knowing that the FDA, in August 1996, had found the drug to be "not approvable for children." "We never knew that," said the father of a three-month old son who died on October 28, 1997, after taking the drug. "To me, that means they took my kid as a guinea pig to see if it would work." By the time the drug was pulled, the FDA had received reports of twenty-four deaths of children under age six who had been given this drug. By then, the drug had generated U.S. sales of over $2.5 billion for the drug company.

✔ An FDA insider said, "People are aware that turning down a drug for approval is going to cause problems with officials higher up in the FDA. Before I came to the FDA, I always assumed things were done properly. I've now lost faith in taking any prescription medication."

✔ According to one *Los Angeles Times* story, seven drugs approved by the FDA were later found to be ineffective and fatal. How the FDA approved these drugs is still a mystery. They obviously relied on misleading and/or false studies. Keep in mind all studies submitted to the FDA are always paid for and produced by the drug company that's seeking approval. These drugs were not needed. They weren't miracle drugs created to save lives. They were simply drugs designed to increase profits of the drug companies. One was for heartburn. Another was a diet pill, and a third was a painkiller. Six of the drugs were never proved to offer any lifesaving benefits and the seventh, an antibiotic, was ultimately deemed totally unnecessary because there were other antibiotics available that had already proven to be safer than this deadly antibiotic. These drugs did not have to be approved, but they were pushed for approval so that the drug companies could market them and make billions of dollars. These seven drugs had to be pulled off the market. The FDA repeatedly allows dangerous drugs to be approved and sold because of the pressure put on it by the drug industry.

✔ According to the *Los Angeles Times*, back in 1988, only 4 percent of new drugs introduced into the world market were approved first by the FDA. Ten years later in 1998, the FDA's first in the world approval spiked to 66 percent. It appears that the easiest agency in the world to approve a new drug, regardless of the safety, has become the FDA. The FDA was once the world's leading organization when it came to the safety of drugs it approved. Now the FDA seems to be more interested in the sales and profits of the drug companies than the safety of consumers.

✔ One particular drug the FDA approved and deemed "safe and effective" was pulled within the first year because it was linked to five deaths, as well as to the removal of many of the patients' colons and other major bowel surgeries. Other drugs called "safe and effective" by the FDA were later proven to cause heart valve damage, liver damage, pancreas damage, prostate cancer, colon cancer, impotency, infertility, heart attack, and stroke.

✔ The *Los Angeles Times* reported that, seven specific drugs that were called "safe and effective" resulted in a minimum of a thousand reported deaths. Other experts say that number is much higher, and could be as high as twenty-thousand deaths. All from drugs the FDA called "safe and effective." What isn't recorded are the potential hundreds of thousands of patients who took these drugs that developed other severe medical conditions such as liver damage, heart problems, cancer, diabetes, digestive issues, etc. The most outrageous thing is that all of these new medical conditions will be treated by the medical doctors with surgeries and/or more drugs. The needless pain and suffering of hundreds of thousands of people, and the deaths of countless more, is being ignored, all in the name of profit.

✔ The *Los Angeles Times* on Tuesday, April 6, 2004, quoted Harvard psychiatrist Dr. Joseph Glen Mullen: "Evidence that the FDA is suppressing a report linking suicide to drugs is an outrage given the public health and safety issues at stake." The FDA has information that antidepressants caused children to be twice as likely to show suicidal behavior. The article shows how the FDA claims that there is no conclusive scientific evidence linking antidepressants and potential suicide behavior. However, the article goes on to say that there is absolute evidence that the FDA is suppressing and hiding the information so that the drug companies can continue to sell drugs.

✔ Nonfatal skin cancers are the number one cancer. The four other most common kinds are breast, prostate, lung, and colorectal, which is cancer of the colon. Research and observations strongly suggest that the people most prone to getting these cancers are those who have taken the most nonprescription and prescription drugs and who have eaten the most fast food, yet the FDA does nothing to inform the public of the dangers of these two activities.

✔ In 2006, the *New York Times* reported that a study found Johnson & Johnson's popular treatment for congestive heart failure, Natrecor, caused reduced kidney function. In 2010, the *Los Angeles Times* reported that a subsequent study dismissed the links to kidney problems, but found that drug was "not effective."

✔ Experts say the drug Zoloft causes dementia.

✔ The *Associated Press* reported that drugs used to treat prostate cancer make men prone to broken bones.

✔ The FDA effectively silenced one of its own drug experts who exposed the safety concerns about the profitable drug Vioxx. This is proof that the FDA is more interested in protecting the profits of the drug companies than the safety of consumers.

✔ A previously unpublished internal survey of FDA scientists points to potentially dangerous gaps in the approval and marketing of prescription drugs. The internal secret survey showed that the FDA does not adequately monitor the safety of prescription drugs once they are on the market, and the majority of FDA scientists do not believe that the labeling decisions adequately address key safety concerns. It also showed that an alarming percentage of FDA scientists themselves were not confident that the final decisions adequately addressed the safety of drugs. The most alarming piece of information to come out of this secret internal survey was the number of scientists that said they have been pressured to approve or recommend drugs despite their own reservations about safety, efficacy, or quality of the drug. This means that the senior executives at the FDA are more interested in protecting the profits of the drug companies than they are about the safety of the consumer.

✔ In 2005 the *Wall Street Journal* reported that too many unproven drugs were getting approved by the FDA.

✔ In 2005, in the wake of the Vioxx scandal, the *Chicago Tribune* reported that the FDA was caught in the middle of a "drug safety conflict." The article suggested that the drug industry actually controls what is happening at the FDA.

✔ The FDA reviewed the drug Celebrex. The FDA's advisory panel recommended that Celebrex stay on the market. The amazing thing is that the members of this advisory panel are all in effect on the payroll of the drug company that sells Celebrex! Can someone stand up, and yell *conflict of interest* please?

✔ The FDA has admitted that two eczema creams cause cancer.

✔ The *Wall Street Journal* reported that cholesterol lowering drugs fail to benefit patients. Cholesterol drugs are the number one selling drugs in the world. They make the most profits for the drug industry, but the fact is cholesterol reducing drugs do not do anything to reduce the potential dangers of heart disease. A study showed that there were no heart health benefits after four months and no significant benefits after two years. However, the study did show that continued use of these cholesterol lowering drugs caused illness and disease.

✔ The *Associated Press* reported that consumer groups blasted the new cholesterol guidelines. Most of the heart disease experts who urged more people to take cholesterol lowering drugs have been exposed to have made huge amounts of money from the companies selling those medicines. "It's outrageous they didn't provide disclosure of the conflicts of interest," said Merrill Goozner with the Center for Science in the Public Interest. Folks, this happens all of the time. Remember, too, that most studies for new and existing drugs are paid for and funded by their own manufacturers.

✔ The New York attorney general sued the pharmaceutical giant Glaxo/Smith/Kline saying it committed fraud by withholding information about the dangers of its antidepressant drugs to children. This should not be the only suit filed. It is important you know that every major pharmaceutical company withholds information about the ineffectiveness and dangers of their drugs. It is important you know that the drug companies and the FDA know that the drugs do not work and are actually dangerous and cause disease, yet they're hiding and withholding this information from the public.

✔ The *Associated Press* reported that the drug Avastin increases the risk of heart ailments including chest pain, strokes, ministrokes, and heart attacks. This means that this drug can kill the people who take it. (It's interesting to note that every article I am reporting on here that talks about drugs also has a heavy emphasis on the stock price and how this news is affecting shareholder value. I cannot emphasize enough that drug companies are *publicly traded companies* whose only objective is to make profit. They do not want to cure or prevent disease.)

✔ *USA Today* reported that a grieving father, Liam Grant, spent a $1 million nest egg to investigate the drug Accutane. He believed that this drug caused his son to commit suicide. Allegedly, Liam was offered hundreds of thousands of dollars to drop the case. After multiple lawsuits Roche Pharmaceuticals stopped selling the drug in 2009. Accutane is no longer available, however its generic version is still available outside of the U.S.

✔ Whistleblowers have reported that internal documents at both the drug manufacturers and FDA show that drugs, both prescription and nonprescription, have no positive effects in over 70 percent of the people who use them. However, these same documents show that all nonprescription and prescription drugs have negative side effects in 100 percent of the people who use them.

7. Still not convinced that the pharmaceutical industry pushes drug sales and usage at all costs, and has an insatiable desire for increasing profits? Then consider this:

✔ Schools get money each month for every child they have on a psychiatric drug, including Ritalin or Adderall. This gives a major incentive for schools to get and keep kids on drugs.

✔ Doctors routinely get visits from pharmaceutical sales reps. These sales reps do not tell doctors how to cure and prevent disease. These sales people have sophisticated presentations designed to tell doctors how they can make more money by prescribing more drugs. These presentations have almost zero information on the safety or effectiveness of these drugs. The concern is not the patient; the emphasis is on how doctors can make more money.

✔ Doctors on government advisory panels make recommendations for drugs while being paid huge sums of money by the manufacturers of those same drugs.

✔ Drug companies routinely sponsor foundations' research. For example, Amgen gave $150,000 for research done by the Kidney Foundation. Remember, all foundations, all charities, and all research conducted on drugs is almost always paid for by the drug companies themselves, which therefore guarantees the results they want.

8. Still not convinced that all over-the-counter nonprescription and prescription drugs are poisons, causing you physical and emotional harm? Then consider this:

✔ Depending on who you listen to, either the third or fourth leading cause of death in America are doctors. This is because doctors routinely prescribe drugs that kill their patients, or perform surgeries that are unsuccessful. Either the patients die, or the doctors misdiagnose the illness and do the wrong thing which causes the person to die.

✔ In 2013, the *Journal of Patient Safety* said that "between 210,000-440,000 die each year" because of mistakes made in hospitals. "Things like unnecessary surgery, medical errors, negative effects of drugs, etc., cause almost as many deaths as heart disease and cancer." This figure does not include people who are permanently maimed, injured, or develop serious other medical conditions due to drugs and surgical procedures.

✔ Lowering cholesterol will not prevent a heart attack.

✔ An aspirin a day can give you gastrointestinal bleeding.

✔ It's been reported that over seven million Americans above sixty-five receive prescriptions for drugs that a panel of experts deemed inappropriate for use by the elderly because of potentially dangerous side effects.

✔ According to a study in the *Journal of the American Medical Association*, every prescription drug has dangerous side effects, and over 20 percent of these drugs come on the market without any warnings.

9. Still not convinced that aspartame (NutraSweet®) is one of the most dangerous food additives available today? Then consider this:

✔ NutraSweet® (aspartame) contains methanol, a wood alcohol which is a deadly poison. Aspartame was approved based on 112 studies submitted to the FDA by the original manufacturer, G.D. Searle, which was acquired by Monsanto. All of these studies were paid for and funded by the drug company. Critics who look at these studies, most notably the fifteen pivotal studies that the FDA based its approval on, are astonished that anyone could deduce that aspartame is safe. It's amazing that one of the subjects in the study died within a year after taking aspartame. Some of the studies showed people who were taking aspartame were having brain seizures. Once the aspartame was withdrawn from the subjects' diets, the brain seizures stopped. All of the studies were brief, (just a few months) and consisted of few subjects. The FDA has received more complaints from people who've consumed aspartame and who've had more major negative side effects than any other approved food, yet no action has ever been taken by the agency. In 2003, a former investigator for the FDA exposed aspartame as a toxin that never should have been approved. In 2013, the dairy industry began petitioning the FDA to allow aspartame in milk.

10. Still not convinced that your thoughts and energy are important to your health, and can have a major impact on physiology? Then consider this:

- ✔ In testing people diagnosed with multiple personality disorder, thought has been shown to do what is otherwise believed to be scientifically impossible. In one case, a person's blood was tested and found to be free of diabetes. Within minutes, when his personality changed, the blood was taken again and the person was tested positive for diabetes. This is physically impossible according to scientists, but the tests confirmed it nonetheless. This shows that the mind can do things to the body, even change body chemistry.

- ✔ An experiment was conducted to determine if thoughts can affect DNA. DNA was placed in a container; it was discovered that the DNA changed its shape according to the feelings, thoughts, and emotions of the researchers. When the researchers felt gratitude, love, and appreciation, the DNA responded by relaxing and the strands unwound; the length of the DNA extended. When the researchers felt anger, fear, frustration, or stress, the DNA responded by tightening up; it became shorter and switched off many of its codes. This could be why people feel shut down when they experience stress and negative emotions. The DNA codes were reversed and switched back on when feelings of love, joy, gratitude, and appreciation were felt by the researchers. This experiment was later followed up by testing HIV-positive patients. It turned out there was a three hundred times increase in resistance to viruses and bacteria when the HIV-positive patients felt love, gratitude, and appreciation. The bottom line is thoughts, feelings, emotions, and "energy" have a positive or negative effect on your DNA structure and can give you disease or cure you of disease.

✔ Ann Harrington, a professor of science at Harvard University wrote an article for *Spirituality and Health* magazine entitled "Miracle Cures—Tapping the Power of Make Believe Medicine." In it, Harrington showed that a placebo actually "cures" disease. She goes on to point out that in reality, the placebo does nothing except help the person believe that his or her disease will be cured and it's the patient's own mind and belief that cures the disease. To demonstrate this, the article gives examples where placebos are moderately effective when given as a little white tablet, but *more* effective when given as a big red capsule, and effective nearly100 percent of the time when the patient has to roll up his or her sleeve and get an injection. In effect, as the belief level increases the power of the mind increases as well and the body heals itself.

✔ In the book *The Hidden Messages in Water*, by Masaru Emoto, it is explained that the structure of water is dramatically affected by thoughts. Candice Pert, Ph.D. says that thought alone can completely change the body. This book shows the pictures so you can see how dramatically the water is changed structurally simply by thoughts.

✔ In research, when a person begins to worry and have stress, the body's pH can go from alkaline to acidic in a matter of minutes. Thoughts can bring on disease faster than any other cause.

11. Still not convinced that organic food is much better for you? Then consider this:

✔ A February 2003 study published in the *Journal of Agriculture and Food Industry* showed organically grown berries contain up to 58 percent more antioxidants than those grown conventionally.

✔ A 1993 study published in the *Journal of Applied Nutrition* showed that over the course of two years organic foods contained up to four times as many trace minerals, thirteen times more selenium and twenty times more calcium and magnesium than commercially grown produce, and also had significantly fewer heavy metals, including 25 percent less lead and 40 percent less aluminum.

12. Still not convinced that we are losing the war on cancer and cancer is getting worse every year? Then consider this:

✔ Every year, over 1.5 million Americans are diagnosed with cancer and the number is increasing. The probability that you will develop cancer is one in every two men and one in every three women, and it's getting worse. The war on cancer has been a total failure. Some scientists estimate that up to 70 percent of all cancers could be prevented simply by dietary change. The only legal remedies for cancer treatment are surgery, chemotherapy, and radiation. You can go to prison if you treat cancer with all natural methods even though they are more effective than surgery, chemotherapy and radiation, and have absolutely no negative side effects.

13. Still not convinced that the FDA suppresses information on natural cures? Then consider this:

✔ The *California Western Law Review* published an article entitled "Why Does the FDA Deny Access to Alternative Cancer Treatments?"

✔ Canadian scientist, Gaston Naessens, created an herbal blend called 714-X. This blend, as of 1991, has cured more than 1,000 people of cancer, as well as several AIDS patients. The FDA has attacked him.

✔ Jason Winters authored the book *Killing Cancer,* which has sold more than a million copies, about how he cured his cancer with herbs. He is quoted as saying, "I must tell you that I was scared about publishing a book talking about how herbs can cure cancer. I was not prepared to take on the billion dollar drug companies, the medical associations and doctors, all of whom would chew up and spit out anyone that would dare to say that possibly, just possibly, herbs can help." Winters outlines the typical fate of natural cancer cures and other cures that are advertised in U.S. publications. Usually the publication gets into a lot of trouble for printing it in the first place, and then all future publicity is stopped. The people selling the products are usually tricked into a phony suit about "practicing medicine without a license," or "selling drugs without a license," or " selling unregistered drugs." If the government can't stop them that way, they usually use another federal agency—the IRS, to attack them with some phony, trumped up income tax charge. Those who practice natural medicine, or sell natural remedies, live with the knowledge that they could be closed down any day.

✔ Virtually all violent acts committed by children in schools over the last ten years were committed by individuals who had been on prescribed psychiatric drugs, including the case in 2012 of the Newtown shooter, Adam Lanza who killed twenty-six people, twenty of them young children. This point was raised quickly after the Newtown event, and then quickly dropped by the mainstream media because (as we've explained) the news outlets are sponsored with advertising from the very drug companies that make these psychiatric drugs. These drugs increase the likelihood of suicide and dramatically increase the propensity for violent acts.

✔ Most drugs are physically addictive. Particularly pain medication, as evidenced by many celebrities who've been given medication by their doctor not knowing the addictive nature of the drugs.

14. Still not convinced that household cleaners are dangerous to your health? Then consider this:

✔ The *Associated Press* reported that deaths show dangers of household chemicals. This article explained how ALL household cleaners are chemicals that are highly toxic. They all can be fatal if they get into your system. They can be absorbed through the skin, through the fumes that you inhale, and of course, by accidentally drinking. Most people won't die immediately by inhaling the fumes, but the article points out that several people *have* died immediately as a result of mixing multiple cleaners together, which created deadly toxic fumes. If these chemicals in high concentrations can cause instantaneous death, then using these chemicals regularly and frequently obviously causes health problems. Exposure to them suppresses the immune system and leads to disease.

15. Still not convinced that the food produced by publicly traded companies and fast food restaurants is giving us disease and making us fat? Then consider this:

- ✔ *Reuters* reported that McDonald's has agreed to pay $8.5 million to settle a lawsuit because they were putting trans fats in their cooking oil. The lawsuit was filed by an activist seeking to raise awareness about the health dangers of trans fats in hydrogenated or partially hydrogenated oils. In 2008, McDonald's switched to a trans fat-free oil. However trans fats were just ONE of the many toxins in fast food and it took activism to change that. These companies will not change their destructive ways by their own volition.

- ✔ Kraft Foods was sued for knowingly putting dangerous trans fats in its food, most notably Oreos.

- ✔ An investigator for an animal rights group captured video showing chickens being kicked, stomped, and thrown against the wall by workers at a supplier for Kentucky Fried Chicken.

- ✔ Beef used for hamburger patties at fast food restaurants now contains enormous numbers of cattle that are being herded, fattened, slaughtered, and ground up together. This means meat from a single cow is not used in the hamburger patty; they are pooling bacteria from as many as a thousand different animals.

- ✔ The magazine *The Ecologist* points out that cosmetically perfect, irresistibly firm, brilliantly colored fruits and vegetables (like those in major supermarkets) taste like nothing because they're genetically modified and contain so many toxins.

- ✔ Samples of nonorganic chicken breasts (like those sold in major supermarkets) were found to be just 54 percent chicken. The rest was essentially fillers, i.e. toxins.

16. Still not convinced that natural remedies cure disease better than drugs, with no side effects? Then consider this:

- ✔ Licensed healthcare practitioners who use natural remedies instead of drugs and surgery report higher success rates than medical doctors using drugs and surgery. They also report virtually no negative side effects from treatments compared to medical doctors, who report negative side effects from treatments in virtually 100 percent of their patients.

- ✔ The *Associated Press* reported that walking may ward off Alzheimer's disease.

- ✔ *Reuters* reported that eating organic is shown to prevent and cure a host of various diseases.

- ✔ *Reuters* reported that the herbal remedy St. John's Wort is as effective, or more effective, in treating depression than drugs.

- ✔ The FDA finally admitted that extra virgin olive oil reduces the chances of coronary heart disease.

- ✔ *BBC* news reported that eating apples wards off colon cancer, and that apples prevent and can potentially cure cancer.

- ✔ The *Associated Press* reported that walking keeps weight in check.

- ✔ *ABC News* reported that relaxation techniques lower blood pressure.

- ✔ *Yahoo News* reported that herbs help ease children's illnesses, such as colds, skin allergies, and sleep problems. It also reported that the herbs worked more efficiently than drugs and had no side effects.

- ✔ Multiple studies have identified green tea as an anticancer agent.

- ✔ There is increased scientific validation for how homeopathy prevents and cures disease.

✔ Mangosteen juice, in studies, has been shown to prevent hardening of the arteries, protect the heart muscle, be beneficial in the treatment of Parkinson's disease, Alzheimer's disease and other forms of dementia, elevate mood and act as an antidepressant, prevent and arrest fungus, prevent bacterial infections, fight viruses, prevent gum disease, lower fever, prevent glaucoma and cataracts, increase energy and fight fatigue, promote anti-aging and weight loss, lower blood fat, have anti-tumor benefits, prevent cancer, lower blood pressure, lower blood sugar, and improve digestion.

17. Still not convinced that electromagnetic energy causes disease? Then consider this:

✔ College researchers believe electric light changes hormone levels in women and makes breast cancer more prevalent. The theory is that exposure to artificial, mostly florescent light, causes cellular damage that can lead to cancer, as well as dozens of other diseases.

✔ A Swedish study showed that people who hold cell phones to their head increase their risk of developing brain tumors. In the last few years evidence has been mounting to corroborate this study. In 2011, the World Health Organization issued a statement reversing its previous claim that no adverse health effects had been established. In its retraction, WHO said: "personal exposure IS possibly carcinogenic to humans."

✔ The cell phone industry has been just as harmful to public health as big tobacco. The similarities are eerily obvious. The cell phone industry was determined to deny any suggestion that its products might be dangerous even though years of negative research proved otherwise. One study showed that mobile phones emanate radio waves that damage the cells in the body, as well as DNA. Most shocking was the fact that the damage extended to the next generation of cells as well. The Cellular Telecommunications & Internet Association headed up a $28 million research program looking into the possible health effects from cellular phone use. Amazingly, the industry's own research showed that heavy cell phone users experience an increased rate of brain cancer deaths, development of tumors, genetic damage in the cells, as well as other negative health issues.

My most recent personal experience of how health care is a monopoly for the pharmaceutical industry was when I requested to take some blood tests. After walking in to a lab and asking for blood work to be performed, I was told it was against the law to do blood work without a prescription. It was appalling to me how the lawmakers created this monopoly for medical doctors. Reluctantly, I acquired a prescription. When I had the blood drawn and paid the bill, I asked when I could have my results. I was told it was against the law for them to release my test results to me. The results must be sent to a medical doctor. This was *my* blood, and *I* paid for the tests with *my* money, yet the law denies me direct access to the results. This is a good example of how lawmakers guarantee profits for medical doctors.

> I was told it was against the law for them to release my test results to me. The results must be sent to a medical doctor.

I could go on and on proving the many points referenced in this chapter and others. The evidence is overwhelming. Volumes of documentation, substantiation, and reports back up everything I say. Can you see why I'm mad as hell and not going to take it anymore?!

CHAPTER 11

Natural Cures for Specific Diseases

Stop! If you just bought this book and flipped to this chapter trying to find the "magic cure" for your specific disease, *please go back and start reading from the beginning*. Many important things are covered earlier and it's essential for you to understand and implement those things before you're ready for this chapter. If you start here you will not *get it*. You must understand how the medical system works and how you've been brainwashed. You must understand the cause of disease and the basic ways to cure yourself and bring your body to a state of balance where disease cannot exist. This chapter is designed *only* to give you suggestions for non-drug, nonsurgical things you can do to potentially address the symptoms that you may have.

If you're experiencing symptoms, the first question to ask is "What is *causing* them?" What most people ask is, "What can I do to *eliminate* the symptoms?" This is jumping the gun. First find out what's causing the symptoms, and then you can address the root cause by making changes. When you do this the symptoms vanish.

As I've mentioned before, the problem with standard drugs and surgery is that they only address the symptoms, they don't address the cause. This is a good modus operandi for the drug manufacturers; it makes them lots of money, but it's bad for you because it doesn't require that you change what created your illness (and the symptoms that come with it), so you're bound to get sick again. Eliminate the *cause* and the illness can't return, because the conditions that led to its creation no longer exist.

If someone approached you and said, "Every time I hit my foot with a hammer it hurts. How do I stop the pain?" You'd laugh and say, "Stop hitting your foot with a hammer!" If you go to a licensed healthcare practitioner and say, "I have acid reflux. What do I do?" What you're really saying is, "Every time I load my body with the chemicals that the food industry is putting into our food supply, I get a burning sensation in my stomach." Well, the simple answer is: "Stop loading up your body with chemicals." Does this make sense?

A man came to me and said, "I have osteoporosis, what should I do?" My answer: "Let's figure out the cause of your osteoporosis. What's causing your body's inability to absorb sufficient calcium? Either (a) you're not getting enough calcium in your diet, or (b) something is blocking the absorption of calcium. It's really pretty simple isn't it?"

He said, "Yes."

I said, "Well, do you know the things that block calcium absorption?" He didn't know. I said, "Carbonated sodas. Do you drink a lot of them?"

His jaw almost hit the ground. He said, "I drink about ten a day."

"Well, if you're drinking ten a day, you're blocking your calcium absorption. It doesn't mean that's the reason for your osteoporosis, but it certainly could be."

I told my friend to visit a licensed healthcare practitioner and suggested that if he stopped drinking the carbonated sodas he would probably start absorbing calcium better. And so he did, and within a few months his condition corrected itself and he no longer had osteoporosis.

Somebody will say, "But not everyone who drinks carbonated sodas has osteoporosis." That's true, and not everyone who smokes cigarettes dies of lung cancer, but 90 percent of the people who die from lung cancer have smoked cigarettes. Get it?

...but more importantly, we're interested in learning what the cause of the symptoms is.

So, if you're experiencing some symptoms right now, our first goal is not to merely suppress those symptoms. Yes, we want them to go away, but more importantly, we're interested in learning what the cause of the symptoms is. We must also understand that since the symptoms did not develop overnight (they probably took years to develop), they may not vanish overnight, either. Like the example of the man hitting himself on the foot with the hammer, if we stop doing the thing that's causing the problem we still may have the current symptom for a while. Even if the man *stops* hitting his foot he may still have lingering pain. Why? Because he hit his foot with a hammer for so long he actually broke bones that need time to heal. Your medical condition may, similarly, need time to heal, before the symptoms subside entirely. So, understand that this approach requires patience.

If you find the cause of your problem while consulting with a licensed healthcare practitioner, together, you'll be able to address that cause. That's what this chapter is really all about.

Chapter 6 addresses the causes of ALL DISEASE. To review, those *causes* are: **(1) toxins in the body; (2) nutritional**

deficiencies; (3) electromagnetic chaos; and (4) emotional and mental stress. If you do all of the things in chapter 6 you'll address all four of these issues and thus be able to cure yourself of virtually any disease, and prevent future disease as well.

However, if you've done little to protect your health in twenty, thirty, forty, or fifty years, there's a good chance you have a serious situation that requires professional attention. This is why I state repeatedly that you must go to a licensed healthcare practitioner who does not only use drugs and surgery. Ideally you should see two or three different practitioners to get multiple opinions. When you go to your licensed healthcare practitioner and receive a personalized treatment for your situation, you can consider some of the following things. Remember, *I am not a doctor*; I have no medical training; I am not even a healthcare practitioner; I am not prescribing medical treatment; I am not treating any medical condition; I do not treat patients; and I am not making any attempt in this book to prescribe, diagnose, treat any illness, or treat any patient. I present this information simply for educational purposes only.

With that said, I'm going to present what I believe to be the best protocol to follow if you are currently sick. This is the procedure I would follow if I were to come down with an illness. Keep in mind that because I do the things in chapter 6, I never get sick.

Go back to chapter 6 and do all of the things recommended there.

I cannot emphasize this enough. The things that I mention in chapter 6, such as seeing a licensed healthcare practitioner, getting energetic rebalancing, doing all of the cleanses, etc. will, in my opinion, and in most cases, cure almost all diseases. Doing the things in chapter 6 can eliminate many, if not all, symptoms in a short period of time, because the recommendations address the root causes of all illness. Simply doing the energetic rebalancing and the various cleanses can cure the "incurable" by bringing the body back into balance. This has been documented by the million-plus reports from around the world confirming that these things effectively cure disease.

In addition to doing the things in chapter 6, there are some specific things you can do to help your body return to a state of "homeostasis" (balance), which will allow your body to heal itself faster. Remember, when given the right conditions, the body heals itself.

In addition to doing the things in chapter 6, I urge you to see a licensed healthcare practitioner. Getting individualized treatment from a licensed healthcare practitioner, which could include essential oils, herbs, homeopathic remedies, chiropractic care, vitamins, minerals, etc., can cure all disease. Getting energetic rebalancing and doing nothing else can virtually cure every disease. Doing a colon cleanse, liver/gallbladder cleanse, kidney cleanse, heavy metal cleanse, parasite cleanse, Candida cleanse, and a full-body cleanse can, in thirty to sixty days, cure any "incurable" disease. *Not* doing these things, in my opinion, makes trying to cure your disease much more difficult and next to impossible.

Yes, you could do some things to reduce your symptoms temporarily, or even eliminate them for a short time, but if you're not addressing the root cause they'll likely reoccur, or diseases will develop elsewhere in your body where there are genetic weaknesses. Therefore, if you want to cure yourself of the illness you have, you must get the toxins out of your body, and stop putting them in; you must start giving your body super nutrition; you must stop or at least neutralize the electromagnetic chaos that you're being exposed to; and you must eliminate any trapped emotional and/or mental stress that you're holding in your body unconsciously. Doing these things will change your body pH from acidic to alkaline where disease cannot exist.

Acid Reflux/Heartburn

Acid reflux is a condition in which food or liquid leaks backward from the stomach into the esophagus.

Main Cause	Natural Cures
Acid reflux can result from a number of issues including: Candida, parasites, nonprescription and prescription drugs, eating too much processed food, overeating, and mental and emotional stress.	• Take raw organic apple cider vinegar—2 to 4 tablespoons in 8 ounces of pure water before meals. • Take digestive enzymes—specifically with betaine hydrochloric acid. • Take probiotics—specifically acidophilus bifidus. • Do a Candida cleanse. • Do a parasite cleanse. • Do a colon cleanse. • Eat more organic raw fruits and vegetables. • Practice stress reduction. • Get alphabiotic alignment. • If symptoms worsen at night when you're reclining, try elevating the top your bed off the floor a couple of inches so that your upper body is lifted and the rest of your body slants down slightly.

Acne

A condition wherein sebaceous glands at the base of hair follicles in the pores of skin become inflamed or impacted with dead skin cells and a proliferation of acne causing bacteria, resulting in pimples.

Main Cause	Natural Cures
There are a number of factors that can result in acne. Some of these may include hormonal imbalances, bacteria in the digestive tract *and* on the skin, Candida, parasites, dehydration, allergies, a high-glycemic diet, and the use of oil-based makeup.	What causes one person's acne may be different for another, so if you're unable to control the condition on your own, see a naturopathic doctor who can evaluate you and determine the triggers specific to you. Two types of bacteria, *Propionibacterium acnes* and *Staphylococcus aureus*, can cause acne breakouts. Eliminating *P. acnes* and/or *S. aureus without* eliminating good bacteria is helpful in controlling acne. *Propionibacterium acnes* can be controlled in the digestive tract as well as topically.

Some suggestions:

- Drink 10 glasses of distilled water daily.

- Drink unsweetened aloe vera juice. (Kills *bad* bacteria.) Start with 2 ounces, build up to 6 ounces per day. Aloe vera juice has been shown to kill acne-causing bacteria in the digestive tract.

- Do a Candida cleanse.

- Do a colon cleanse.

- Do a liver/gallbladder cleanse.

- Do a parasite cleanse.

- Do a full-body fat cleanse.

- Exfoliate the skin regularly—skin brushing, microdermabrasion, and other forms of exfoliation can slough off the dead skin cells that may mix with sebum and contribute to clogged pores.

- Apply tea tree oil topically to affected areas.

- Internally, take 2 to 4 tablespoons of raw organic apple cider vinegar in 8 ounces of pure water before meals.

- Drink unsweetened, organic green tea (kills bad bacteria).

- Take probiotics.

- Take omega-3s.

- Eat organic plain yogurt (controls bad bacteria while maintaining good bacteria).

- Use an infrared sauna.

- Practice stress reduction.

- Eliminate sugar, white flour, milk products, and processed foods from the diet. These foods create acne-causing bacteria in the digestive tract.

- Coconut oil is an effective moisturizer for those suffering with acne breakouts. It is antibacterial and will not clog pores. Applying coconut oil will, over time, help *control* oily skin. While this seems counter-intuitive, the reason is that the skin responds to the oil by minimizing its own production of oil.

ADD/ADHD

Attention deficit disorder (ADD) also known as attention deficit hyperactivity disorder (ADHD) is a persistent pattern of inattention and/or hyperactivity or impulsivity that is noticeably more frequent and severe than is typically observed in individuals at a comparable level of development.

Main Cause	Natural Cures
ADD and ADHD can result from a number of things including the presence of Candida in the body, ingesting food additives like monosodium glutamate, aspartame, and other artificial sweeteners, high fructose corn syrup, allergies, heavy metal toxicity, electromagnetic chaos, essential fatty acid deficiency, sensitivity to the chemicals in dairy and meat, nitrites, and blocked calcium absorption.	If you or your child has been diagnosed with ADD or ADHD, harsh medications may have been prescribed. See a naturopathic doctor for an evaluation and assistance in coming off harsh medications. While it can be difficult to change a child's diet dramatically, relief can come from dietary adjustments. Some suggestions: • Do a Candida cleanse. • Do a liver/gallbladder cleanse. • Take omega-3s. • Eliminate dairy. • Eliminate nitrites. • Eliminate high fructose corn syrup. • Eliminate artificial sweeteners. • Eliminate fast food. • Get alphabiotic alignment (alleviates stress). • Get cranial sacral therapy. • Practice stress reduction.

Allergies

An allergy is an immune response to something that either enters the body, or comes in contact with the body and causes hypersensitivity. The substance is usually harmless, however in sensitive individuals, the body responds to the substance as if it were a pathogen and tries to destroy it.

Main Cause	Natural Cures
Allergies are caused by a variety of things that are specific to individuals. Triggers may include a weakened immune system, Candida, clogged liver, weak adrenal glands, and lack of exposure to irritants in early childhood.	Though allergic reactions are unique to the individual, in using natural cures the first goal should be to assist the body in ways that will reduce its tendency to produce antibodies that result in allergic reactions. See a licensed naturopathic doctor who can assist you in strengthening your adrenal, digestive, and immune systems.

	Some suggestions:
	• Drink 10, 8-ounce glasses of distilled water daily.
	• Do a liver/gallbladder cleanse.
	• Do a Candida cleanse.
	• Do a colon cleanse.
	• Consult with a certified NAET practitioner. (NAET is an allergy elimination technique.)
	• Practice stress reduction.
	• Take bee pollen (do *not* take if you're allergic to bees or pollen).
	• Take bioflavonoids.
	• Take flaxseed oil.
	• Take probiotics.
	• Take the herbs dong quai and gingko biloba.
	• Dietary adjustments: eliminate alcohol, caffeine, artificial food colorings, processed sugar and wheat.
	• Eat: leafy greens, yellow vegetables, onions, garlic, ginger, cayenne, and kimchi.

Anxiety/Stress

Stress can be the result of a situation that is frustrating, or that provokes anger, or creates nervousness. Anxiety is the feeling of intense worry, unease, or fear.

Main Cause	Natural Cures
The cause of anxiety and/or stress is unique to each individual. However, there are physiological conditions that can contribute to stress and anxiety. For example, many people report feeling relief from stress and anxiety after doing a fast or a cleanse, which would suggest that diet and the state of the body can contribute to, or exacerbate stress and anxiety.	• See one or more licensed healthcare practitioners. Consider a chiropractor, herbalist, acupuncturist, hypnotist, Thought Field Therapy specialist (Callahan technique), or Emotional Freedom Technique specialist.
	• Practice stress reduction.
	• Get alphabiotic alignment.
	• Get massages.
	• Exercise.
	• Meditate.
	• Do rebounding.

	• Walk for an hour each day. • Drive less. • Don't talk on a cell phone and drive. • Get adequate sunlight. • Get adequate rest. • Reduce usage of cell phones, computers, tablets etc. • Reduce or eliminate caffeine. Excess caffeine can cause an anxiety attack. • Do an organic juice fast. • Do a heavy metal cleanse. • Do a colon cleanse. • Do a liver/gallbladder cleanse.

Arthritis

Arthritis is degeneration or inflammation and/or stiffness of the joints.

Main Cause	Natural Cures
Arthritis can result from loss of collagen, Candida, heavy metal toxicity, parasites, and viruses.	See a naturopathic doctor who can determine the specific type of arthritis you have (there are over a hundred types), and then create a plan to address it. In some cases herbs may be beneficial. If your naturopath doesn't prescribe herbs, you may want to visit an herbalist. Homeopathy may benefit the condition as well. A "homeopathic" doctor is different from a naturopathic doctor, although some naturopaths practice homeopathy. Anti-inflammatory drugs which may have provided pain relief can actually reduce the body's ability to repair cartilage and make the condition worse, so you will need to stop taking over-the-counter pain killers if you've been using them. Some suggestions: • Drink 8 to 10 glasses of pure water daily. • Eliminate foods in the "nightshade" family: tomatoes, potatoes, peppers, eggplant and tobacco. These contain alkaloids that can increase inflammation.

	• Eliminate: sugar, processed foods, caffeine. • Eat: kale, celery, mustard greens, almonds, figs, limes, olive oil, unflavored gelatin. • Supplements: cetyl myristoleate (CMO), dimethyl sulfoxide (DMSO), methyl-sulfonylmethane (MSM), glucosamine, copper, evening primrose oil, royal jelly, omega-5e, SierraSil, flaxseed oil. • Herbs: black cohosh, burdock, larrea, devil's claw. • Homeopathy: Bryonia, Ruta graveolens. • Do a parasite cleanse. • Take crocodile protein peptide. • Drink organic bone broth (provides collagen). • Use castor oil packs (cotton flannel soaked in castor oil, placed on the body with a heating pad or hot water bottle on top). • Remove all metal from the mouth.

Asthma

A disorder wherein the airways of the lungs swell and narrow, leading to wheezing, shortness of breath, chest tightness, and coughing.

Main Cause	Natural Cures
A number of circumstances can lead to asthma, including trapped mental and emotional stress, allergies, hormonal imbalance, Candida, lack of early exposure to bacteria preventing immune system stimulation, environmental irritants, poor diet, reaction to lactose, having been fed a breast milk substitute in infancy that was an allergen, use of antibiotics in early childhood, insufficient stomach acid production.	See a naturopathic doctor who can develop a comprehensive approach to the condition. Rather than plying you with drugs that only treat the symptoms, a good N.D. will work on a variety of aspects of the condition. These may include reducing allergic exposure, reducing the sensitivity and spasticity of the airways of the lungs, addressing nutritional deficiencies and imbalances, and addressing the inflammatory pathways of the body. Some suggestions: • Do a colon cleanse. • Do a Candida cleanse. • Do a liver cleanse. • Do a heavy metal cleanse.

- Remove metal from the mouth.
- Eliminate wheat.
- Take probiotics.
- Supplements: hyrdrochloric acid (helps replace stomach acid often lacking in asthma sufferers), magnesium, omega-3s, vitamin C, vitamin B6.
- Avoid cow's milk and high lactose products.
- Practice stress reduction.
- Do oxygen therapy.

Autism
A systemic body disorder affecting the brain with developmental disabilities that appear within the first three years of life. Social and communication skills are impaired.

Main Cause	Natural Cures
Autism is a complicated disorder, which may result from environmental toxins, genetics (the toxins trigger a genetic response in those susceptible), viral infections, heavy metal toxicity, mercury, Candida, and adverse reaction to prescription and nonprescription drugs.	Find a naturopathic doctor who specializes in treating autism. An N.D. will likely recommend detoxification of heavy metals, viruses and bacteria, and once the detox has been achieved, further treatment may include neurological healing. Recommendations: • Heavy metal cleanse, Candida cleanse, colon cleanse. • Drink pure, un-fluoridated water. • Test for food allergens and eliminate those allergens from your diet. • Eliminate processed foods. • Eliminate GMOs. • Take probiotics. • Take digestive enzymes. Vaccines are the controversial culprits in autism. According to medical science the theory that vaccines cause the disorder has been debunked. However, there are people who continue to believe that vaccines do contribute to autism in children who are genetically predisposed to mercury sensitivity.

Back Pain

Back pain usually originates from the muscles, nerves, bones, joints or other structures in the spine.

Main Cause	Natural Cures
Mental and emotional stress, trauma, dehydration, viral infections, improper posture, and movements that lead to misalignment can all contribute to back pain.	• See a chiropractor and/or an acupuncturist; both can be especially helpful with back pain. • Drink 8 glasses of pure water daily. • Get alphabiotic alignment. • Get rolfing. • Get cranial sacral therapy. • Get deep-tissue massage. • Use a magnetic mattress pad. • Practice stress reduction.

Bad Breath

Chronic unpleasant odor of the breath that is not due to something one has eaten.

Main Cause	Natural Cures
Lack of digestive enzymes, toxic overload, Candida, parasites, heavy metal toxicity, prescription and nonprescription drugs, constipation, and a sluggish liver are among the many contributing factors to bad breath.	A change in diet to include more raw fruits and vegetables and eliminating processed foods will help with this condition. People who eat high protein diets with a lot of meat and few live foods will tend to have bad breath. Some suggestions: • Drink at least 8 glasses of pure water daily. • Do a colon cleanse. • Take digestive enzymes. • Do a liver/gallbladder cleanse. • Do a Candida cleanse. • Drink aloe vera juice. • Take organic raw apple cider vinegar in pure water (2 to 4 tablespoons in 8 ounces) twice daily. • Take probiotics. • Use an infrared sauna. • Drink green juice containing parsley or cilantro, which acts as a deodorizer.

Bladder Infection
A bacterial infection in the urinary tract, also called cystitis.

Main Cause	Natural Cures
When germs or bacteria enter through the urethra the result may be a bladder or urinary tract infection.	If you're experiencing recurring symptoms see a naturopathic doctor. Without proper treatment, bladder infections can lead to more serious conditions. Some suggestions: • Alkalize urine by drinking 1/2 teaspoon of baking soda in 8 ounces of pure water. • Take raw organic apple cider vinegar (2 tablespoons) mixed with 1 tablespoon of raw honey in 8 ounces two to three times daily before meals. • Drink organic *unsweetened* pure cranberry juice (up to a quart a day)—best if made fresh with a juicer at home. Cranberry juice is very strong; dilute with pure water as necessary, or juice with another organic fruit like apples: one part apple to two parts cranberries. • Homeopathic remedies can be helpful. See a homeopathic doctor for treatment. Some homeopathic remedies to consider include Belladonna, Berberis Vulgaris, Cantharis, and sarsaparilla. • Take larrea. • Take bee propolis.

Bloating/Gas
Feeling that the abdomen is enlarged, sometimes includes actual intermittent distention of the abdomen generally caused by intestinal gas.

Main Cause	Natural Cures
There are many things that can cause gas, including intestinal bacteria, Candida, parasites, nonprescription and prescription drugs, processed foods, sugars (lactose, sorbitol, fructose in particular), artificial sweeteners	Chronic gas can signal a more serious issue with your digestive tract, so visit a naturopathic doctor if your bloating/gas persists after eliminating what you believe to be the source. Some suggestions: • Take digestive enzymes with betaine hydrochloric acid.

(especially mannitol and xylitol), polysaccharides (wheat in particular), fruits and vegetable that are high in sugar and/or polysaccharides.	• Take raw organic apple cider, 2 to 4 tablespoons in 8 ounces of pure water before meals. • Eliminate wheat. • Eliminate sugars and artificial sweeteners that cause a reaction. • Drink aloe vera juice, 4 ounces before breakfast. • Drink ginger tea: peel and chop a large piece of ginger, boil in a pot of,16 to 20 ounces of water, cool and drink the "ginger tea." • Take liquid sage in pure water. • Take probiotics. • Do a Candida cleanse. • Do a parasite cleanse. • Do a colon cleanse.

Blood Clots

Blood clots are abnormally formed semi-solid masses of coagulated blood. They can be life threatening.

Main Cause	Natural Cures
Blood clots can result from nonprescription and prescription drug use, mental and emotional stress, trans fats (hydrogenated oils), homogenized dairy products, vitamin E deficiency, obesity, and being immobile for long periods of time, for example on long flights or drives.	See a naturopathic doctor if you've been diagnosed with a blood clot, if you suspect that you have one, or know that you're prone to them. Some suggestions: • Take raw apple cider vinegar, 2 to 4 ounces in 8 ounces of pure water, add a dash of cayenne pepper. • Add ginger to your diet. • Walk daily. • Take natural vitamin E. • Take nattokinase. • Take oral chelation. (Both nattokinase and oral chelation improve circulation.)

Cancer
An uncontrolled growth of abnormal cells in the body.

Main Cause	Natural Cures
Cancer results from toxins in the body, nutritional deficiencies, electromagnetic chaos, mental and emotional stress.	See a licensed healthcare practitioner. Start with a naturopathic doctor. An N.D. may recommend other healthcare practitioners to assist with your treatment. Some suggestions: • Do all of the things recommended in chapter 6. It's very important that you eliminate toxins, improve your body's ability to absorb nutrients, eliminate electromagnetic chaos and eliminate stress. • Drink fresh, unpasteurized, organic juices made with low-sugar vegetables and low-sugar fruits. • Eat more raw fruits (low-glycemic) and vegetables. (Improves your nutritional intake.) • Eliminate sugars, including natural sugars from the diet. Fructose promotes the growth of cancer cells. • Eliminate processed vegetable oils. (Soy, corn, canola, and margarine are chemically altered and toxic to the body.) • Take omega-3s. • Take vitamin D. • Take linseed oil. • Take food grade hydrogen peroxide (35%). • Take oxygen therapy. • See a specialist in Chinese medicine. • Practice stress reduction. Laugh, get massages, meditate, and walk in nature. • Get plenty of sleep.

Cardiac Arrhythmia
Irregular heartbeat.

Main Cause	Natural Cures
A weakened or damaged heart, excessive caffeine, smoking, alcohol abuse, drug abuse, and mental stress can all cause cardiac arrhythmia.	See a licensed healthcare practitioner, beginning with a naturopathic doctor. This can be a serious condition and not one that's appropriate for self-treatment. Some recommendations: • Get acupuncture. • Take fish oil. • Take magnesium—tends to stabilize the heart. • Take potassium. • Take vitamin C. • Take the herb hawthorn berry. • Avoid caffeine. • Take nattokinase. (Improves circulation, strengthens the heart.) • Reduce stress.

Chemical Sensitivity
Multiple chemical sensitivity (MCS) is a response to chemical, biological or physical agents, manifesting in a number of symptoms including headache, fatigue, nausea, diarrhea, muscle pain, sneezing, itching, sore throat, rashes, gas, bloating, confusion, concentration and memory problems and mood swings. These responses can be due to chemical spills, or to things as minor as new carpet, bedding, ventilation systems, cleaning products, perfumes, automobile exhaust or anything with some sort of chemical residue.

Main Cause	Natural Cures
Toxic chemicals are generally the cause, although some believe that there's an immune response similar to allergies that causes people with the condition to be highly sensitive to low levels of chemicals deemed safe and that do not cause discomfort in others.	• Detox—to rid your body of any ingested toxins. • Do all of the cleanses recommended in chapter 6. • Stop using any chemical cleaners. • Avoid plastics in food preparation. • Use air purifiers with HEPA filters. • Use a vacuum with a HEPA filter.

Chronic Fatigue Syndrome (CFS)

Extreme fatigue that doesn't improve with rest, often accompanies by achiness and swollen lymph nodes.

Main Cause	Natural Cures
CFS may be caused by Candida, viruses—in particular the Epstein-Barr virus, parasites, heavy metal toxicity, hypoactive thyroid, and allergies.	• Do all of the things in chapter 6. • Test body pH and if too acid, alkalize the body. • Practice yoga and/or meditation. • See a homeopathic doctor. Homeopathic remedies may include muriatic acid, Gelsemium, Kali Phosphoricum, picric acid, and Stannum. • Eliminate wheat. • Eliminate caffeine. • Eliminate alcohol. • Eat raw foods. • Eat/use extra virgin coconut oil—use in cooking and mix into fruit/vegetable smoothies.

Crohn's Disease

Crohn's is a form of inflammatory bowel disease that involves the intestines, but may affect any part of the gastrointestinal tract and range anywhere from the mouth to the anus.

Main Cause	Natural Cures
What causes Crohn's is unclear, but diet and stress aggravate the situation. In people with Crohn's the immune system responds to normal bacteria like harmful invaders and produces chronic inflammation in the intestines.	Some suggestions: • See a naturopathic doctor who can evaluate you and create a treatment plan specifically designed for you. • Acupuncture is helpful for some Crohn's sufferers. • Take probiotics, specifically acidophilus and bifidus organisms, which help restore healthy bacteria to the intestines. • Take fish oil. • Consider biofeedback treatment, which has been shown to improve the condition in some. • Drink aloe vera juice.

	• Eliminate gluten.
	• Eliminate lactose.
	• Avoid fried foods.
	• Reduce caffeine consumption.
	• Reduce alcohol consumption.

Circulation Problems
Restricted blood flow in the body that can lead to more serious conditions.

Main Cause	Natural Cures
Blockages in the arteries due to chlorine in drinking and/or bathing water, homogenized dairy products, trans fats, Candida, heavy metals, allergies and viruses can all contribute to circulation problems.	See a naturopathic doctor who can evaluate the causes for your particular circulation issues. Some suggestions: • Drink at least 8 glasses of pure water daily. Filter your drinking water and bathing water. • Avoid chlorinated pools. • Avoid dairy that is pasteurized and homogenized. • Take oral chelation. • For severe cases take intravenous chelation. • Take food grade hydrogen peroxide therapy (35%). • Take natural vitamin E. • Take omega-3s. • Get massages. • Walk for an hour daily.

Cold Sores
Often called "fever blisters," they are small sores that appear on the lips or outer edges of the mouth. Also known as herpes simplex virus type 1 (HSV-1).

Main Cause	Natural Cures
Viral infection is the cause of cold sores. If you've had the chicken pox, you have been exposed to HSV-1. (Not the same virus that causes genital herpes.)	See a licensed healthcare provider. A naturopathic doctor, a homeopathic doctor and an herbalist all may be helpful in controlling and even eradicating the condition. (Despite medical science's claim that there is no cure.) Some suggestions: • Do all of the things recommended in chapter 6, particularly the cleanses.

	• Strengthen the immune system; a weakened immune system is what allows the virus to attack.
	• Some suggestions for immune support:
	• Take echinacea, vitamin C and zinc.
	• Take reishi mushroom.
	• Take larrea.
	• Take red marine algae.
	• Take lysine.
	• Take food grade hydrogen peroxide (35%).
	• Use dimethyl sulfoxide (DMSO) topically to heal lesions.
	• Consider the following anti-viral herbs: thyme, lapacho, astragalus, licorice, galangal, cat's claw, ligustrum, pansy, cayenne and myrrh. These are suggestions, but rather than self-prescribing, see a professional herbalist who can determine which of these is best for your particular situation.
	• Homeopathic remedies to consider include Natrum muriaticum, Rhus toxicodendron and Sepia. Again, rather than self-medicate, get an evaluation from a trained herbalist.
	With all of these suggestions, you must first do the things in chapter 6. You need to bring your body into balance and remove toxins from your system before any treatment will eradicate the virus.

Colds

Common viral infection affecting the upper respiratory system, wherein the mucus membranes of the throat and nose become inflamed.

Main Cause	Natural Cures
Colds are the result of a viral infection, usually the "rhinovirus," which infiltrates the cells that line the nasal passages and then proliferates.	If you do the things in chapter 6 you should not come down with colds. It's possible to go for years without contracting viruses if the immune system is strong and the body's pH is alkaline.

Some suggestions:
• Bed rest. |

	• Make a nasal spray or flush with pure warm water, sea salt and baking soda. Mix 1 teaspoon of sea salt, 1 teaspoon of baking soda, and 1 cup of warm water in a bowl. You can inhale it drawing the water into your nose, which is not comfortable, but will help clear congestion. OR, you can use a bulb syringe and spray it into your nose. • Take Oscillococcinum—a homeopathic remedy that's easy to find in drugs stores. • Take green papaya extract. • Take digestive enzymes. • Take probiotics. • Take crocodile protein peptide. • Use an infrared sauna. • Get sunlight. • Drink ginger tea made with raw ginger boiled in water.

Colitis
Colitis is a swelling of the large intestine.

Main Cause	Natural Cures
People of Ashkenazi heritage are more prone to colitis leading to the conclusion that genetics may play quite a large role in the condition. However, lifestyle choices are also a factor. Poor diet—sugars, processed foods, wheat, white flour, and too much linoleic acid which is found in red meat, margarine, processed foods and vegetable oils including soybean oil, corn oil, and safflower oil, can lead to colitis.	See a naturopathic doctor who can put together a program specifically for you. Some suggestions: • Drink aloe vera juice. The amount will vary from person to person. Aloe vera juice has an anti-inflammatory effect on the intestine. • Take probiotics. • Take omega-3s. • Take boswellia extract. • Do a Candida cleanse. • Eliminate sugar. • Eliminate wheat. • Eliminate flour (white and whole wheat). • Take bromelain. • Practice stress reduction.

Constipation

A condition where there is difficulty emptying the bowels and one may experience bowel movements less than three times per week and with hardened stools.

Main Cause	Natural Cures
A number of lifestyle choices will result in conditions that cause constipation. Eating food without living enzymes, white flour, white sugar and refined foods that cause poor gut flora, Candida, taking nonprescription and prescription drugs, not eating enough fibrous foods, mental and emotional stress, and not drinking enough water (dehydration) all contribute to constipation.	Short-term constipation can be addressed on one's own, but long-term or chronic constipation is serious and requires the help of a licensed healthcare practitioner such as a naturopathic doctor. Doing the recommendations in chapter 6 will alleviate constipation. Some suggestions: • Drink 10 glasses of distilled water daily. • Eat 5 organic apples a day. • Eat prunes. • Eat ginger—raw in smoothies and/or cooked in vegetable stir-fry dishes. • Get colonics. • Drink aloe vera juice. • Drink 2 to 4 tablespoons of raw organic apple cider vinegar in 8 ounces of pure water before meals. • Take probiotics. • Take digestive enzymes. • Do a colon cleanse. • Do a Candida cleanse.

Cough

Coughing is a natural reflex that protects the lungs, however a prolonged or persistent cough can indicate infection or disease.

Main Cause	Natural Cures
Candida, bacterial or viral infections, and allergies may cause coughs.	• Gargle with warm water (pure or distilled) and sea salt. • Gargle with colloidal minerals. • Drink hot tea with organic lemon and raw honey. • Make a mixture of melted coconut oil, raw honey (1 tablespoon of each) and 1/2 an organic lemon and sip slowly letting it coat the throat.

Dandruff

Dandruff is a scalp condition in which skin flakes off. It can be due to dry scalp or it can be due to eczema, psoriasis, seborrheic dermatitis, or fungal infection.

Main Cause	Natural Cures
Dandruff can result from a number of things including Candida, toxic overload, allergies, dehydration and parasites.	• Wash the scalp with baking soda (mix one part baking soda with two parts water and pour over the scalp, follow with a rinse made of equal parts of raw apple cider vinegar and water and then rinse with water thoroughly. • You can also mix equal parts raw apple cider vinegar and pure water, add to a spray bottle, spray on the scalp and allow it to sit for 20 minutes and then wash out. • Massage scalp with extra virgin coconut oil, leave in either for 15 minutes or overnight and wash out the next day. • Do all of the cleanses recommended in chapter 6. • Take probiotics. • Take omega-3s. • Drink 10 glasses of distilled water daily.

Depression

Feelings of severe despondency accompanied by feelings of hopelessness and inadequacy that persists over a period of time.

Main Cause	Natural Cures
The causes of depression are unique to each individual. Candida can contribute to depression in some people. Poor diet, poor sleep habits, chronic dehydration, and hormonal imbalance can also contribute to depression.	• See a licensed healthcare practitioner for a treatment plan specifically designed for you. A naturopathic doctor can advise on natural remedies as well as make recommendations for other kinds of therapies. • See an acupuncturist. • Suggested supplements: St. John's wort, S-Adenosylmethionine (SAM-E), omega-3s. Some suggestions: • Get adequate sleep. • Walk for an hour daily.

	• Spend more time in the sun, 20 minutes per day when possible.
	• Do rebounding.
	• Eliminate all prescription and nonprescription drugs.
	• Eliminate aspartame.
	• Drink 8 to10 glasses of pure water daily.
	• Do a Candida cleanse.
	• Do all of the cleanses recommended in chapter 6.
	• Do a week-long juice fast using fresh, organic, non-pasteurized low-sugar vegetables and fruits.
	• Practice stress reduction.
	• Do Thought Field Therapy (TFT) or the Emotional Freedom Technique (EFT).

Diabetes

A metabolic disease in which the body's inability to produce insulin results in high levels of sugar (or glucose) in the blood.

Main Cause	Natural Cures
Genetics *and* behavioral factors play a part diabetes, type 1 and type 2. Type 1, early onset, seems to be inherited, while type 2 appears to result primarily from lifestyle choices. Prescription drugs, Candida, artificial sweeteners, too much white sugar and white flour, trans fats, obesity, and being sedentary contribute to type 2 diabetes, but because the disease may run in families some believe there may be a genetic link there as well. Though, generally this can be attributed to the dietary and exercise	See a naturopathic doctor who can develop a plan for you. Type 1 and type 2 diabetes can be treated successfully. Some suggestions: • Lose weight if you're overweight. • Eliminate aspartame. It's toxic and makes weight loss more difficult. • Eliminate all prescription and nonprescription drugs. • Eliminate all processed foods. • Eliminate sugar and white flour. • Reduce consumption of grains. • Consume raw vegetables and low-glycemic fruits. • Eat probiotic foods: kimchi, sauerkraut, organic plain yogurt.

habits in families being similar. Doing the things in chapter 6 will help both forms of diabetes.	• Consider adding these to the diet: cinnamon, ginger, aloe vera, and bilberry extract. • Take omega-3s. • Take vitamin C. • Take vitamin D—cod liver oil is a good source. • Walk for an hour daily. • Do a Candida cleanse.

Diarrhea

A condition involving the frequent passing of loose or watery stools.

Main Cause	Natural Cures
Parasites, Candida, prescription and nonprescription drugs, flu virus, and bacteria are all causes of diarrhea.	• Drink 8 to10 glasses of distilled water daily. • Take digestive enzymes. • Take fenugreek seeds. • Take probiotics. • Eat probiotics, in particular, organic plain yogurt with active cultures. • Do a Candida cleanse. • Do a parasite cleanse. • Do a colon cleanse. • Do a liver/gallbladder cleanse.

Eczema

Eczema is a skin condition wherein patches of skin become rough and inflamed with blisters that cause itching and bleeding.

Main Cause	Natural Cures
Eczema is believed to be a genetically inherited condition. Allergies, hormonal imbalance, and stress can trigger flare-ups.	• Do all of the things in chapter 6. • See a naturopathic doctor. • Homeopathy, hypnosis and acupuncture should also be explored as all have been helpful among eczema sufferers. Some suggestions: • Eliminate wheat and all gluten. • Consider eliminating milk, eggs, nuts and soy, which can be triggers. • Take gamma-linolenic acid (GMA).

	• Take evening primrose oil.
	• Take fish oil.
	• Take vitamin A.
	• Take vitamin B complex.
	• Take vitamin E.
	• Take zinc.
	• Take the Bach flower essence Rescue Remedy (drops). Rescue Remedy also comes in a topical ointment that may be applied to the affected areas.
	• Use aloe vera gel topically.
	• Use coconut oil topically as a lotion.
	• Practice stress reduction.

Edema

Edema is fluid retention that leads to bloating or swelling in the body's tissues.

Main Cause	Natural Cures
There are a number of causes for edema, including general lack of physical activity, standing or sitting for too long, surgery, burns, menstruation, menopause, prescription and nonprescription drugs, and poor diet. A number of illnesses and conditions can cause edema as well, including head injury, heart failure, diabetes, allergies, arthritis, liver disease, kidney disease, thyroid disease and chronic lung disease.	• Do all of the things in chapter 6. • See a naturopathic doctor. Some recommendations: • Take dandelion leaf (a natural diuretic). • Take vitamin B complex. • Take vitamin C. • Take vitamin D. • Take pantothenic acid. • Take potassium. • Reduce salt intake.

Fibromyalgia

A syndrome in which there is long-term body-wide pain and tenderness in the joints, muscles, tendons and other soft tissues.

Main Cause	Natural Cures
Causes vary from person to person. Stress and toxic overload can contribute to	• See a naturopathic doctor who can determine the cause of your fibromyalgia and create a treatment plan specifically for you.

| the condition. Some people develop fibromyalgia after an accident or trauma. | • Do all of the cleanses in chapter 6.
• Eliminate wheat, dairy, sugar and processed foods.
• Take oral chelation.
• Take crocodile protein peptide.
• Use a magnetic mattress pad. |

Gallbladder Problems

Most gallbladder issues are due to inflammation of the organ resulting when gallstones obstruct the ducts leading to the small intestines.

Main Cause	Natural Cures
Prescription and nonprescription drugs, excessive intake of trans fats, Candida, genetic weaknesses exacerbated by chemicals in food (primarily meat and dairy), food allergies, hypothyroidism, and lack of exercise all contribute to gallbladder issues.	See a naturopathic doctor for a treatment plan. Some suggestions: • Do a liver/gallbladder cleanse. • Do a heavy metal cleanse. • Do a Candida cleanse. • Do a colon cleanse. • Do a parasite cleanse. • Do a heavy metal cleanse. • Take digestive enzymes.

Gout

A type of arthritis that occurs when uric acid builds up in the blood and leads to inflammation of the joints, or often one joint in particular.

Main Cause	Natural Cures
Eating too many foods rich in "purines." Organ meats are particularly high in purines. Other causes include consuming high fructose corn syrup, excess protein in the blood, poor circulation, being overweight, and excessive alcohol consumption. Some people are genetically predisposed to gout. Some prescription and nonprescription drugs can cause gout such as diuretics, aspirin, cyclosporine, and levodopa.	• Lose weight if you're overweight. • Drink 8 to 10 glasses of pure water daily. (Will assist the body in flushing out uric acid.) • Eliminate alcohol. • Eliminate organ meats and high fructose corn syrup. • Exercise regularly. • Eat organic strawberries. Strawberries help the body get rid of excess uric acid. • Both oral and intravenous chelation therapy can help with gout.

Heart Disease

Any type of disorder that affects the heart. It is distinct from cardiovascular disease, which affects disorders of the blood vessels *and* the heart. Heart disease refers only to the heart. More specifically, these diseases include angina (heart muscle doesn't get enough oxygen), arrhythmia (irregular heartbeat), congenital (birth defects of the heart), coronary artery disease (diseased coronary arteries), dilated cardiomyopathy (heart chambers dilated due to weak heart muscle), myocardial infarction (heart attack or interrupted blood flow), heart failure (heart doesn't pump blood around the body efficiently), hypertrophic cardiomyopathy (wall of left ventricle too thick, making it harder for blood to leave the heart), mitral regurgitation (when mitral valve doesn't close tightly enough and blood flows back into the heart), mitral valve prolapse (when valve between left atrium and left ventricle does not fully close; it bulges upwards back into the atrium), pulmonary stenosis (when pulmonary valve is too tight making it difficult for the heart to pump blood from the right ventricle to the pulmonary artery).

Main Cause	Natural Cures
Smoking, being overweight, excess sugar consumption (damages the arteries), Candida, bacterial infections, viral infections, parasites, heavy metal toxicity, trans fats, homogenized dairy products, chlorinated drinking and bathing water, nonprescription and prescription drugs, lack of exercise, magnesium deficiency, and mental and emotional stress can all contribute to heart disease.	See a naturopathic doctor to devise a plan specifically for you. Some suggestions: • Weight loss if needed. Being overweight strains the heart. • Eat a primarily plant-based diet. If your arteries have plaque, eliminate the foods that contributed to that. • Eliminate processed meats. • Exercise regularly to get your heart rate up. 30 minutes per day—walk, rebound, dance— *move.* • Eliminate processed foods and sugar. In recent years, a connection between sugar's inflammatory effect and artery damage has been discovered. • Take probiotics. Heart disease has been linked to unhealthy gut flora. You can also eat probiotic foods such as kimchi, sauerkraut, and plain organic yogurt. • Take omega-3s. • Take natural vitamin E. • Take magnesium.

	• Take oral chelation and in extreme cases intravenous chelation, which will improve circulation.

Hepatitis C
A viral disease that leads to inflammation of the liver.

Main Cause	Natural Cures
Hepatitis C is a viral infection one can contract via sharing needles with someone who has the virus. It is generally contracted when one is exposed to contaminated blood. Years ago, people receiving blood transfusions were at risk, however, blood used for transfusion is now screened for hepatitis C to prevent spread of the condition.	• If you have hepatitis C see an herbalist and/or an expert in Chinese medicine. • Herbal treatments may include milk thistle, schizandra, bupleurum, scutellaria, isatis, licorice root, astragalus, and white peony.

Herpes
A viral infection affecting the skin. We discussed cold sores (type 1) above. Type 2 is genital herpes.

Main Cause	Natural Cures
Genital herpes results from contact with someone who has the virus.	See a healthcare practitioner who can evaluate you and develop a treatment plan specifically for you. Consider a naturopathic doctor, an herbalist, and/or homeopathic doctor. Some suggestions: • Detox. Do a colon cleanse, a Candida cleanse, a liver and gallbladder cleanse. This will strengthen your immune system. A weakened immune system allows the virus to flare up. • Remedy nutritional deficiencies. Consider a fresh, organic juice fast. • Eat raw, organic fruits and vegetables. • Address energetic frequency imbalances. Homeopathy deals with frequencies.

	• Consider an energetic balancing program. With the AIM program (www. AIMprogram.com) you can have your energetic frequencies balanced twenty-four hours a day. • Take lysine. Lysine is an amino acid that helps suppress the virus. • Take red marine algae. This product appears to eliminate the herpes virus. • Use dimethyl sulfoxide (DMSO). Applied topically, it kills the virus. • Take food grade hydrogen peroxide therapy (35%). • Drink liquid oxygen. The virus cannot live in an oxygen rich environment. • Take larrea. This plant is anti-viral and can kill the herpes virus in 30 days. • Herbal remedies include thyme, lapacho, astragalus, licorice, galangal, cat's claw, ligustrum, pansy, cayenne, and myrrh. • Homeopathic remedies include Natrum muriaticum, Rhus toxicodendron, and Sepia.

High Blood Pressure
When blood pressure is 140/90 or higher most of the time.

Main Cause	Natural Cures
Mental and emotional stress, nutritional deficiencies, a diet high in sodium, a diet high in fructose, Candida, being overweight, and smoking all contribute to high blood pressure.	• Do a Candida cleanse. • Eliminate processed sugar, white flower, white rice, and white potatoes. These foods elevate insulin levels and also keep blood pressure elevated. • Eliminate caffeine. Caffeine exacerbates hypertension. • Take omega-3s—fish oil, flaxseed. • Take natural vitamin E. • Take calcium and magnesium. (Both have been shown to lower blood pressure.) • Eat organic extra virgin coconut oil.

	• Reduce omega-6s (corn oil, soy oil, canola oil.) • Consume probiotic fermented foods such as kimchi, sauerkraut, natto, miso, organic, plain yogurt. Bad bacteria in the gut is linked to heart disease. • Get more vitamin D via sun exposure. (Helps regulate blood pressure.) • Exercise—walk daily. • Practice stress reduction.

High Cholesterol
The presence of high levels of fats in the blood.

Main Cause	Natural Cures
For some, genetics play a part in high cholesterol. For others, it's lifestyle choices— eating too many foods that are high in saturated fats and trans fats, smoking, stress, being overweight and being sedentary.	• Doing the things in chapter 6 can help those with a genetic predisposition to high cholesterol as well as those afflicted as a result of behavioral choices. • See a naturopathic doctor who can pre-scribe a treatment plan specifically for you. Some suggestions: • Eliminate foods high in saturated fat such as red meat, processed meat, most cheese, and lard. • Eliminate pastry, cakes, biscuits, cream, and anything with trans fats. • Eat more raw foods—organic fruits and vegetables. • Eat more whole grains, particularly oats, which reduce cholesterol. • Eat good quality fats with omega-3s—fish oil, walnuts, hemp seeds, and chia seeds. • Eat garlic. • Replace corn oil and soy oil with olive oil. Coconut oil is also a good oil for cook-ing and contrary to what was previously believed, coconut oil does not raise choles-terol. • Take garlic supplements. • Take red yeast rice.

	• Drink mangosteen juice.
	• Lose weight if overweight.
	• Exercise regularly.
	• Avoid excessive alcohol. Red wine in moderation, however, is helpful in reducing cholesterol.
	• Stop smoking.
	• Practice stress reduction.

Inflammation/Pain (chronic)

Inflammation is the body's attempt to remove harmful stimuli, including damaged cells, and/or pathogens and begin the healing process.

Main Cause	Natural Cures
Inflammation is the body's response to infection or injury. *Chronic* inflammation is an over-response resulting from a variety of issues that may include dehydration and blockage of electromagnetic impulses between cells.	• See a licensed healthcare practitioner who can treat your pain without pharmaceutical drugs. Pharmaceutical pain medications are highly addictive and harmful. • Depending on the source of your inflammation, acupuncture can be especially helpful. • Chiropractic adjustments are also recommended. Some suggestions: • Drink 10 glasses of pure water a day. • Use a magnetic mattress pad. • Get alphabiotic adjustments. • Do a Candida cleanse. • Do a heavy metal cleanse. • Take oral chelation. • Do ozone therapy.

Insomnia

Persistent difficulty falling asleep, or staying asleep through the night.

Main Cause	Natural Cures
Many different things result in insomnia and each person's cause may be different from the next. Among the many triggers are anxiety/ stress, excess caffeine, alcohol	• Practice stress reduction, including relaxation exercises, and deep breathing. • Meditate. • Get massages.

consumed too close to bedtime, hormonal imbalance, lack of exercise, pain, prescription and nonprescription drugs, electronics in the bedroom, and medical conditions.	• Exercise regularly, preferably daily. Walk for one hour a day. • Eliminate prescription and nonprescription medication. • Do a Candida cleanse. • Do a liver cleanse. • Do a parasite cleanse. • Take magnesium. • Take melatonin. • Take valerian root or drink valerian root tea. • Take kava kava. • Adjust your sleep/rise schedule. Get up at 6 a.m., retire at 10 p.m. and keep the schedule consistent, even on weekends.

Irritable Bowel Syndrome (IBS)

A functional gastrointestinal disorder with symptoms associated with changes in how the gastrointestinal tract functions. It's not the same as colitis. In IBS the structure of the bowel is not abnormal, but it typically includes chronic abdominal discomfort.

Main Cause	Natural Cures
Several factors contribute to IBS, including stress, taking antibiotics, bacterial overgrowth, Candida, nonprescription drugs, and for some people, a disruption in the way the brain and digestive system interact.	• Do a colon cleanse. • Do a Candida cleanse. • Take probiotics. • Eat probiotic foods such as kimchi, organic plain yogurt, sauerkraut, and miso. • That omegas-3s. • Take digestive enzymes. • Drink aloe vera juice, 2 to 4 ounces at a time.

Kidney Stones

Hard masses formed in the kidneys made up of tiny crystals, typically formed by calcium compounds.

Main Cause	Natural Cures
Kidneys stones are often the result of lifestyle choices, most commonly neglecting to drink enough water. The lack of water results in an acidic environment in the	• If you have stones, consider the following: drink one gallon of distilled water combined with the juice of five organic lemons and two cups of apple cider vinegar every day for two weeks. • Do a colon cleanse.

kidneys, (too much uric acid) putting one at risk for the development of the stones. Fluoride in drinking water can lead to some types of stones. Some prescription and nonprescription medications can cause kidney stones. Being overweight increases one's risk. Recently it's been discussed that eating raw leafy greens and other vegetables can contribute to the formation of kidney stones because of their high oxalate content. Cooking removes a small percentage of oxalates. If you're getting enough water, there's little need to be too concerned about the oxalates from leafy greens unless you're consuming excessive amounts, or you've been diagnosed with a condition requiring the restriction of oxalates.

- Do a liver/gallbladder cleanse.
- Do a kidney/bladder cleanse.
- Do a parasite cleanse.
- For prevention:
- Drink plenty of pure water. Not tap water, which may be fluoridated. Drink 8 to 10 glasses a day of pure or distilled water.
- Eliminate sugar. Sugar can disrupt calcium and magnesium absorption.
- Eliminate all sodas. Sodas block calcium absorption and calcium deficiency can contribute to kidney stones.
- Eat calcium-rich foods. Calcium *supplements* can lead to stones, but eating calcium-rich foods helps prevent them. Plain, organic yogurt, sardines, wild salmon, and soy are some good choices.

Liver Problems

Liver diseases can include cirrhosis, fatty liver, jaundice, and hepatitis. Cirrhosis is when normal liver cells are replaced with scar tissue. Fatty liver is the accumulation of certain fats in the liver. Jaundice is an excess of bilirubin in the blood, usually due to obstruction of the bile duct. Hepatitis is inflammation of the liver.

Main Cause	Natural Cures
Cirrhosis: the end result of chronic liver disease.	If you have a liver condition, see a licensed healthcare professional. A naturopathic doctor can evaluate you and come up with the right plan to restore your liver.
Fatty liver: obesity, diabetes, and poor diet.	Some suggestions:
Jaundice: too much bilirubin (formed by the breakdown of dead red blood cells in the liver).	• Manage your weight. Obesity can result in fatty liver.
	• Do not smoke.

Hepatitis: a viral infection. The following can lead to different types of liver problems: nonprescription drugs, prescription drugs (cholesterol reducing drugs in particular), Candida, parasites, and trans fats (hydrogenated oils).	• Do a colon cleanse. • Do a liver/gallbladder cleanse. • Do a Candida cleanse. • Do a heavy metal cleanse. • Do a parasite cleanse. • Reduce salt intake. • Eliminate processed foods. • Eliminate excessive alcohol. • Eliminate prescription and nonprescription drugs. • If you're taking vitamin A, be sure that you're not taking too much. Excessive vitamin A is toxic to the liver. • Exercise to burn fat.

Lupus

An autoimmune disease where the body's immune system becomes hyperactive and begins to attack normal healthy tissue resulting in chronic inflammation and damage to skin, joints, kidneys, the blood, heart, and lungs.

Main Cause	Natural Cures
The cause of lupus is unknown. Hormones, genetics, and environmental factors are all possible contributors to the condition.	See a naturopathic doctor. With treatment, remission can be achieved. Doing all of the things in chapter 6 will suppress the condition. Some suggestions: • Consider taking DHEA, however, do so only with the guidance of a licensed healthcare practitioner. • Practice stress reduction. • Hypnosis has been shown to help people with the stress from lupus. • Exercise regularly. • Get adequate sleep. • Take omega-3s.

Male Erectile Dysfunction
A condition wherein a man is unable to get or maintain an erection firm enough to have intercourse.

Main Cause	Natural Cures
There are a number of things that can cause erectile dysfunction, including mental and emotional stress, poor circulation, nonprescription and prescription drugs, vaccines, vitamin E deficiency, calcium deficiency, diabetes, hormonal imbalance, Candida, heavy metal toxicity, and prostate problems.	• Address diabetes as discussed under the diabetes section. • Get intravenous chelation (via a licensed healthcare practitioner). • Take oral chelation—increases blood flow. • Get regular exercise. • Practice stress reduction. • Take nattokinase (for circulation). • Take natural vitamin E. • Take omega-3s. • Take ginseng. • Take Peruvian maca root. • Consider the following herbs: horny goat weed, muira puama, tribulus terrestris, gingko biloba. • Do a Candida cleanse. • Do a heavy metal cleanse.

Melanoma
A tumor of melanin forming cells that is typically cancerous.

Main Cause	Natural Cures
There is debate over the cause of melanoma. Many in the medical community say that it's due to exposure to the sun, however, that is not conclusive, as some melanomas occur in parts of the body that receive little or no sun exposure. The causes of disease are: (1) Toxins in the body. (2) Nutritional deficiencies. (3) Electromagnetic chaos. And (4) Emotional and mental stress.	• See a licensed healthcare practitioner. • Do the things in chapter 6. • Use eggplant extract cream. • Take fish oil containing vitamin D. • Eat garlic or take garlic as a supplement. • Drink green tea. • Take magnesium. • Take vitamin C. • Take vitamin D. • Take vitamin E.

One or more of those must be present to cause melanoma. Toxins in the body are one likely cause. Many types of sunscreens contain toxins and may contribute to melanoma. There are other kinds of lotions, creams, soaps, etc. people use that could contribute to melanoma. Some people may be more genetically susceptible to developing melanoma.	

Migraine Headaches
Migraines are throbbing headaches that typically appear on one side of the head and are often accompanied by nausea and sensitivity to light.

Main Cause	Natural Cures
A number of things can cause migraines, including dehydration, stress, hormonal imbalance, Candida, food allergies, parasites, heavy metal toxicity, environmental allergies, and TMJ (temporomandibular joint and muscle disorders).	• Do all of the cleanses recommended in chapter 6. • Take organic apple cider vinegar (2 tablespoons in 8 ounces of pure water before meals). • Eliminate artificial sweeteners. • Practice stress reduction. • Get cranial sacral therapy. • See a chiropractor for adjustments.

Multiple Sclerosis (MS)
A chronic and typically progressive autoimmune disease that affects the brain and spinal cord.

Main Cause	Natural Cures
Heavy metal toxicity, aspartame, mental and emotional stress, viral infections, and Candida are among the factors that can cause MS.	• Do all of the things in chapter 6. • See a naturopathic doctor. • Eliminate ALL metal dental work. There have been many reports wherein removing the metal in a person's mouth has resulted in a reversal of MS. • Do a heavy metal cleanse. • Eliminate all artificial sweeteners.

	• Eliminate monosodium glutamate (MSG).
	• Use a magnetic mattress pad.
	• Do a liver/gallbladder cleanse.
	• Get alphabiotic treatments.
	• Change diet to eliminate processed foods, grains, starches, and sugar. Replace with organic foods, raw foods, and increase consumption of organic leafy greens, sulfur-rich organic vegetables (onions, broccoli, mushrooms), and bright colored organic fruits like berries. Consume wild fish high in omega-3s.
	• Improve vitamin D levels with supplement and sun exposure.

Obesity

The state of having too much body fat. An adult with a body mass index (BMI) of 30 or greater is considered obese.

Main Cause	Natural Cures
Many factors contribute to obesity, including low metabolism, mental and emotional stress, inactivity, Candida, hypoactive thyroid, inefficient pancreas, processed foods, and chemical additives in food.	• Eliminate processed foods. Anything in a box, can, or package from a major supermarket chain is likely to be processed which means it contains chemical additives. Switch to organic foods and shop in a health food store or store that contains non-processed, non-GMO food.
• Never eat in fast food restaurants. It is not the calories and fat content that causes obesity, it is the chemical additives.
• Do a juice fast—with guidance of a licensed healthcare practitioner.
• Eat more raw foods and consider going for periods of time where you eat raw food exclusively.
• Eliminate processed sugar and high fructose corn syrup. Read food labels, because high fructose corn syrup is in many foods that you might not suspect.
• Do a colon cleanse.
• Do a liver/gallbladder cleanse.

	• Do a parasite cleanse.
	• Do a Candida cleanse.
	• Do a heavy metal cleanse.
	• Take oral chelation.
	• Walk for an hour daily.
	• Drink at least 8 glasses of pure water daily.
	• Use extra virgin coconut oil in place of other cooking oils.
	• Take raw,organic apple cider vinegar, 2 to 4 tablespoons in 8 ounces of pure water before meals.
	• Take digestive enzymes.
	• Take probiotics.
	• Drink aloe vera juice, 2 to 4 ounces on an empty stomach.
	• Eat a balanced breakfast daily.
	• Get on a regular sleep schedule, close to rising at 6 a.m. and going to bed at 10 p.m.

Phobias
Extreme fear of, or aversion to something.

Main Cause	Natural Cures
A definitive cause of phobias is unknown and they are unique to each individual, however some phobias may run in families or have cultural connections. Phobias usually begin in childhood and can be the result of traumatic experiences. Recent studies have revealed that fears and phobias can be passed to subsequent generations via DNA, which means they can be inherited.	• If you suffer from a phobia consider hypnosis. Hypnosis reprograms the subconscious and has been shown to be a successful treatment for phobias.
	• Look into Callahan Thought Field Therapy (TFT) techniques. Tapping and TFT were developed by Robert Callahan. You can find TFT practitioners around the country via an online search. Many people find relief from all kinds of issues via tapping.
	• Consider Emotional Freedom Technique (EFT)—As with TFT, you may find EFT practitioners in various parts of the country via an online search. Gary Craig was a student of Robert Callahan and developed EFT.

PMS
Period prior to menstrual cycle wherein uncomfortable symptoms arise, including bloating, breast tenderness, food cravings, fatigue, sadness, tension, irritability, and mood swings.

Main Cause	Natural Cures
Calcium and magnesium deficiency, hormonal imbalance, thyroid abnormality, heavy metal toxicity, Candida, nonprescription and prescription drugs, mental and emotional stress.	• A change in diet may help PMS symptoms. Reduce sugar and caffeine. Eat raw organic fruits and vegetables. Drink fresh organic juices. • Take calcium and magnesium supplements. • Do a colon cleanse. • Do a liver/gallbladder cleanse. • Do a heavy metal cleanse. • Do a parasite cleanse. • Use stress reduction techniques—deep breathing, yoga, meditation. • Eat and/or cook with extra virgin coconut oil—helps with hormones.

Peripheral Vascular Disease
A condition of the blood vessels that can lead to narrowing and ultimately hardening of the arteries.

Main Cause	Natural Cures
Plaque buildup in the arteries, smoking, high cholesterol, obesity, and diabetes contribute to peripheral vascular disease.	• See a licensed healthcare practitioner. • If you're overweight, lose weight. • Quit smoking. • Walk regularly, preferably daily. This stimulates the opening of blood vessels in lower legs. (Symptoms of this condition include lower leg pain.) • Take vitamin C—helps with inflammation and keeps lining of arteries strong. • Take vitamin E—helps thin the blood. • Take and/or eat garlic—helps thin the blood. • Take ginkgo biloba—enhances blood flow. • Take oral chelation.

Snoring
Hoarse or harsh breathing sound during sleep.

Main Cause	Natural Cures
Dehydration, Candida, excess weight (which puts pressure on airways), blockage in the nose resulting from a deformed nasal septum, nasal polyps, allergies, sleeping pills, antihistamines, and alcohol consumed close to bedtime may all cause snoring.	• Use essential oil throat spray. • Change sleeping position. Sleeping on the back promotes snoring. Try sleeping on the side. • If overweight, losing weight can help. • Avoid alcohol, especially within 4 hours of going to sleep. • Open nasal passages either with steam from a hot shower or with "Breathe right" strips.

Sore Throat
Painful inflammation of the pharynx.

Main Cause	Natural Cures
Bacterial and viral infections cause sore throats. Candida and parasites are other possible causes to consider.	If a sore throat continues for more than a few days, see a licensed healthcare practitioner because the condition could be the result of a more serious illness. Some suggestions: • Gargle with colloidal silver or colloidal minerals. • Gargle with Himalayan pink sea salt and warm purified water. • Gargle with goldenseal root powder and warm purified water. • Mix coconut oil (1 tablespoon) with raw honey (1 teaspoon) and 2 tablespoons of organic lemon juice. Heat if necessary. Sip slowly and let the mixture coat the throat. All three ingredients are antibacterial and will help heal the inflammation. • Do a Candida cleanse. • Do a parasite cleanse. • Do a heavy metal cleanse. • Take the herbs cat's claw and larrea.

Tumors
An abnormal growth of body tissue.

Main Cause	Natural Cures
Toxic overload, electromagnetic chaos such as cell phones or laptop computers, mental and emotional stress, Candida, and viral infections are causes of tumors.	• Do all of the things in chapter 6, particularly the cleanses. • See a licensed healthcare practitioner. Some suggestions: • Take food grade hydrogen peroxide therapy (35%). • Get ozone therapy. • Take oral and/or intravenous chelation therapy. • Take flaxseed oil. • Take shark cartilage. • Use infrared saunas. • Practice stress reduction. • Get energetic rebalancing (AIM program, www.AIMprogram.com).

Varicose Veins
Varicose veins are veins that have become enlarged due to being filled with an abnormal collection of blood.

Main Cause	Natural Cures
Nonprescription and prescription drugs, mental and emotional stress, trans fats, homogenized dairy products, vitamin E deficiency, and being overweight contribute to varicose veins.	• See an herbalist who can prescribe an herbal remedy specifically for you. • Some herbs to consider are horse chestnut extract, grape seed extract, and butcher's broom, all of which have been shown to be helpful in eliminating varicose veins. Some suggestions: • Take natural vitamin E. • Take omega-3s. • Take nattokinase. • Take oral chelation and/or intravenous chelation.

It's important to understand that while specific cures are excellent information to have, they're only *one part* of what needs to be done to restore the body to health. The conditions I've covered above can and should be addressed by implementing the things in chapter 6. It's important to know that people who are looking for a "specific cure" for a "specific disease" are completely missing the point of this book. You must undergo an entire lifestyle change in order to be fully cured and that's why you must absorb this book in its entirety, not just this chapter.

> You must undergo an entire lifestyle change in order to be fully cured...

A disease is nothing more than a label put on a series of symptoms. The symptoms could be caused by hundreds of factors, or combinations of factors. This is one of the things that medical science does not want you to know about. In order for the medical community to make money, they must "isolate" a specific something so they can find a drug that can be patented to treat it. The medical community would prescribe that one expensive drug to treat the symptoms of all kinds of people without understanding each individual's *cause* for developing those symptoms. If you were to take a hundred people who were experiencing the exact same symptom, a migraine headache for example, each person's migraine headache could have a different cause. This means every person's treatment should be different. What will work for one person might not work for another.

This is why when you ask, "What's the cure for X?" the answer is I don't know, because no one knows until you're looked at by a healthcare practitioner, analyzed, and the cause is determined. Once the cause is determined, then the right treatment will be discussed. For example, if you have genital herpes, we all know the cause is a virus. What we don't know is why the virus became active in you. Everyone gets exposed to the virus, but not everyone develops breakouts and succumbs to it. So even though we do know that it's a virus, if you had five people with a genital herpes breakout, each person's reason for succumbing to the herpes virus could be different; therefore, the treatment that would work for each of the five people could be slightly different. In one person red marine algae may completely kill the virus and he or she would never have an outbreak again. In another person it could be the herb larrea; in another person hydrogen peroxide applied to the breakout could kill the virus; in another person dimethyl sulfoxide (DMSO) applied to the breakout area could kill the virus; in another person lysine could suppress the symptoms. In some people, they may need to use a combination of treatments. This is why individualized treatment is necessary.

When you look at a hundred sick people with different illnesses, you do find some common denominators. Most sick people are dehydrated; most sick people need a colon cleanse; most sick people need a liver/gallbladder cleanse; most sick people have a Candida yeast overgrowth; most sick people have parasites; most sick people have nutritional deficiencies; most sick people's bodies are loaded with toxins; most sick people have some type of emotional or mental stress that has been trapped in their physical body; most sick people have heavy metal toxicities; most sick people have environmental and food allergies and don't even realize it. This is why I always tell people who have any physical problems to do the things in chapter 6, and then reevaluate their condition in three to six months. It is amazing that the majority of people see their symptoms diminish dramatically, or even vanish.

A few years ago, I received a call from a seventy-eight year old woman who told me she'd been on five different prescription drugs for over ten years. Her symptoms continually got worse. Then she read my book and started implementing the things in chapter 6. She did this under the care of a licensed healthcare practitioner who didn't use drugs and surgery. Within three months she got completely off of all her prescription medications, and told me that she did about half of the recommendations in chapter 6. She said she felt twenty-five years younger and full of energy, full of vitality, and all of her symptoms and conditions were cured.

This is not an isolated incident. I'm constantly hearing stories from people who read the first version of this book and implemented the cures.

Larry said, "I was on a number of medications—anti-depressants, acid reflux medication, I had high blood pressure, high cholesterol, arthritis, I was forty to fifty pounds overweight, always tired, and had no energy. I read *Natural Cures*. Now I don't go to the doctor and I don't get sick. I don't have acid reflux, I don't have high cholesterol, I don't have high blood pressure, I don't have gout or arthritis anymore. I am drug free."

Dan said, "Before I read the book, I was diagnosed with incurable cancer. Stage 3B melanoma. Didn't have a good prognosis— less than a 2% chance survival rate. With that type of cancer, chemo and radiation weren't options. So I was really looking into some recommendations for treatments. I mentioned to my doctors that I'd hold off on the surgery and try some things on my own. They told me I was making a big mistake. 'There's no proof that's going to help and you'll waste a lot of money. ' So I said, 'Well, wish me luck anyways. I'm going to check it out.' So we started eating organic and started to detox and we jumped in. A four year journey, full-time, did some crazy things, and in the end, I'm cancer free."

Julianne said, "*Natural Cures* saved my life. I had a genetically passed down heart condition, and the doctors one day looked at me and said, 'You have about a month to live.' I was around fifteen, sixteen years old. I had no awareness that the food I was eating had GMOs and was literally destroying my body at such a young age. I picked up the book, my mom had it, and was able to change my diet, change the way I was living my life and within months, my heart was strong."

These kind of "miraculous " cures continue to happen to thousands of people all over the world every week. It could happen for you.

...if you're sick, you must see a licensed healthcare practitioner who does not use only drugs and surgery.

Let me emphasize again, if you're sick, you must see a licensed healthcare practitioner who does not use only drugs and surgery. In my opinion, you must be on an energetic rebalancing program. You must do a colon cleanse, a liver/gallbladder cleanse, a kidney/bladder cleanse, a Candida cleanse, a parasite cleanse, a heavy metal cleanse, and, ideally, a full-body cleanse. You must stop all nonprescription and prescription drugs. You must stop eating poisons such as fast food and artificial sweeteners. You must be drinking at least eight to ten glasses of purified water every day. You must use some technology to eliminate the stress your body is holding on to. If you don't do these basic things, it's impossible, in my opinion, for you to truly get your body back in a state of balance, eliminate your symptoms, and cure yourself of disease.

To return to good health, the most important thing you can do is take personal responsibility and decide that you *are* going to find the cause and cure for your disease. In order to do this, in my opinion, you must seek out licensed healthcare practitioners to assist you. Please do not attempt to treat yourself without guidance from a professional. Though I have copious knowledge about the causes, cures, and prevention of disease, I still seek the advice and opinions of licensed healthcare practitioners regularly. I do this to prevent disease, gain knowledge, and to get other people's perspectives. I don't believe I'm the smartest guy in the world. And I believe that two heads are better than one. If you truly want to prevent and/or cure disease, it's vital that you seek advice. That said, it's equally important that you not look at these people as "all-knowing gods." Get several opinions and understand that what you're getting are just that—*opinions*. You must gather the information yourself, listen to the various points of view, review them, and decide the course of action that *you* feel is most beneficial. Remember, it's your body, your health, and your life. You take responsibility.

To find a licensed healthcare practitioner you can go to your local Yellow Pages (if you still use it), or do an online search. I recommend that you start with a naturopathic doctor (N.D.). An N.D. is highly trained and able to treat a wide variety of health problems. An N.D. will also be able to direct you to other healthcare professionals that are appropriate for your situation. These may include chiropractors, massage therapists, colon therapists, herbalists, etc. You can do your own online searches for any of those and also for other modalities in the "natural healthcare arena" such as oriental medicine, homeopathy, acupuncture, iridology, holistic medicine etc. But if you begin with being evaluated by a naturopathic doctor, he or she will likely be helpful in advising what treatments will be useful to you. Even if you're not sick, or experiencing any negative symptoms, I encourage you to visit a variety of licensed healthcare practitioners now, for the maintenance of optimum health. Better to *prevent* disease than to worry about trying to cure it once you have it.

CHAPTER 12

Frequently Asked Questions

Since this book was published, millions of people have been exposed to the fact that: (a) drugs and surgery are ineffective and cause most diseases, (b) the food produced by the publicly traded food corporations and fast food restaurants causes illness and disease, and (c) there are natural non-drug and nonsurgical ways to prevent and cure virtually every disease. Because of the success of this book, many health advocates who promote organic food and health experts who promote non-drug and nonsurgical ways to prevent and cure disease, are now becoming more mainstream. With so many voices talking about the subject, there are obviously different opinions regarding natural remedies. This is good. As I mentioned early on, nobody has a monopoly on the truth, including me. There are no such things as "facts," there are only *opinions* based on the information we currently have. Health experts may therefore come up with slightly different perspectives on what a person should do for his or her best health outcome.

That said, I'd like to address some of the most frequently asked questions I receive regarding health and nutrition, and the concepts covered in this book. Even if you don't think a question is relevant to you, please keep reading, because the answer may be more relevant than you thought.

Question: My doctor says I need drugs and/or surgery. What do I do?

Answer: First, I would encourage you to stop going to medical doctors who only prescribe drugs and surgery. I'd encourage you to also get advice from licensed healthcare practitioners who don't prescribe drugs and surgery. Get three or four opinions. This way you can make an informed decision. Your condition may be past the point of no return, where only drugs and surgery would be effective in keeping you alive a little longer. However, I believe that anyone who says that you "need" drugs and surgery is either misinformed, not knowledgeable about natural methods, or simply trying to make money on your illness.

Question: Can I ever eat a cheeseburger again, or go to a fast food restaurant?

Answer: You can eat cheeseburgers and French fries as long as you make them at home with organic ingredients. People always ask me what I eat. I eat anything and everything (with some exceptions) as long as it's certified organic. You can eat beef, cheese, butter, milk, cream, eggs, lamb, chicken, duck, mashed potatoes, French fries, onion rings, ice cream, chocolate, you name it, as long as it's organic. No, you cannot eat in fast food restaurants if you want to cure yourself of disease and remain healthy. Fast food restaurants use chemical ingredients to grow, process, and manufacture their so-called food. The chemicals, the lack of nutrients and the out-rageous number of free radicals in their energetically altered food is making you sick.

Question: So, is fast food really that bad?

Answer: Yes. Fast food absolutely causes illness and disease, including cancer, diabetes, and a host of other major health problems. Fast food makes you fat. Fast food is purposely produced with chemical additives that are designed to increase your appetite, get you physically and chemically addicted, and make you fat. The fast food industry is knowingly causing illness and disease. McDonald's itself stated that it's a matter of common knowledge that any processing that its foods undergo serve to make them more harmful than unprocessed foods. An example is McNuggets. These were originally made from old chickens that could no longer lay eggs. Now they're made from chickens that have unusually large breasts, a kind of genetically altered and produced animal. The manufacturing process includes stripping the meat from the bone and grinding it up in a mash. It is then combined with a host of preservatives, stabilizers, and other chemicals, pressed into shapes, breaded, deep fried, freeze-dried, and then shipped to McDonald's. Judge Robert Sweet called them "a McFrankenstein creation of various elements not utilized by the home cook."

I encourage you to view the documentary *Supersize Me*, which is available on DVD. This is a must watch for anyone who eats at fast food restaurants. This film examines the **question:** *What if a person ate nothing but McDonald's food for thirty days?* Could thirty days of eating nothing but McDonald's cause medical problems? Could just thirty days of eating McDonald's food cause massive weight gain? Could thirty days of eating McDonald's food cause disease and illness? This documentary shows the truth. The man had his blood work tested before, during, and after his experiment. He had his weight checked. In just thirty days, the medical doctors were astonished by what happened to his body. In just thirty days of eating McDonald's food he gained twenty-five pounds. No doctor could believe it. I can believe it because I know that McDonald's, like every other fast food restaurant, in my opinion, is purposely putting ingredients in the food to get you physically addicted to it, to increase your appetite, and make you fat. This movie certainly substantiates this opinion. From a health standpoint, the doctors were shocked that his liver virtually turned to fat and his cholesterol shot up sixty-five points. His body-fat percentage went from 11 percent to over 18 percent. He nearly doubled his risk of coronary heart disease. He said he felt depressed and exhausted most of the time. His moods swung on a dime, and his sex life suffered. He craved McDonald's food, and got headaches when he didn't eat it. The doctor said if he stayed on this diet, he would develop coronary artery disease, inflammation, hardening of the liver, and probably develop dozens of other illnesses and die an early death.

The doctors who did his blood work could not believe how he was, in effect, *dying* after just thirty days. They couldn't believe it because they were only looking at calories, carbohydrates, protein, fat, and sodium. They weren't considering the "trans fats." They weren't considering how the food has been genetically produced. They weren't considering how the food was energetically destroyed and toxic. They weren't considering all of the food processing chemicals and additives. That's the reason this man became so sick in such a short time. This is why you need to know that if you're sick and you're eating fast food, or food from publicly traded corporations, they are in fact making you sick. It is the poisons, chemicals, additives, and energetic altering of the food that's making you ill.

Fast food restaurants, like all food manufacturers, have one objective and that is to increase profits. They increase profits by getting more of your money. One of the ways they get you to buy more food is by increasing the portion size.

When French fries were first sold at McDonald's there was one size. That size French fries is now the "small." McDonald's also has a medium, a large, and a super-size. The original size is still there, but few people order it. The difference is the original size is 200 calories, but the super-size is over 600 calories.

When Burger King first opened they sold a twelve-ounce small soda and a sixteen-ounce large soda. Today, the twelve-ounce soda is called "kiddy" size, the sixteen-ounce is no longer a large; it's now the "small." They have a medium, which is thirty-two ounces, and a forty-two ounce size. This is pretty much across the board at all fast food restaurants.

In 2013, New York City's then Mayor Bloomberg tried to ban these outrageously large sodas, however, the ban was struck down as a violation of principle of "separation of powers." In *Supersize Me* it was mentioned that cars have introduced larger cup holders to accommodate those huge 7-Eleven double gulps, which are sixty-four ounces, a full half gallon, and hold anywhere from six-hundred to eight-hundred calories. Just imagine, a half gallon of soda for one person. That's forty-eight teaspoons of sugar!

Fast food restaurants also are involved in some of the most devious advertising campaigns ever. This is similar to what happened in the tobacco industry. As discussed in *Supersize Me*, a secret study by one of the tobacco companies was about brand imprinting for later acquisition in life. What this means is the tobacco companies would produce things such as toy cigarettes, so that a child at age four, five, or six would "play smoke" them. The theory was that even though the little child had no understanding of what they were doing, they were imprinting their memory with the act of smoking. So when they grew to the age where they were allowed to smoke, without realizing it, they would be going for that pack and recognize it because they had those nice feelings when they were a kid.

The same goes for children at the playgrounds at fast food restaurants like McDonald's and Burger King. They bring the children in, they have fun, they have warm fuzzy feelings, and later in life they relive those feelings when they go to their fast food restaurant. This is being done purposely by the fast food industry to increase sales down the road. You have to understand, the fast food industry is spending millions of dollars researching ways to get people hooked on their products. Kids who eat in fast food restaurants as little as three times a week have elevated abnormal liver function tests. Under a microscope there is evidence of scarring of the liver, fibrosis of the liver, and early states of sclerosis. This is all caused by fast food.

In addition to viewing *Supersize Me,* I also encourage you to read the book *Fast Food Nation* and or watch the film of the same name so you can see just how bad fast food really is, not only for your health, but for society in general. Think about this: The average American child sees ten-thousand food advertisements per year on TV alone. Ninety-five percent of those are for sugared cereals, soft drinks, fast food, and candy. It's not a fair fight. The food industry has the money to brainwash children into buying their products. Sadly, when children are shown pictures of people like George Washington, Abraham Lincoln, and Jesus Christ, they often have no idea who these people are. But when they're shown a picture of Ronald McDonald, every single one knows his name. And what's even sadder is they believe that he's a "good man" who's helping children. This is how the food industry misleads and brainwashes our kids.

Think about this, as discussed in the movie *Supersize Me,* companies spend billions of dollars making sure you know about their product. In 2001, on direct media advertising alone (radio, television, and print) McDonald's spent $1.4 billion worldwide getting you to buy their products. On direct media advertising Pepsi spent more than $1 billion. To advertise its candy, Hershey Foods spent almost $200 million. In its peak year, the five-a-day fruit and vegetable campaign had a total advertising budget, in *all* media, of just $2 million. That's a hundred times less than the direct media budget of one food company. We're being bombarded by the food industry with lies and deceptions that brainwash us into believing that their products are healthy for us, and it's working. Think about the way food is marketed: T-shirts, coupons, toys for children, giveaways in fast food places, etc. The most heavily advertised foods are the most consumed. That's no surprise. Whoever spends the most money on advertising sells the most food.

Think about this scary fact—the majority of people tested could not recite the "Pledge of Allegiance," however almost all of them could sing the Big Mac song, "Two all-beef patties, special sauce, lettuce, cheese, pickles, onions on a sesame seed bun." You're probably singing it right now.

> All fast food companies and junk food manufacturers want you to be physically addicted to their food...

One of the scariest things is how fast food is being sold in schools. When you look at the school lunch programs, the most appalling observation is about junk food companies that make huge profits off of the schools. Junk food companies don't want to get kicked out of the school system. They want to be there to addict the children so they'll have them as customers for life. This points out that food manufacturers know their foods are dangerous and cause harm to the body. They don't care. They specifically target children, demanding that soda machines and junk food be sold in schools, which guarantees that these kids will have illness and disease, because as publicly traded corporations they have one objective: To increase profits. Therefore, they'll do anything, hurt anyone, and destroy people's lives by giving them disease, all in the name of making more money.

All fast food companies and junk food manufacturers want you to be physically addicted to their food, just like drug dealers want you to become physically addicted to their drugs. This is why these companies have spent millions in secret laboratories producing chemical additives that get you physically addicted to the food, increase your appetite, and make you fat. The chemical-laden products that McDonald's and other fast food companies sell are essentially drugs. Internal documents at McDonald's refer to the people who eat their food at least once a week as "heavy users." Seventy-two percent of people who eat at McDonald's are heavy users. They also have another category, the "super heavy user." These people eat their food three, four, five times a week and up. Twenty-two percent of the people who eat at McDonald's are super heavy users. *Supersize Me* states that if you look at the menu at a fast food restaurant they use all of the addicting components. They'll take a slab of meat, cover it with cheese, and then serve it with a sugary soda, which has the addictive powers of sugar with plenty of added caffeine. Give this to a twelve year old and his or her brain is no match for that chemical combination.

I wondered about the health of the 22 percent of people who ate at McDonald's three, four, five times a week and up. In my observations, I found that these people are riddled with disease. I found that people who eat at McDonald's three times a week or more have the highest chance of getting cancer, diabetes, obesity, heart disease, acid reflux, constipation, sleep disorders, depression, eczema, dandruff, and a host of other medical disorders. McDonald's will, of course, disagree with my observations. In my opinion, they are the new "evil empire." Remember, the food industry uses lobbyists in Washington to make sure that no government agency ever says *eat less* of its products, and to make sure that the government never passes legislation that could hurt the industry's profits.

So the bottom line answer to the question is absolutely *never* eat in a fast food restaurant.

Question: Why don't you talk about calories, fats, protein, or carbohydrates?

Answer: While those things are important, they're not as important to discuss as the chemicals and poisons put into our food supply. The chemical fertilizers and the pesticides used in the food, the fact that the food is picked too early and then gassed, and the fact that the food is genetically modified and manufactured in natural ways is far more important than the number of calories, or the fat and carbohydrate content, because the unnatural, chemical-laden food will make you hungry, addicted, and fat. That's what everyone is missing.

Question: How are you qualified to write this book when you're not a medical doctor?

Answer: The number one qualification I have to write this book is precisely the fact that I am not a medical doctor. If I were a medical doctor, I'd be unqualified to write it. Think about it. If you're a medical doctor, you spent the majority of your training on traditional medical practices, including prescribing drugs and surgery. How can you wake up one day and say that everything you've been taught is wrong; everything that was drilled into your head, that you were forced to believe, is false? It would be next to impossible. How can medical doctors be qualified to talk about health and nutrition when they have little to no training in natural methods of prevention and curing disease?

My qualifications are that I'm logical, I use common sense, and I can see the truth. I've also done extensive research, traveled around the world, interviewed thousands of patients and doctors, been treated by hundreds of licensed alternative healthcare practitioners, studied volumes of books, research papers, and other documents; and I've made billions of dollars in business, which has put me in corporate boardrooms all around the world dealing with the most powerful people on the planet. I know the inner workings of government and of corporations, and I know the greed. I also know about the insatiable appetite to make money at all costs. I know about the fraud and deception that goes on behind closed doors. I've been a part of it, such a part of it that I spent two years in federal prison. I understand more about the inner workings of the moneymaking machines and political machines around the world than most people. I also live everything I talk about. I've experienced it and I've seen the results in my friends, my family, and myself. Plus, I'm 156 years old and have virtually never been sick. (Just kidding!)

Question: How come I never hear about the stuff you say on the radio or on TV, and I never see it in newspapers and magazines?

Answer: As I've mentioned, newspapers, magazines, radio, and television are outlets owned by publicly traded corporations whose main interest is in making a profit, not in providing truthful information. They'll produce stories that get the best ratings, because good ratings mean good profits. Unfortunately, the sponsors of these media outlets (the advertisers) also control the message you hear on television and radio, and read in newspapers and magazines. And since the majority of advertisers are pharmaceutical companies and major food companies, you're never going to get the truth that the food industry and pharmaceutical industry are making you ill.

Question: Is there a difference between fitness and health?

Answer: Absolutely. A person can be exceptionally fit, yet also unhealthy. Jim Fixx was a well-known runner who wrote *The Complete Book of Running*. He dropped dead of a heart attack at age 52 after inspiring many people to become fit. He ran daily, and appeared to be very fit, but his arteries had blockages and he was *not* healthy. There are other people who may be slightly overweight, and they may not be strong or flexible, yet they're very healthy and may even live to be a hundred years old. Generally speaking, there's a balance between fitness and health. In order to be super healthy you have to be at least moderately fit; but you can be exceptionally fit and still develop diseases and die young. It is more important to be healthy than fit, but for those who want to look good in a bathing suit, being fit is more important. I believe in both fitness and health, but health should take priority over fitness. If health is your number one priority, your fitness level is probably going to be better than average anyway.

Question: How do I change my body pH from acid to alkaline?

Answer: Do all of the things in chapter 6.

Question: Why is a liver cleanse so important?

Answer: The liver is the only organ that can pump fat out of the body. The liver is also the filter and cleanser of the bloodstream. Most people, in my opinion, have a sluggish liver. If your liver is sluggish, you can't burn fat properly, and you can't filter and clean your blood properly. That means you're setting yourself up for illness and disease. Your liver is sluggish because of all of the chemicals and toxins in the food you eat, as well as all of the nonprescription and prescription drugs you've taken. If you're taking cholesterol-reducing drugs, you definitely have a sluggish liver. If you've ever taken an antibiotic in your life, that antibiotic has killed the friendly bacteria in your intestine, causing a Candida yeast overgrowth, which always attacks the liver. When most people do a liver cleanse, they feel so much better and can't believe the difference.

Question: Are we really full of toxins, and will doing cleanses really prevent and cure diseases as serious as cancer, diabetes, or heart disease?

Answer: Yes. Every person has toxic material in his or her body causing illness and disease. Yes, by doing a colon cleanse, a liver/

gallbladder cleanse, a kidney/ bladder cleanse, a heavy metal cleanse, a parasite cleanse, a Candida cleanse, and a full-body fat cleanse you can prevent yourself from getting sick, as well as cure yourself of even the most horrible diseases. Yes, doing the recommended cleanse is one of the "natural cures" that they don't want you to know about. Here's a questionnaire to ascertain just how toxic you are. Answer each question yes or no. If you answer yes to over twenty questions, you are highly toxic.

1. I've received vaccines.

2. I've taken antibiotics in my life.

3. I've taken prescription drugs in the last five years.

4. I've taken aspirin, Tylenol, ibuprofen, or other over-the-counter pain medication.

5. I've taken over-the-counter nonprescription drugs.

6. I shower and/or bathe in regular tap water.

7. I drink water out of the tap.

8. I have been in a swimming pool where chlorine was used.

9. I use a cellular telephone without any electromagnetic chaos protection.

10. I use a laptop computer with a wireless device.

11. I watch TV.

12. I own and watch a high-definition television.

13. I use a wireless telephone in my house.

14. I use a remote control for my television or other electronic appliances.

15. I have a satellite television.

16. I drive in a car every day.

17. I drive in heavy traffic.

18. I use hair dyes.

19. I use fingernail polish.

20. I use makeup and cosmetics.

21. I use moisturizers, body lotions, and sunscreens on my skin.

22. I use air fresheners in my house.

23. I use bug spray in my house.

24. I use standard cleaning products in my house.

25. I use standard soap and detergent for my skin and my clothes.

26. I use toothpaste with fluoride.

27. I eat in fast food restaurants at least once a month.

28. I eat in restaurants at least once a month.

29. I eat products produced by large publicly traded corporations.

30. I buy brand name food products that are heavily advertised on TV.

31. I eat food that is not certified 100 percent organic.

32. I eat beef, lamb, poultry, eggs, and dairy products that are not organic.

33. I eat pork and shellfish.

34. I use artificial sweeteners such as NutraSweet or Splenda.

35. I drink sodas at least several times a week.

36. I drink diet sodas at least several times a week.

37. I don't have at least one large bowel movement each day.

38. I use nonstick pans to cook with.

39. I use deodorant and antiperspirant.

40. I do not drink eight glasses of purified water every day.

41. I have never had a colonic or enema.

42. I live near high-tension power lines.

43. I live within a few miles of a manufacturing plant of some kind.

44. I live within a hundred miles of an agricultural area where produce is grown.

45. I live within a hundred miles of ranches where livestock, cattle, chickens, or other animals are raised.

This is a quick list that I hope will open your eyes to the fact that simply living a "normal life" results in a lot of toxins going into your body. Keep in mind this is a relatively new phenomena. A hundred years ago people were not exposed to so many toxins in the environment. A hundred years ago people weren't loading their bodies with huge amounts of toxins the way we are today. Every single year the level of toxins we're exposed to increases. The level of toxins in the air, in the water supply, and the food supply are constantly rising. The level of toxins surrounding our environment and our living spaces are rising. The level of electromagnetic chaos is increasing. The amount of nonprescription and prescription drugs is going up. The amount of chemicals used in the production of our food is going up. The amount of toxins being force-fed to us by large publicly traded corporations continues to rise. So yes, you are absolutely toxic, and yes, by cleaning the toxins out of your body you *can* produce miraculous cures.

Question: Can we really get disease just by breathing the air?

Answer: Sadly, yes we can. The *Associated Press* reports that toxic dust is a household threat. The article states that Americans are exposed to a variety of potentially dangerous chemicals in their homes from products such as computers, frying pans, shower curtains, cleaning chemicals, bug sprays, etc. A study found thirty-five hazardous industrial chemicals in household dust samples. This brings home the fact that hazardous chemicals are in our daily lives. All of these chemicals are known to be harmful to the immune, respiratory, cardiovascular, and reproductive systems. Infants and children are especially vulnerable. The lobbying group, the American Chemistry Council, which represents major chemical companies, made the insane statement: "Just because a toxic substance is found in dust or in the body doesn't necessarily mean it causes health problems." This is why you need air filters and air cleaners and you must start using nontoxic, organic cleaning products in your home.

Question: Are all brand named popular foods sold by publicly traded corporations bad?

Answer: Yes. Remember, natural food, organic food, is fine. It's when the profit motive becomes the main objective that those foods stop being natural and are in effect manufactured. This is when the situation causes obesity and disease. Think about the average farmer. He wants to produce some vegetables and make a profit. The problem is chemical companies bombard him with sales pitches telling "Farmer Joe" how he can increase his yield and increase his profits by using their fantastic chemicals. So Farmer Joe buys genetically modified seed that he's told will produce more crops faster and also be germ resistant. Farmer Joe also uses chemical fertilizers to make the vegetables grow at an unnaturally, unhealthy fast rate. He then sprays poisonous pesticides and herbicides on his vegetables. These are all absorbed into the vegetables and cannot be washed off. In order to make the vegetables look beautiful and last longer, they are picked before they are ripe and put into a gas chamber and sprayed with more chemicals. They are then shipped to the grocery store where they can last for days or weeks without spoiling. You then eat them. The problem is that the product is genetically modified, full of toxins and chemicals, devoid of any nutrients and, because of the irradiation, energetically changed, causing the food to be toxic to the body.

Question: Can something as serious as multiple sclerosis be cured with natural methods?

Answer: Yes. A few months ago I met a woman who had multiple sclerosis. She had a cane and couldn't walk very well. She recognized me from television and asked if I was the author of the *Natural Cures* book. I said yes. She then said that she read the book and didn't understand how anything in it could help her with her multiple sclerosis. As she said this I noticed that she had a diet soda in her hand. I explained that MS, like all diseases, is caused by too many toxins in the body, nutritional deficiencies, electromagnetic chaos, and/or stress. I asked her how long she had been drinking diet soda. She said most of her life. I asked her if she had a lot of dental work. She said her mouth was filled with dental work and various kinds of metal. I told her that the majority of MS sufferers who I'd seen had experienced tremendous results by eliminating aspartame, the artificial sweetener in diet sodas, getting rid of all of the metal in their mouth, and sleeping on a magnetic mattress pad. Most also have Lyme disease, which can be cured with homeopathies, intravenous hydrogen peroxide therapy, and other natural therapies. Usually sufferers see tremendous relief in just a matter of weeks or months. She said it didn't sound like it would help, but she'd give it a try. I gave her my number and told her to call me, as I was curious about her results. I also let her know that I was not a doctor or a licensed healthcare practitioner and could not treat her, and that she must seek professional help. Three months later she called to tell me that she could not believe the spectacular results she had experienced; she said she felt like a new woman and she felt fifteen years younger. This is a good example of how simple "natural cures" work.

Question: Will "natural cures" work for everybody?

Answer: I believe "natural cures" will work for everyone, but the specific *natural cure* that works for one person's symptoms may not work for another. An example is not everyone who smokes cigarettes comes down with lung cancer, but 90 percent of the people who develop lung cancer smoke cigarettes. What this means is not every single person who drinks diet soda will come down with multiple sclerosis, but almost everyone who comes down with multiple sclerosis probably is adversely affected by the aspartame in the diet soda. This is an important aspect to understand. The reason for this apparent inconsistency is that everyone's genetic strengths and weaknesses are different. The four causes of all disease (too many toxins in the body, nutritional deficiencies, electromagnetic chaos, and/or stress) affect the genetically weak areas in a person. Therefore, two people could do exactly the same things and one person could come down with a disease and another person may not. This is also why two people can do the exact same "natural cure" and one person will see spectacular results and another person may not see the same exceptional results. However, there is a "natural cure" that the second person could use that would lead to great results. That is why doing the things in chapter 6 is so vitally important for prevention and curing of disease.

Closing Thoughts

Throughout this book I've repeatedly made the statement, "I'm mad as hell and I'm not going to take it anymore." Many who read this feel my outrage at the lies and deceptions perpetrated against people by our government, the FDA and the FTC, as well as large, publicly traded corporations, all in the effort to increase their power, influence, and money. I am doing this because it's a calling. I believe it's my mission to help educate people and make society a better place. I'm sincerely grateful to know that my mission is having a positive impact on millions of people's lives, while also having a negative impact on the power, influence, and profits of the "Goliaths" around the world.

I've been offered tens of millions of dollars to stop saying what I'm saying. One organization offered me $100 million dollars if I would stop my consumer advocacy work, stop blowing the whistle on insider information, and simply live a quiet life. Prominent and powerful people, who will remain nameless, have assured me that if I continue my mission I will be repeatedly sued, attacked, debunked, ridiculed, persecuted in the media, the press, and in the courts. I've been threatened in every way you can imagine.

All of these things only bolster my resolve.

I refuse to be bribed or bought. I refuse to cave in to pressure. I will not live my life operating from fear.

It's gratifying to know that the work I'm doing is having a positive impact. Every week I receive correspondence from people telling me how they're off drugs and how their symptoms and illnesses have been cured. When I listen to how people's lives have changed for the better, how they're saving money, and how the pain in their bodies is gone, I know that what I am doing is right. Every time I speak publicly or do a presentation, I close my eyes and wish for at least one person to be positively impacted by the information. That's what makes my mission worth it. I hope you are that person. I hope this book has made a difference in your life. I hope that it helps you to begin an exciting and beautiful journey. I invite you to stay updated with new natural cures through my newsletter (which you can order through my website at www.NaturalCuresBook.com/newsletter) and to share your success stories by emailing me at mystory@ NaturalCuresSuccess.com. May your family be happier, healthier, and wealthier because you apply the knowledge I've shared. We've all heard the phrase "knowledge is power," but in actuality, knowledge is only power *if* you *use* it. The knowledge you've gained will only benefit you and your family when you use it. The wonderful author Leo Buscaglia once said, "To know and not to do is not to know." Apply these techniques in your life and as I mentioned in the beginning of this book, I *know* you'll never be the same.

> ...knowledge is only power if you use it.

Humbly yours in health,

Kevin Trudeau

Resources

Websites:

Acupressure
www.acupressure.com

Acupuncture
www.acupuncture.com
www.medicalacupunture.com

Aromatherapy
www.naha.org

Callahan Technique
www.rogercallahan.com

Ayurvedic Medicine
www.ayurveda.com

Bioenergetic Bodywork
www.bioenergetic-therapy.com

Biological Dentistry
www.biologicaldentistry.org
www.holisticdental.org
www.hugginsappliedhealing.com

Bowen Therapy Technique
www.bowendirectory.com
www.boweninfo.com

Cancer
www.centurywellness.com

Candida Cleansing
www.candidaplan.com

Chelation Therapy
www.angelmedcenter.com/chelationtherapy
www.centurywellness.com

Chiropractic
www.chiropractic.org
www.americanchiropractic.org

Colon Therapy
www.i-act.org

Craniosacral Therapy
www.upledger.com

Detoxification and Cleansing
www.wecarespa.com
www.hippocratesinst.com

Energetic Rebalancing
www.aimprogram.com

Feldenkrais
www.feldenkrais.com

Hakomi
www.hakomiinstitute.com

Healing Touch
www.healingtouch.net

Heller Work
www.hellerwork.com

Herbal Medicine
www.herbalgram.org
www.ahpa.org

Homeopathic Medicine
www.homeopathyusa.org
www.homeopathic.org
www.homeopathy.org

Iridology
www.iridologyassn.org

Kinesiology
www.uskinesiologyinstitute.com
www.icak.com

Magnetic Field Therapy
www.polarpowermagnets.com

Massage Therapy
www.abmp.com
www.amtamassage.org
www.aobta.org

Music Therapy
www.musictherapy.org

Naturopathic Doctors
www.naturopathic.org
www.calnd.org
www.findnd.com
www.hanp.net

Neuro-Emotional Technique
www.NetMindBody.com

Organic Information
www.organic-center.org
www.organicconsumers.org
www.ota.com

Orthomolecular Medicine
www.orthomed.org

Osteopathic Medicine
www.academyofosteopathy.org
www.holisticmedicine.org
www.cranialacademy.com

Reflexology
www.reflexology-usa.net

Reiki
www.reiki.org

Rolfing
www.rolf.org

Rosen Method
www.rosenmethod.com

Sound Therapy
www.soundlistening.com

Sunlight Therapy
www.solarhealing.com
www.sungazing.com

Total Integration Therapy
www.touch4health.com

Organic/Kosher Meats
www.kolfoods.com

Trager Approach
www.trager.com

Other Helpful Websites:
www.dreammoods.com
www.drrathresearch.com
www.themeatrix.com
www.eatwellguide.com
www.davidwolfe.com
www.sunfood.net
www.mercola.com
www.thetruthaboutsplenda.com
www.healthfreedom.net

www.naturalcuresbook.com
www.whatthebleep.com
www.thesecret.tv
www.thecorporation.com
www.corporatewatch.org
www.prwatch.org
www.tvnewslies.org
www.foxbghsuit.com

Books:

I call this my Still Not Convinced? recommended reading list.

1. Not convinced that pasteurized and homogenized milk is deadly? Then read:
   - *Homogenized Milk May Cause Your Heart Attack: The XO Factor by Kurt A. Oster, M.D.*
   - *Don't Drink Your Milk! by Frank A. Oski, M.D.*
   - *Milk-The Deadly Poison by Robert Cohen*

2. Not Convinced That Aspartame (Nutrasweet®) And Monosodium Glutamate (MSG) Are Deadly? Then Read:
   - *Aspartame (NutraSweet®) Is It Safe? by H. J. Roberts, M.D.*
   - *Excitotoxins-The Taste that Kills by Russell L. Blaylock, M.D.*
   - *In Bad Taste: The MSG Symptom Complex by George R. Schwartz, M.D.*

3. Not convinced that you have a candida yeast overgrowth causing all types of medical problems including excess

weight, arthritis, depression, pms, acne, migraines, stress, constipation, bloating, skin rashes and more? Then read:

- *Lifeforce by Jeffrey S. McCombs, D.C.*

4. Not convinced that subtle energy therapies can cure virtually all disease? Then read:

- *Sanctuary by Stephen Lewis and Evan Slawson*
- *Vibrational Medicine by Richard Gerber, M.D.*
- *Energy Medicine-The Scientific Basis of Bioenergy Therapies by James L. Oschman and Candace Pert, Ph.D.*

5. Not convinced that food additives are a leading cause of illness? Then read:

- *Hard to Swallow by Doris Sarjeant and Karen Evans*

6. Not convinced the food industry is purposely creating foods that make you physically addicted, increase your appetite, make you fat and give you disease? Then read:

- *Fast Food Nation-The Dark Side of the All-American Meal by Eric Schlosser*
- *The Crazy Makers by Carol Simontacchi*
- *Genetically Engineered Food-Changing the Nature of Nature by Martin Teitel, Ph.D. and Kimberly A. Wilson*
- *Food Politics by Marion Nestle and Michael Pollan*
- *Restaurant Confidential: The Shocking Truth About what You're Really Eating When You're Eating Out by Michael F. Jacobson, Ph.D.*
- *Fat Land by Greg Critser*

7. Not convinced that vaccines are deadly, cause disease and should not be used? Then read:

- *A Shot in the Dark by Harris L. Coulter and Barbara Loe Fisher*
- *Vaccines: Are They Really Safe & Effective? by Neil Z. Miller*
- *What Your Doctor May Not Tell You About Children's Vaccinations by Stephanie Cave, M.D., F.A.A.F.P., with Deborah Mitchell*

8. Not convinced that cancer can be cured without drugs and surgery? Then read:

   • *The Cancer Cure That Worked! Fifty Years of Suppression by Barry Lynes*
   • *The Cancer Conspiracy by Barry Lynes*
   • *How to Fight Cancer & Win by William L. Fisher*
   • *The Breuss Cancer Cure by Rudolf Breuss*
   • *The Cancer Industry by Ralph W. Moss, Ph.D.*
   • *The Cure for All Cancers by Hulda Regehr Clark, Ph.D., N.D.*
   • *The Healing of Cancer-The Cures-the Cover-ups and the Solution Now by Barry Lynes*

9. Not convinced that your thoughts can make you sick or heal you? Then read:

   • *Anatomy of an Illness as Perceived by the Patient by Norman Cousins*
   • *Head First-The Biology of Hope and Healing Power of the Human Spirit by Norman Cousins*

10. Not convinced that you should never eat meat or poultry that is not organic? Then read:

    • *Slaughterhouse by Gail A. Eisnitz*
    • *No More Bull!: The Mad Cowboy Targets America's Worst Enemy: Our Food by Howard F. Lyman with Glen Merzer*
    • *Prisoned Chickens, Poisoned Eggs by Karen Davis, Ph.D.*

11. Not convinced that our food is loaded with chemicals causing illness and disease? Then read:

    • *The Chemical Feast by James S. Turner*
    • *A Chemical Feast by W. Harding Le Riche*
    • *Sowing the Wind by Harrison Wellford*

12. Not convinced that electromagnetic pollution is bombarding your body, causing all kinds of medical problems? Then read:

- *Cross Currents-The Promise of Electromedicine by Robert O. Becker, M.D.*
  - *Electromagnetic Fields by B. Blake Levitt*

13. Not convinced that we all have an energetic field around us that is adversely affected by magnetic pollution? Then read:
    - *The Unseen Self, Revised: Kirlian Photography Explained by Brian Snellgrove*
    - *Kirlian Photography-A Hands-On Guide by John Iovine*

14. Not convinced that drugs are poisons and cause most disease? Then read:
    - *Over Dose: The Case Against the Drug Companies Prescription Drugs, Side Effects, and Your Health by Jay S. Cohen, M.D.*
    - *Bitter Pills: Inside the Hazardous World of Legal Drugs by Stephen Fried*

15. Not convinced that the pharmaceutical industry is purposely selling ineffective dangerous drugs, and working tirelessly to suppress natural, effective cures for disease? Then read:
    - *Racketeering in Medicine-The Suppression of Alternatives by James P. Cater, M.D., Ph.D.*
    - *The Drug Lords: America's Pharmaceutical Cartel by Tonda R. Bian*
    - *The Big Fix by Katharine Greider*
    - *The Assault on Medical Freedom by P. Joseph Lisa*
    - *Disease-Mongers: How Doctors, Drug Companies, and Insurers Are Making You Feel Sick by Lynn Payer*
    - *Under the Influence of Modern Medicine by Terry A. Rondberg, D.C.*
    - *The Social Transformation of American Medicine by Paul Starr*
    - *Medical Blunders: Amazing True Stories of Mad, Bad and Dangerous Doctors by Robert Youngson and Ian Schott*

16. Not convinced that psychiatry, and all psychiatric drugs harm patients and actually cause depression, suicide, violent acts, and disease? Then read:

- *Psychiatry: The Ultimate Betrayal by Bruce Wiseman*
- *Your Drug May Be Your Problem by Peter R. Breggin, M.D. and David Cohen*
- *Talking Back To Ritalin by Peter R. Breggin, M.D. and Dick Scruggs*
- *Talking Back To Prozac by Peter R. Breggin, M.D. and Ginger Ross*
- *The Antidepressant Fact Book by Peter R. Breggin, M.D.*
- *The Myth of Mental Illness by Thomas S. Szasz, M.D.*
- *The Manufacture of Madness by Thomas S. Szasz, M.D.*
- *Mad in America by Robert Whitaker*

17. Not convinced that calcium is a nutrient that most people are depleted in? Then read:

- *The Calcium Factor: The Scientific Secret of Health and Youth by Robert R. Barefoot and Carl J. Reich, M.D.*

18. Not convinced that if your body pH is alkaline you can virtually never get sick? Then read:

- *Alkalize or Die by Theodore A. Baroody*
- *Dynamic Health by Dr. M. Ted Morter, Jr.*
- *The Acid-Alkaline Diet for Optimum Health by Christopher Vasey and John Graham*
- *The pH Miracle by Robert O. Young, Ph.D. and Shelly Redford Young*

19. Not convinced that magnets can heal, alleviate pain, and cure disease? Then read:

- *Magnet Therapy: Discover the Powerful New Force in Health and Recovery by Gloria Vergari and Tony Cowell*
- *Healing with Magnets by Gary Null, Ph.D. with Vickie Riba Koestler*

20. Not convinced that aids is one of the greatest hoaxes and deceptions perpetrated on the american public? Then read:

- *Inventing the AIDS Virus by Peter H. Duesberg, Ph.D.*
- *AIDS: What the Government Isn't Telling You by Lorraine Day*
- *Infectious AIDS: Have We Been Misled? by Peter H. Duesberg, Ph.D.*
- *The AIDS War by John Lauritsen*
- *Do Insects Transmit AIDS? by Lawrence Miike*
- *Why We Will Never Win the War on AIDS by Bryan J. Ellison and Peter H. Duesberg, Ph.D.*

21. Not convinced that your digestive system is dysfunctional if you live in america? Then read:

- *Restoring Your Digestive Health by Jordan S. Rubin, N.M.D. and Joseph Brasco, M.D.*

22. Not convinced that stress, anxiety, and emotional problems can be cured almost instanty? Then read:

- *7 Steps to Overcoming Depression and Anxiety by Gary Null, Ph.D.*
- *Dianetics by L. Ron Hubbard.*

23. Not convinced that pain in any part of your body can be eliminated easily without drugs or surgery? Then read:

- *Pain Free: An Evolutionary Method for Stopping Chronic Pain by Peter Egoscue*
- *Instant Relief: Tell Me Where it Hurts and I'll Tell You What to Do by Peggy W. Brill, P.T. and Susan Suffes*
- *Pain Free at Your PC by Peter Egoscue*
- *Natural Relief from Aches & Pains by C. J. Puotinen*

24. Not convinced that women are being exploited by the medical establishment? Then read:

- *The Politics of Stupid by Susan Powter*
- *Hormone Replacement Therapy: Yes or No? by Betty Kamen, Ph.D.*

- *Alternative Medicine Guide to Women's Health by Burton Goldberg*
- *Male Practice: How Doctors Manipulate Women by Robert S. Mendelsohn, M.D.*

25. Not convinced that tap water containing fluoride, chlorine and other contaminants is a major cause of illness and disease? Then read:

- *Fluoride: The Aging Factor by John Yiamouyannis, Ph.D.*
- *Your Body's Many Cries for Water by F. Batmanghelidj, M.D.*
- *Don't Drink the Water by Lono Kahuna Kupua A'o*
- *Water-The Foundation of Youth, Health, and Beauty by William D. Holloway, Jr. and Herb Joiner-Bey, N.D.*
- *The Water We Drink by Joshua L. Barzilay, M.D., Winkler G. Weinberg, M.D., and J. William Eley, M.D.*
- *The Drinking Water Book by Colin Ingram*
- *Water: For Health, For Healing, For Life by F. Batmanghelidj, M.D.*
- *Water Wasteland by David Zwick with Marcy Benstock*

26. Not convinced that arthritis can be eliminated without drugs or surgery? Then read:

- *Arthritis Defeated at Last! The Real Arthritis Cure by Len Sands, N.D., Ph.D., ACRP*
- *Arthritis Beaten Today! by Len Sands, N.D., Ph.D., ACRP*

27. Not convinced that rebounding exercises strengthen every cell in the body, and lead to vibrant health and weight loss? Then read:

- *Looking Good, Feeling Great by Karol Kuhn Truman and Alan Parkinson*
- *Rebounding to Better Health by Linda Brooks*
- *Urban Rebounding: An Exercise for the New Millennium by J. B. Berns*
- *Harry and Sarah Sneider's Olympic Trainer by Harry and Sarah Sneider*

28. Not convinced that the FDA Is purposely suppressing natural cures for diseases and allows drug manufacturers to sell ineffective and dangerous drugs? Then read:

- *Innocent Casualties: The FDA's War Against Humanity by Elaine Feuer*
- *Stop the FDA: Save Your Health Freedom by John Mogenthaler and Steven W. Fowkes*
- *Hazardous to Our Health? by Robert Higgs*
- *Protecting America's Health: The FDA, Business and One Hundred Years of Regulation by Philip J. Hilts*

29. Not convinced that using oxygen can reverse aging, speed healing, and potentially cure many diseases? Then read:

- *Flood Your Body with Oxygen by Ed McCabe*
- *Stop Aging or Slow the Process: How Exercise With Oxygen Therapy (EWOT) Can Help by William Campbell Douglass II, M.D.*
- *Oxygen Healing Therapies by Nathaniel Altman*

30. Not convinced that yoga has amazing health benefits? Then read:

- *Ancient Secret of The Fountain of Youth by Peter Kelder and Bernie S. Siegel*
- *Bikram's Beginning Yoga Class by Bikram Choudhury with Bonnie Jones Reynolds*
- *Power Yoga by Beryl Bender Birch*

31. Not convinced that you can eliminate phobias, traumas, addictions and compulsions in as little as five minutes? Then read:

- *Tapping the Healer Within by Roger J. Callahan, Ph.D. with Richard Trubo*
- *Next Generation Herbal Medicine by Daniel B. Mowrey, Ph.D.*
- *Herbal Tonic Therapies by Daniel B. Mowrey, Ph.D.*

- *Prescription for Herbal Healing: An Easy to Use A-Z Reference by Phyllis A. Balch*

32. Not convinced that homeopathic medicines are a safe natural alternative to drugs and surgery and can cure disease and keep you healthy? Then read:
    - *Everybody's Guide to Homeopathic Medicines by Stephen Cummings, M.D. and Dana Ullman, M.P.H.*
    - *The Complete Homeopathy Handbook by Miranda Castro*

33. Not convinced that fibromyalgia can be eliminated naturally? Then read:
    - *The Fibromyalgia Relief Handbook by Chet Cunningham*

34. Not convinced that there are natural remedies for virtually every disease? Then read:
    - *The Cure for All Diseases by Hulda Reghr Clark, Ph.D., N.D.*
    - *Encyclopedia of Natural Medicine by Michael Murray, N.D. and Joseph Pizzorno, N.D.*
    - *Health and Nutrition Secrets That Can Save Your Life by Russell L. Blaylock, M.D.*
    - *The Natural Physician's Healing Therapies: Proven Remedies That Medical Doctors Don't Know About by Mark Stengler, N.D.*
    - *Alternative Medicine: The Definitive Guide by Larry Trivieri and Burton Goldberg*
    - *Dr. Duarte's The Most Common Diseases & Their Alternative Natural Therapies by Alex Duarte, O.D., Ph.D.*

35. Not convinced that you never have to get sick? Then read:
    - *You Can Be...Well At Any Age: Your Definitive Guide to Vibrant Health & Longevity by K. Steven Whiting, Ph.D.*
    - *How to Get Well: Dr. Airola's Handbook of Natural Healing by Paavo Airola, Ph.D.*
    - *Death by Diet: The Relation Between Nutrient Deficiency and Disease by Robert R. Barefoot*
    - *The Food Revolution by John Robbins and Dean Ornish*

36. Not convinced that proper deep breathing is one of the most beneficial things you can do? Then read:

- *Super Power Breathing for Super Energy, High Health & Longevity* by Paul C. Bragg, N.D. and Patricia Bragg, N.D., Ph.D.

37. Not convinced that your liver is clogged and needs cleansing? Then read:

- *The Liver Cleansing Diet* by Dr. Sandra Cabot, M.D.
- *The Amazing Liver and Gallbladder Flush* by Andreas Moritz
- *The Healthy Liver & Bowel Book* by Dr. Sandra Cabot, M.D.

38. Not convinced that there is an all natural cure for diabetes, and that the pharmaceutical industry offered $30 million to take it off the market? Then read:

- *The Natural Solution To Diabetes* by Richard Laliberte, Pat Harper and William Petit

39. Not convinced that juicing is absolutely needed if you want to get the nutrition your body needs? Then read:

- *The Juice Lady's Juicing For High-Level Wellness and Vibrant Good Looks* by Cherie Calbom, M.S.
- *The Juice Lady's Guide to Juicing for Health* by Cherie Calbom, M.S.
- *The Ultimate Smoothie Book* by Cherie Calbom, M.S.
- *The Joy of Juicing* by Gary Null, Ph.D.
- *Power Juices Super Drinks* by Steve Meyerowitz

40. Not convinced juice fasting is the most effective way to lose weight, cleanse the body of impurities, increase energy, and stimulate the immune system? Then read:

- *Juice Fasting & Detoxification* by Steve Meyerowitz
- *The Miracle of Fasting* by Paul C. Bragg, N.D. and Patricia Bragg, N.D., Ph.D.

41. Not convinced that colon cleansing is absolutely needed by every single person, and that doing so can alleviate illness and disease, increase metabolism and potentially slow or reverse aging? Then read:

- *Cleanse & Purify Thyself. Book One: The Cleanse by Richard Anderson, N.D., N.M.D.*
- *The Detox Diet: Third Edition by Elson M. Haas, M.D. and Daniella Chace*
- *How to Cleanse and Detoxify Your Body Today! by Elson M. Haas, M.D.*
- *Internal Cleansing by Linda Berry, D.C., C.C.N.*
- *The Master Cleanser by Stanley Burroughs*
- *Healthy Living: A Holistic Guide to Cleansing, Revitalization and Nutrition by Susana Lombardi*

42. Not convinced that toxins lodge in the fatty tissues of the body and are causing a host of physical and mental problems? Then read:

- *Clear Body, Clear Mind by L. Ron Hubbard*

43. Not convinced that proper diet can cure illness and lead to vibrant health and wellness? Then read:

- *The 7 Steps to Perfect Health by Gary Null, Ph.D.*
- *The Ultimate Healing System by Donald Lepore*
- *Diet for a New America by John Robbins*
- *Ultimate Lifetime Diet by Gary Null, Ph.D.*
- *Fell's Official Know-It-All Guide: Health & Wellness by Dr. M. Ted Morter, Jr.*

44. Not convinced that energy exists, and energy healing works? Then read:

- *The Healing Energy of Your Hands by Michael Bradford*
- *Quantum-Touch: The Power to Heal by Richard Gordon*
- *Wheels of Light: Chakras, Auras, and the Healing Energy of the Body by Rosalyn L. Bruyere*

45. Not convinced that hydrogenated oil and trans fats cause heart disease and a host of medical problems? Then read:
    * *Trans Fats by Judith Shaw*

46. Not convinced that watching too much television causes the body to become acidic, leading to disease? Then read:
    * *Four Arguments for the Elimination of Television by Jerry Mander*

47. Not convinced that lack of smiles, love and affection can cause illness and a host of emotional disorders? Then read:
    * *A Cry Unheard: New Insights Into The Medical Consequences of Loneliness by James Lynch*

48. Not convinced that what you say and how you say it have a powerful impact on your health and success? Then read:
    * *Should: How Habits of Language Shape Our Lives by Rebecca Smith*
    * *What You Say Is What You Get by Don Gossett*
    * *The Tongue: A Creative Force by Charles Capps*

49. Not convinced that writing things down causes them to happen? Then read:
    * *Write it Down, Make it Happen by Henriette Anne Klauser*

50. Not convinced that you can easily live to be over a hundred years old, never get sick, and that virtually everything i'm saying in this book is true? Then read:
    * *How Long Do You Choose to Live? A Question of a Lifetime by Peter Ragnar*
    * *Gary Null's Power Aging by Gary Null, Ph.D.*
    * *The 100 Simple Secrets of Healthy People by David Niven, Ph.D*
    * *Stopping the Clock by Ronald Klatz and Robert Goldman*
    * *The Longevity Strategy by David Mahoney and Richard Restak*
    * *Successful Aging by John W. Rowe, M.D. and Robert L.Kahn, Ph.D.*

- *The Okinawa Program by Bradley J. Willcox, M.D., Craig Willcox, Ph.D., and Makoto Suzuki, M.D.*
- *On My Own at 107: Reflections on Life Without Bessie by Sarah L. Delany with Amy Hill Hearth and Brian M. Kotsky*
- *Having Our Say: The Delany Sisters' First 100 Years by Sarah L. Delany and Elizabeth Delany with Amy Hill Hearth*
- *Living to 100 by Thomas T. Perls, M.D., M.P.H. and Margery Hutter Silver, Ed.D with John F. Lauerman*
- *Centenarians: The Bonus Years by Lynn Peters Alder, J.D.*
- *If I Live to be 100 by Neenah Ellis*
- *On Being 100 by Liane Enkelis*
- *Centenarians by Dale Richard Perelman*

51. Still not convinced that it's always all about the money, and corruption is permeating corporations and government in america and around the world? Then read:

- *The Informant: A True Story by Kurt Eichenwald*
- *Serpent on the Rock: Crime, Betrayal and the Terrible Secrets of Prudential Bache by Kurt Eichenwald*
- *Rats in the Grain: The Dirty Tricks and Trial of Archer Daniels Midland, the Supermarket to the World by James B. Leiber*
- *Funny Money by Mark Singer*

About the Author

KEVIN TRUDEAU is widely regarded as one of the nation's foremost consumer advocates. He's a New York Times bestselling author who has sold over thirty million books, including six million copies of the original *Natural Cures* book. Adopting as both his business and personal mission statement a vow to "positively impact the whole person," Kevin has built a global business empire that has marketed or sold products he personally uses and believes in 100 percent. Kevin knows from personal experience how big business and government try to debunk individuals who promote products that could hurt the profits of the giant multinational corporations. Kevin is also dedicated to the formation of various foundations to pursue these goals, and has donated part of his fortune for that purpose.

Books by David Halberstam

The Noblest Roman

The Making of a Quagmire

One Very Hot Day

The Unfinished Odyssey of Robert Kennedy

The Unfinished Odyssey
of Robert Kennedy

The Unfinished Odyssey of Robert Kennedy

David Halberstam

 Random House

New York

973.923
K386Yha

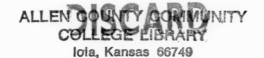

Acknowledgments

Many people assisted in the writing of this book; a list of everyone who cooperated would be hopelessly long. From Senator Kennedy's staff I am particularly indebted to Frank Mankiewicz and Fred Dutton; among colleagues, Dick Harwood, Jimmy Breslin, and Pete Hamill for their coverage of incidents where I was not present. At *Harper's Magazine* Willie Morris and Bob Kotlowitz provided aid and encouragement; Lucille Beachy of *Newsweek* was generous in providing material on the campaign. In addition, William Shannon's *The Heir Apparent* and Dick Schaap's *R.F.K.* were particularly helpful.

18288

This book is for

Bill Barry

and Dick Tuck

Odyssey: . . . 2. . . . A long series
of wanderings, esp when
filled with notable experiences,
hardships, etc.

The Random House Dictionary of the
English Language, Unabridged Edition

The Unfinished Odyssey
of Robert Kennedy

I

In the late summer of 1967, a time of growing social turbulence and dissatisfaction in America, a young liberal named Allard Lowenstein went to visit his senator from New York, Robert Kennedy. A few years before, no two men in the Democratic party could have been more dissimilar: Lowenstein was a reformer, indeed an almost promiscuous reformer. A protégé of Eleanor Roosevelt and quick to enter her name in every conversation, he was identified with a vast list, perhaps too vast a list, of good and decent causes. Indeed it was not a liberal cause unless it were championed by Al Lowenstein. He was exactly the kind of person that Robert Kennedy, just a few years before, had most despised. Then Robert Kennedy had been the tough guy, ramrodding through his brother's nomination and election, and the reformers, God, at the beginning the reformers were almost worse than the Republicans. They hemmed and hawed; they talked too much and said too little; and they loved Stevenson. The reformers were too soft; too issue-prone; too—and this was the worst word yet—predictable. In 1960 Kennedy had exploded before New York's finest and purest reformers, saying, "Gentlemen, I don't give a damn if the state and county organizations survive after November and I don't give a damn if you survive. I want to elect John F. Kennedy President." And they loved that, though in later years when they thought warm thoughts about the Kennedy Presidency they would not remember Robert Kennedy's hard work and vital contribution to that end, but rather the harshness of his words.

Kennedy would have considered Lowenstein one of the worst of them. He was very closely associated with the old New Dealers, always running around Mississippi with black people, and had gone to South Africa and written a book about it. Indeed his liberalism was so pure and so all-encompassing that his friends gently and affectionately mocked it. According to Lowenstein legend, a friend once called his house and asked for him—"Al just left for Spain," replied his mother. "You know he never did like that General Franco. . . ."

By 1967, however, the intensity of social upheaval had brought Lowenstein and Kennedy closer together. Lowenstein was devoting himself to heightening and sharpening the protest against Lyndon Johnson. Ambitious and deeply committed, a rare moralist-activist, and a member of the board of the ADA (though more radical and less anti-Communist than men ten years older than he), he would appear on campus after campus, a veteran student leader, perhaps the oldest in America, giving a focal point to the growing discontent. Whenever *The New York Times* ran a full-page ad saying "Rhodes Scholars Oppose War in Vietnam," or "Mister President, Peace Corps Returnees Oppose Your War," or "College Editors Oppose," etc., it was sure to be the work of Al Lowenstein. He had become truly evangelical on the campus, taking the dissenting and the alienated, telling them, really beseeching them, that yes, they could still work within the system, it could still be done, that protest against the war could be effectively registered within the system. Anyone who saw him during those days would remember the almost feverish quality to his work and remember asking him if it were hard to get kids interested in his crusade, and his answering that the only problem was bringing them back into the system; that no one knew how deeply alienated they were. Then he would excuse himself and fly off to Berkeley for two days and from there to Oregon and from there to Idaho. Al Lowenstein had gone everywhere in 1967, haunting Lyndon Johnson, and he had been properly smeared by Government officials. Peace Corps public-information officers had gone as far as to leak material insinuating that he was very left wing. Now, in the late summer, Lowenstein was trying to convince Robert Kennedy to run for President against Lyndon Johnson.

Kennedy, once a conservative, then an unannounced and reluctant liberal whose credentials were regularly challenged by more orthodox liberals, was by 1967 pursuing a course of increasing radicalism—proffering more radical ideas and taking on, from people like Lowenstein, more radical advice. His course was not so much a consistent philosophy as it was the application of his puritanism (what one friend called his perpetual sense of outrage) to a changing America. The more he looked, the more his vision of the country changed; darkening as he saw more of the inequities and more of the failures. The country was in transition politically, and curiously, so was he.

By both intent and heredity Kennedy had become the leader of the honorable opposition in the Democratic party; the leading critic of the administration's treatment of the ghettos, the leading critic of a great Pandora's box of social problems, and if not the leading critic of the war, the most important politically. When J. William Fulbright attacked the war it annoyed the President, but when Robert Kennedy attacked the war it meant that armies might march. The young liberals and radicals in their thirties and forties, and the college students, those who were staying within the system, no longer turned to Hubert Humphrey for their leadership, but to Robert Kennedy.

Lowenstein, this day, was telling Kennedy that the

time had come when the speeches on Vietnam in the Senate, and the articles for *Look* magazine on the ghetto were no longer enough. It was 1967-going-on-1968 and the army, the vast network of conspirators, was ready to march. It had decided that despite the foremost myth of American politics—Rule One: You cannot unseat a sitting president of your own party—Johnson must and, more important, could be beaten. Lowenstein felt that the issues were far too great to let traditional party loyalty and regulations dominate. Times were different now. The network was in action and was very strong within the Democratic party; Johnson's invincibility was a myth, he could be beaten. The polls showed otherwise, but the polls reflected the mythology. The politicians said otherwise, but as John Kenneth Galbraith, the head of Americans for Democratic Action and another pioneer in the Bust Johnson movement, had said with great insight and accuracy early in 1967, "This is a year when the people are right and the politicians are wrong." It would be a new and different coalition, Lowenstein told Kennedy; it would have to be done outside the party machinery. It would make powerful enemies for Kennedy, but they would be older men; men who, given the changing nature of American politics, would be less influential politically year by year; whereas the friends he would make would be young people and increasingly influential. But it could be done. Johnson was a hollow man politically; no one, and this was crucial, was for him or liked him. The war in the year ahead would get worse, turning more and more hawks to doves, making the opposition more and more respectable. Indeed doing the right thing would be politically advantageous. But the important thing, Lowenstein emphasized, was the nature of the issues —the war and the ghettos. They were issues of moral imperative, so serious that they did not permit waiting until 1972.

They were good friends now, and had been since 1966 when Kennedy, planning to take a trip to South Africa, had prepared a speech with which he was not totally satisfied. Someone recommended Lowenstein as a South African expert and he, as was the Kennedy wont, was summoned imperiously. He could not come, he said, because he was taking Norman Thomas, who was almost blind, to the Dominican Republic. For God's sake, Norman Thomas!, Kennedy said, exasperated—for to him Norman Thomas was *then* and this was *now*—get someone else to take Norman Thomas to the Dominican Republic. It was only at Kennedy Airport that Lowenstein did find someone to escort the old man; and he left to join Kennedy. He looked at the South Africa speech and did not hesitate to tell the Senator that he found it appalling, representing basically the view of the South African Bureau of Tourism—a totally white viewpoint —the conclusion of which was that the South Africans must do a little better by their Kaffirs. Lowenstein criticized the speech sharply and bluntly, and got on the phone to call some South African students attending colleges in the East. When they were assembled, they too rallied, testifying to the fact that it was a disastrous speech; it was accordingly changed, though much to the regret of the South African government. Disliking sycophants, Kennedy was delighted with Lowenstein and his display. They became friends. Kennedy came to value Lowenstein as an extra-intelligence operative, admiring his commitment and idealism, and appreciating the fact that Lowenstein was well connected among some radicals and students. He could help Kennedy interpret the relative merits of the tribes in that particular jungle; a jungle in which he was particularly interested.

But Allard Lowenstein was not the first to tell him to run for the Presidency. Half the people Kennedy met were telling him to run, and the other half, of course, were telling him not to. The dilemma had been with him for some time.

At an ADA meeting in 1967, he had sat with a group of distinguished liberals, all frustrated by the war and their party's control of the presidency. One of the men had said that the great strategy for 1968 would be to have a peace plank in the platform; yes, Lyndon Johnson running on a peace plank. Kennedy had turned and said, "When was the last time you heard of rallying millions of people to a plank?" Robert Lowell, the poet, had bitterly challenged him earlier in the year, saying that Kennedy's ambivalent behavior was disgraceful, and asking what it really was that Kennedy was running for, the presidency of Harvard? Kennedy agreed thoroughly, noting that the way things were going he would be very lucky to get even that.

Kennedy in fact had thought about the race a great deal and had talked to many people; friends from the Kennedy administration, the bosses who had helped put John Kennedy in office. Though he was getting active and enthusiastic encouragement from friends whom he associated with social issues and whose judgment he trusted on these issues, he was getting just the opposite from people whose judgment he trusted on political matters—the people he had always turned to in the past, the professionals. They told him that first: no, it couldn't be done, and second: he would destroy himself in the party if he tried—he would never be forgiven by the party faithful, and would be charged with dividing the party (which was of course already hopelessly divided: the party regulars vs. virtually everyone else). Though this was to be a year in which social issues and new social forces would finally surface politically, Robert Kennedy had not yet realized that; and he sided with the political judgment of the pros. He admired the moral judgment, the sincerity, of people like Lowenstein, but he had talked with Mayor Daley, and Governor Y, and Chairman Z, and they had all said the same thing: you

can't do it, it's not the year, you must wait. We like you; we
loved your brother; and we think favorably of you for 1972,
but you can't do it. And so Robert Kennedy passed this on to
Lowenstein: I'm sorry, he said, I can't do it. And Lowenstein, an intense and consummately serious young man,
looked at him for a long time and then answered: "The
people who think that the future and the honor of this
country are at stake because of Vietnam don't give a shit
what Mayor Daley and Governor Y and Chairman Z think.
We're going to do it, and we're going to win, and it's a
shame you're not with us, because you could have been
President." Then they shook hands rather sadly and parted.

That was how the 1968 campaign began for Robert
Kennedy: it began badly. Later he realized this as his
natural constituency slipped away. In late March, after he
had finally entered the race, he was on a bus with Lowenstein in upstate New York. Overhearing someone say that
Lowenstein had left Eugene McCarthy and had come over
to him, Kennedy excitedly grabbed Lowenstein, anticipating
that this move might bring some of the kids around to his
side, but only to find that he had heard incorrectly. Impressed with Lowenstein's loyalty to McCarthy, and feeling
somewhat sad for himself, later during that ride he took up
a pad and scribbled a note to his friend:

> For Al, who knew the lessons of Emerson and taught it to
> the rest of us: "They did not yet see and thousands of young
> men as hopeful, now crowding to the barriers of their
> careers, do not yet see that if a single man plant himself
> on his convictions and then abide, the huge world will
> come round to him." From his friend Bob Kennedy.

The coalition which was forming in the country in mid-1967
was a loose one, people like Lowenstein and Galbraith,

some of the key officials of the California Democratic Councils, a few eggheads here and there, and occasionally a dissenting party official. The coalition was strong on the campuses, for it was there that the issue of Vietnam had first bloomed politically. It had started with the teach-ins in 1965. The issue had been taken up by white middle-class kids and intensified by the fact that it was not just an intangible moral issue, but indeed a very tangible one—the draft having given it great immediacy. In 1967 the issue had not yet touched some of the traditional centers of the Democratic party such as the labor unions or the party apparatus itself. Though there were places where party officials sensed its presence, they remained silent, for fear that discussion would heighten the issue and the Republicans would end up exploiting it. The party professionals by and large would not accept the fact that it was already an expanding issue. They would sample the temperature of the water as they always had, largely by talking to people very much like themselves, and they would find little if any dissent among what they considered real people. The average non-intellectual American at that time may have felt doubts about the war, but he was being extremely cautious about expressing them. He might have suspected that the war was one great, terrible, stupid disaster, but when asked would perhaps mumble something about protecting Thailand. The professionals, in 1967, did not talk to students, nor to the middle class in the suburbs; they saw little of what was happening.

But the coalition was convinced that this was not a lost cause. The country was ripe for an unorthodox political movement. They believed Johnson to be a war president who could only drag the country deeper into the war and they vowed that their party would not be his vehicle if they could help it. These men were driven by their own moral imperative. They saw the war as a quagmire, the country hopelessly bogged down in a useless, hopeless conflict which could not be won, and they felt that the longer the war went on, the more dangerous and more isolated Johnson became. Writing now, in 1968, it is hard to re-create the atmosphere. They saw a steady migration of doubters from Washington's official circles, and when McNamara left in 1967, they were terrified. Though McNamara had earlier been the symbol of the war, McNamara's War, they thought that he had, by the end, become a voice of sanity. It was rumored in dark corners that McNamara was a dove in hawk's clothing, and the departure of the Good McNamara proved to them the insanity of the administration. They also witnessed the steady ascension of the sycophants, the people who told the President what he wanted to hear. It was no longer a credibility gap, but rather a reality gap, which existed in Washington. The President had never been known as a man to honor those who brought him bad news, and that most human weakness of his—under the pressure of the war's becoming a dangerous one—was becoming worse daily. At a small dinner party for Everett Martin, a distinguished *Newsweek* correspondent just back from two years in Vietnam, Walt Whitman Rostow, the man who chose what the President would see on Vietnam and chose it very carefully indeed, managed to spend a full evening without ever once acknowledging that Martin had been to Vietnam—no small feat. The dissenters in late 1967 were not normal political opponents, they were men genuinely terrified about the course of American action. They were frightened by Johnson's personal identification with the war—he chose every bombing site, he flew every mission—and were uneasy not only with where their country was, but where it was going.

They were also convinced that the alleged hawkish orientation of the country was misleading; that a lot of hawks were only skin deep; and once dovishness was given any kind of serious political outlet, there would be an exodus from hawk to dove. "Our advantage," said Galbraith, "was that even if there were more hawks than doves, the hawks didn't really believe what they said. It was easy to turn them around."

The coalition had sought Kennedy first for he was the ideal candidate. He was not only the logical leader on many of the vital issues, but he was by far the candidate with the broadest base of power. He had the Kennedy name, the Kennedy glamour, and he would be able to hold some of the blue-collar people who might otherwise be outside their coalition because of anti-Negro or pro-war feeling. (Significantly, Lyndon Johnson received his biggest ovations in 1967 at labor-union meetings whereas it was almost impossible for him to visit any campus.) The choice of Kennedy was not an instance of Camelotism or Kennedyism. The Camelot people, the people who had had it very good in the early sixties and who wanted a restoration, were as yet uneasy about the race. They wanted the restoration, but they didn't want to blow it. They were willing to wait until 1972 and thought the country should also be willing. Most of the people pulling for Kennedy to make the race were doing so not because it was Camelot, but precisely because it was not—because Robert Kennedy, in the past few years, had very deliberately taken over the leadership of the disenfranchised and the dissatisfied in America. These people were tough minded. They traveled throughout the country and saw glimmers of political responsiveness that others, sitting in Washington talking to themselves, did not see. For if in those days the average political reporter scorned and underestimated what Lowenstein and Galbraith and others were doing, it was also true that they did not travel as much as these men; and when they did, they talked more often with other political reporters and professional politicians rather than with the people on the campuses and in the middle-class suburbs.

Failing with Kennedy, the coalition started looking around for another candidate. There was the possibility of General James Gavin, the ex-paratrooper who had been making dovish noises, but when they spoke with him, Gavin said he was a Republican. There were some well-known doves in the Senate such as Frank Church and George McGovern and Wayne Morse, but all three had tough fights for reelection on their hands. McGovern, one of the most decent men in the Senate, suggested Lowenstein go out to South Dakota to sample the waters and decide whether he could run for both the Senate and the presidency. Lowenstein did, and reluctantly concluded that McGovern would have to run two different races with two different tones, something that might prove at best embarrassing, and at worst, disastrous. McGovern did say, however, that if no one else would do it they should come back and see him. Then they turned to Eugene McCarthy of Minnesota, perhaps not as outspoken as some of the others on the war, but nonetheless a member of the liberal Senate group, and a man, and this was crucial, who was not up for reelection. McCarthy, when approached by the Turks, was neither messianic nor coy. Yes; he thought someone should make the race, but no; he did not think he was the best choice. He suggested Robert Kennedy as a likelier candidate, a man with a broader base, but he did say that if no one else would run, he would make the race. "There comes a time when an honorable man simply has to raise the flag," he said.

McCarthy seemed an unlikely man to challenge the most active, restless President in recent history. He was a particularly calm, low-keyed man, and even his friends sometimes suspected he had something of an energy gap. He was a liberal (with a few bad marks from the ADA for some of his oil-depletion votes—"Gene is a little soft on minor issues," explained one friend), an ex-professor, and a devout, almost mystic, Catholic. Later in the campaign his aides sometimes complained to each other that he was not available; he could not be reached either physically or spiritually; he was in one of his mystic moods. He was witty; sharp and acid in his comments. Describing the government in South Vietnam, he said it was "not a dictatorship, but a public-relations job." When asked by a reporter what he would do if elected, he mimicked the Eisenhower vow of 1952, saying, "I will go to the Pentagon." He obviously looked down upon most of the men he dealt with in politics, including his colleagues in the Senate, and regarded much of the press with considerable distaste. He was also obviously bright: he would listen to someone for a minute or two and then turn off, having absorbed as much as he thought he wanted to and having become bored. Yet it was part of his particular appeal that his admirers and his critics were equally divided as to whether he was the humblest man ever to enter American politics, or the most arrogant. Indeed it was a distinction that McCarthy himself was well aware of: "There is a fine line," he said once, "between humility and the ultimate arrogance." He could be caustic and witty, and at times his humor bordered on bitterness and one sensed in him a certain petulance; as if the American system had never really given him his due. He was at once the kind of man who could inspire the youth of America with his New Hampshire campaign, bringing them to a feverish pitch of activity, and then note afterward that this primary had proved that all one needed in American politics was a candidate and someone to drive him—a statement which did not endear him to these thousands of young volunteers.

McCarthy had had national ambitions before and, for a variety of reasons, he was not unreceptive when, in late 1967, he was asked to run. In 1960 he had told friends, in one of those half jokes which are much more serious than anyone really intends, that he was a better candidate than Hubert Humphrey, Jack Kennedy, or Stuart Symington, "because [he was] twice as liberal as Hubert, twice as Catholic as Jack and twice as smart as Stu." He never favored the Kennedy candidacy before the nomination, looking down upon Kennedy, as many of the Stevenson disciples did at that time, as something of an intellectual lightweight. In addition, McCarthy, a serious lay intellectual and a not entirely secular man, tended to look down on Kennedy's religious feeling which he thought was less serious than his own. This angered the Kennedys, and Robert Kennedy in particular. The bad feeling was sharpened by McCarthy's behavior at the Los Angeles convention. He arrived there as a supporter of Lyndon Johnson and yet, when the Stevenson boom started, it was he who made the nominating speech. It was probably the best of his career: "Do not turn your back on this man who made us proud to be Democrats." The moment was regarded by most liberals as the high point of the convention—a moment of the heart and brain working together—but was regarded by the Kennedy camp as part of a cynical Johnsonian cabal; a move to halt Jack Kennedy and nominate Lyndon Johnson. Indeed it was a deliberate part of Johnson's strategy to use Stevenson to stop Kennedy on the first ballot. Recalling this incident, in 1967, McCarthy remembered that he preferred Johnson to Kennedy but recalled some of his doubts. "I told people I was for Johnson for prime minister which is a pretty good indication of my reservations. I was sure he could get as much out of a given situation as any man could, but I had doubts about whether he could project the country into a certain direction. That's why I said prime minister—

the prime minister operates within the pattern of his party, subject to his cabinet and the path the party sets, and thus tries to get the most out of that path. It's not as personalized as the presidency. I was wrong about Kennedy though; he did have an institutionalized sense of the presidency, whereas with Johnson you have this terribly personalized presidency—'they're all my helicopters.' (A reference to an incident during which a young airman said 'this is your helicopter, sir,' as the President was about to board the wrong one. The President explained to the airman the error of his ways; 'they're all my helicopters, son.')"

McCarthy and Johnson had stayed reasonably good friends during the Kennedy administration (neither was an insider in those days), and in 1964, when Johnson was dangling the vice-presidency all over Washington, McCarthy was one of those interested. Indeed Senate aficionados attribute one of McCarthy's soft oil votes to vice-presidential hopes. McCarthy was convenient for Johnson in those days too; the President could keep Robert Kennedy off the ticket and still end up with a liberal Catholic. McCarthy rose to the bait. Johnson delighted in playing Humphrey and McCarthy against each other; there was one particularly banal television show in which they outdid each other flattering the President. There was a certain quality of low-level humiliation to it and finally McCarthy, realizing what was happening, sent a telegram to the President, withdrawing. Thus he spared himself, as Senator Thomas Dodd did not, being a puppet in the very last minute of the marionette show. (William S. White, Johnson's favorite columnist, later wrote that McCarthy was still bitter over the incident and that this had made him more willing to run in 1968. "What meat then is feeding this improbable Caesar, Eugene McCarthy?" intoned White, no small authority on Caesars himself, ". . . a fierce fire of ambition, fanned by the hot, fanatic thirst that now grips the throats of the American peacenik movement.)"

But now in 1968, after McCarthy entered, the feeling between Kennedy and McCarthy—the two key men who would be in opposition to Johnson—was still surprisingly hostile. This became a vital factor as the campaign developed and minor points became major ones, and the uneasiness and mutual suspicion developed into genuine hard feeling. At the start, when McCarthy first went in, they wished each other well and spoke well of one another. Though Kennedy still talked ambivalently about supporting Johnson, he gave McCarthy good advice about New Hampshire; enter and run against the machine. And McCarthy spoke well of Kennedy, regularly denying that he was his stalking horse. However McCarthy did concede, as he told this reporter in early December, that, because the issue involved was so great, if Kennedy finally did enter, he would probably move aside. There would be no problem there; Kennedy had a larger base. But underneath there was considerable hostility. McCarthy regarded Kennedy as an intellectual inferior, an arrogant and pushy young man cashing in on his brother's myth and his family's money. One always sensed that a good deal of McCarthy's hostility toward the American political system, and this hostility existed, came from the advantages he felt it gave the rich. He felt his own natural resources were greater than Kennedy's, and if wealth were not a factor, there would be no comparison.

Robert Kennedy, for his part, retained a blind spot as far as John Kennedy was concerned. Those who had helped him (such as Hubert Humphrey; there was a curious sense of sympathy and friendship for Humphrey because after the Kennedy's had fought him, and had broken him in West Virginia, Humphrey had rallied to campaign for Jack Kennedy and had wept at the news of his death) had a special place, and those who had downgraded him were rarely reprieved; and McCarthy had downgraded him. But it went deeper; Kennedy, the evangelist, thought McCarthy a cynical man, a lazy man; and the part of Kennedy which loved power was uneasy about McCarthy's course. Sometimes he saw in it elements of another Henry Wallace campaign (a curious aspect of Kennedy, for he himself sought the very people that McCarthy had), and he wondered whether McCarthy was stronger than some of the people swirling around him. In late December their relationship was still cordial but suspicious; Kennedy was still playing Hamlet on whether or not to run. The Kennedy people suggested to McCarthy that he enter New Hampshire and run there and stay out of Massachusetts, which might prove more difficult and which, of course, was regarded as their very own preserve. McCarthy, hearing that, immediately entered Massachusetts. He had not intended to enter New Hampshire until his arm was virtually twisted into it by his own people. There was no mutual ease, and it was to get worse between them. One remembered Kennedy, several months later, preparing to go on *Face the Nation* and going through a mock press conference with aides. Someone, posing as a reporter, asked him, "Senator Kennedy, would you support President Johnson if he is the nominee?" "That's easy," Kennedy said smiling, "but don't ask me whether I would support McCarthy." Fortunately for him no one asked.

The race seemed on the surface a dubious honor in the first place. In late December and early January, Lyndon Johnson appeared to be supreme. He dominated his own party and though his own party was restless, it appeared paralyzed and bound to him by loyalty and tradition. The Republicans might run against him, but it was hard to imagine a Republican candidate running to the left of him on the war and on the ghettos. Johnson appeared to be a war president who would somehow hold the center. Anyone to the left of him would be a super-dove, anyone to the right of him would be a super-hawk. He would try and hold the Negroes with one hand (behind his back), while he would softly work the crime-in-the-streets issue with the other hand. Though the war was not going well, it did not appear to be going badly either, and again, the dissent was within his own party and thus not serious dissent. But Lyndon Johnson was tied to the war, and it was becoming a bitterly unpopular war. Both the nature of the war and the nature of Lyndon Johnson would combine in 1968 to destroy him, and destroy him where he was supposed to be unbeatable, within his own party.

The war. Nothing dominated American life in 1967 and 1968 like the war. It flashed across the television sets each night; it sapped the financial resources of the country and more, it sapped its moral fiber. In a country consumed by serious social problems everything eventually led back to the war; nothing could be done until the war was over. Much of the tension between black and white was directly traceable to the war and the breakdown of poverty programs it had effected; much of the intensifying division between young and old stemmed from youth's opposition to the war. At a time of growing disillusion with American life, a younger generation found many of the inequities of this country difficult to accept. The war somehow seemed to them to symbolize the thrust of American life; and it was Lyndon Johnson's war.

Curiously enough it had been a minor issue in the election of 1964. Vietnam was simply a distant country which Barry Goldwater wanted to defoliate and which Lyn-

don Johnson thought unworthy of the lives of American
boys, particularly because Asian boys should be doing the
job. So it was a muffled issue, overshadowed by the overall
issue of Goldwaterism: Was Goldwater safe? Wouldn't he
just lob one into the Kremlin men's room? Did you want
Goldwater's finger on the button? Johnson would ask, and
then he'd gnash his own thumb on an imaginary button,
and one knew with great relief that Johnson would not do
anything foolish, would not push buttons, would not send
the Marines anywhere, would not lob grenades into anyone's men's rooms. (The post-election Republican joke was:
"They warned me if I voted for Goldwater we would get in a
big war, and the Marines would be sent out, and we would
bomb North Vietnam; and I voted for Goldwater and they
were right.")

But the atmosphere was curiously relaxed in 1964. A
reporter just back from Vietnam and covering the political
campaign found a surprising lack of interest among the
candidates and their staffs about the war, though fateful
decisions were near at hand. Everyone seemed to assume
that it was going badly or at least not very well, but that
somehow it would go away. The campaign went its way;
Vietnam was not the issue, Goldwater was. Goldwater destroyed himself as a candidate. Johnson was elected by a
landslide on a mandate of peace. The words hawk and dove
did not exist together in the modern political lexicon. The
thrust of the right wing seemed terminated; they had finally
run their very own candidate, with disastrous results for the
Republican party. Now the country seemed curiously
united; ready, after many years of delay, to turn this great
restless powerhouse of a President loose on long neglected
urban and racial problems. Johnson, though not beloved by
the liberal columnists, was respected by them. They described him as a healing man and America, God knew, had
enough things to heal. Yet the day after his landslide victory

aides placed on his desk a list of targets to be bombed in the north—thus assuring, at its very beginning, the end of the Great Society, the destruction of Johnson's presidential years, and his downfall in 1968. For though the issue had been avoided during the campaign, the problems had not gone away; they were all there. All the agonizing decisions of Indochina, delayed ten years, finally had to be confronted —whether the president be Lyndon Johnson, Barry Goldwater or John Kennedy. The proxy war, itself a desperate measure, had been going badly for more than a year and a half. Our proxies could barely hold out (indeed that they had held out that long was itself astounding). The Vietcong had reached the point where they were ambushing not just platoons at night, but now battalions, and even regiments, and often in the daytime. Despite all the calm and placid assurances of Secretary McNamara and General Maxwell Taylor, it was obviously only a short time before the whole proxy effort would collapse.

The war in Vietnam is different from other wars, it is not a war for control of terrain. The side with the greater armament, with all the airplanes, could appear for a long time to be stronger than it really was, its kill statistics would be greater, and its political liabilities barely visible (except in the cold sullen eye of a peasant) and for these reasons it had been possible to sweep the problems of Vietnam under the rug. It had made it possible for men in high places to fool themselves and fool men in even higher places, and for the reality to be delayed, again and again, until finally, one day, the problems surface. When they surface to the insider, they do so only after he has already been caught out on a limb—made too many rash statements, too many easy promises and predictions—and gotten himself in a position where he and his vanity are terribly trapped. When they surface to the general public, it is with a deadly finality.

The American commitment to Vietnam began in 1954

after the French had lost their war and the country was divided. It was the time of Dulles' containment, and the idea was to create an anti-Communist, anti-colonialist state in the South. But from the start the idea was doomed; the Communists had taken over the nationalism of Indochina during their eight-year war, and now all the dynamism, all the talent and drive, all the best young men were on their side, and it would be only a matter of time before that showed militarily and politically in the South. Frustrated by the U.S.-Diem decision against holding free elections (Eisenhower had noted very simply at the time that had the elections been held, Ho Chi Minh would have won in the South), Hanoi, in 1959, began to use its proxies in the South in the second Indochina war. The American proxy was the Diem regime, suspicious, increasingly isolated from all other elements in the country, its base narrowing all the time. Diem's situation did not improve with the American aid. In 1962 Bernard Fall interviewed Pham Van Dong, the North Vietnamese prime minister, and asked about Diem's personal position. "It is quite difficult," Dong said. "He is unpopular and the more unpopular he becomes, the more American aid he will need to remain in power. And the more American aid he gets, the more of an American puppet he'll look and the less likely he is to regain popularity."

"That sounds pretty much like a vicious circle," commented Fall.

"No," said Pham Van Dong, "it's a downward spiral."

The Kennedy administration had come into office in 1961. It immediately suffered a series of foreign policy setbacks—a particularly difficult position for a young president with a razor-thin margin of victory. There was the Bay of Pigs, Laos, the Berlin Wall, Khrushchev's bullying at Vienna, and now it looked like Vietnam was about to go down the drain. Its government clearly could not hold out much longer despite its own predictions. In addition to their setbacks there was one other quite separate force which drove the Kennedy administration into Vietnam, and this was a basic contempt for the Eisenhower administration. The Kennedy people looked upon their predecessor as flabby, unaware of a changing world, and far too dependent upon military response. It had been ignorant of the subtleties and possibilities of guerrilla warfare in the third world. The Communists, they felt, had been using this effectively against us, and now it would be used against them. They believed that the failure of the Eisenhower administration in Vietnam lay in the fact that the South Vietnamese army had been trained for a conventional war, while it was fighting in reality an unconventional one. There was a certain arrogance to this, a feeling that they were tougher, brighter and more contemporary than the Eisenhower people, and Robert Kennedy was one of the worst offenders. He became the New Frontier's leading student on guerrilla warfare and Green Beretism, the latter being something of a Washington fad.

Kennedy increased the American commitment to Vietnam—there were now 15,000 advisers as opposed to 600 and Americans were now flying dangerous combat missions in helicopters and old World War II fighter bombers. The flag was planted just that much more (Eisenhower, despite all the Dulles bombast, or perhaps precisely because of it, had never bothered to plant the flag; coming back from World War II he had never felt the political pressure to be a hero or to prove his anti-communism that his two successors might feel). The Kennedy escalation was an action taken out of weakness more than anything else. We had escalated to keep from being driven out of Indochina, and at a price— we had involved ourselves that much deeper; it was no longer a highly avoidable war. We had gone in on the

recommendation of Maxwell Taylor, Kennedy's special en-
voy in Vietnam. Galbraith, Kennedy's all-purpose critic,
had read the Taylor report at the time, in 1961, and had
told the President that it was "a most curious document. It
calls for certain changes and aids to the government but
notes that given the nature of the government these changes
cannot be achieved." Robert Kennedy was always to have
ambivalent opinions about the origins of the war in which
he was involved, and particularly the role of Taylor who
had become a close family friend. In 1964, while covering
his campaign for the Senate, I remember Maxwell Taylor's
name having come up in conversation. Ethel Kennedy
asked, with her usual enthusiasm, "Don't you just love
Max Taylor?" I said rather bitterly that I did not, that I
thought him one of the most overrated men in American
life and that I thought he was one of the men most responsible for a growing tragedy. Ethel turned white, hurt and
offended, and moved away. Ed Guthman, the normally
good-natured press secretary, grabbed me angrily and said
"Goddamit, don't you know better than to criticize Max
Taylor to her. What the hell's wrong with you?" We argued
sharply and it was a chilly evening the rest of the way. Even
in 1968, when Robert Kennedy was one of the major critics
of the war, some of the ambivalence remained. When asked
about Taylor, he would say with a certain sadness, "Well he
was very helpful to President Kennedy. . . . "

There is a particular quality about this war, a quality
which was to have a very considerable political effect,
albeit a delayed one. For this is a war in which you can
fake it. It is not like desert warfare where if one side is
stronger than the other, it is painfully apparent the very
next day; nor even like conventional war where the evidence

is slower to come, but comes nevertheless—an army inching ahead, holding terrain, a mile or two a day. But in guerrilla warfare, military-political warfare, the stronger side, in military-*political* terms, does not hold terrain, it lacks airpower and heavy artillery and thus does not produce statistics which can match those of the weaker side. Indeed most of what it does best is invisible to the Western eye, and particularly to the Western military eye, which is accustomed and trained to look for something entirely different—in this case, something highly misleading. Thus the weaker side can and did, in Vietnam, delude itself into believing that its charts and predictions were true, and that it was winning. Powerful men with powerful vanities were sucked deeper into avoidable mistakes.

This happened in 1962 and 1963 in Vietnam. Slowly in this proxy war our proxies began to lose and lose badly at an ever intensifying rate; the Vietcong becoming more audacious by the day. Thus the booster-shot commitment had, in late 1963 and 1964, come to an end. Very soon a president would have to make the most basic decision of all; a decision which had been postponed through four administrations—all the way in, or all the way out. But this was a subsurface dilemma, it was still not evident to the American public. Nor was it evident to the American politicians— whether by August of 1964 the White House realized it or wanted to realize it is a matter for conjecture; people at a certain point believe what they want to believe. There was a handful of reporters in Vietnam in 1964 and, though the best of them were pessimistic, they hardly represented a major political voice. On the theory that any news was bad news, the administration had long ago decided to tell the public as little as possible about Vietnam. Any candid admission about where the U.S. stood would point to the fact that all previous predictions had been highly fallacious and would be highly embarrassing to the men already in power. An administration can talk candidly about the errors of American foreign policy only if those errors were made by a previous administration. So, in 1964, the administration kept the reality of the war hidden. What should have been the dominant issue of the 1964 campaign was shelved. Johnson was the peace candidate, peace being but a general thing, and Goldwater was the war candidate. Had he known of the onrushing dilemma in Vietnam, Goldwater might have campaigned vigorously for escalation and Johnson might have moved to the left. Had it been as such, he would have entered the presidency with Vietnam an issue, with himself a partial dove, and would have still been elected by a landslide. He had no such luck.

Thus Johnson was elected by a landslide, but on the key issue of the time he had gotten a free ride, and now he was afraid of his own mandate. He had postponed the decision, and he had postponed it at the price of his own credibility. From the very moment he escalated, his credibility was to be put seriously in doubt, particularly within his own party. He was to start his first full term by creating an issue which would eventually cost him his second term. He had not trusted the American people, and this set a pattern which was to haunt him. Now, newly elected, he had to deal with the immensity of the problem. He was elected a peace candidate and yet he had a special vision of himself; he saw himself somehow as a figure in *High Noon*. "Sell the Johnson image as one of a big tall tough Texan," he told Pierre Salinger in 1960. In truth he was not a particularly good rider, and his World War II Silver Star was a bogus one. As for the war, he did not see it in terms of the modern world, as a struggle in an underdeveloped country in which Communists had taken over the nationalism and where the arrival of Caucasian soldiers might aid the enemy politically, but rather in terms of his own reckoning of the domino theory. "I am not going to be the President who saw Southeast Asia go the way China went," he said. In military terms, he saw the war not as an extension of the French war— what one reporter later described as dreaming different dreams than the French, but walking in the same footsteps —but as an extension of the Alamo. He told the National Security Council: "Hell, Vietnam is just like the Alamo. Hell, it's just like if you were down at that gate and you were surrounded and you damn well needed somebody. Well by God, I'm going to go—and I thank the Lord that I've got men who want to go with me, from McNamara right on down to the littlest private who's carrying a gun." Tom Wicker, of *The New York Times,* quotes Johnson talking about his Mexican neighbors in his excellent book on Johnson and Kennedy. "They'll come right in your yard and take it over if you let them. And the next day they'll be right on your porch barefoot, and weighing one hundred and thirty pounds, and they'll take that too. But if you say to 'em, 'hold on, wait just a minute,' they'll know they're dealing with someone who'll stand up. And after that, you can get along fine." "The enemy in Vietnam," noted Wicker, "was barefoot and weighed one hundred and thirty pounds. He was the kind of man who might be fine in his place, who could be a useful citizen and a good friend if he let you train him right and help him a little, but who would take over your front porch if you didn't stand up to him. Lyndon Johnson was not about to let little brown men who skulked in the jungle do that to him and the United States of America. . . ."

Badly advised by his immediate aides, most of whom were Kennedy men, Lyndon Johnson, who had helped deny John Foster Dulles the air strikes he had sought for Dienbienphu in 1954, now plunged the country into what would be a major, useless, tragic and divisive war. He did it with a totally unnecessary miscalculation of the nature of the war, of the enemy, and of his own popular mandate. He did it at a time when America's domestic problems were in desperate need of a solution, or at least the beginning of a solution. He listened to the military whom he had traditionally mistrusted, and who had already been proven consistently wrong on Vietnam. He had entered the office with an extraordinary mandate for social progress in America, intent on going down as a great president. Now the war was to destroy his presidency, destroy his hopes for social reform, cloud his chances for any serious historical recognition and, perhaps most bitter of all, the divisions and unrest the war was to create would rebound to the political advantage of the Democratic politician he disliked the most, Robert Kennedy. The Johnson years would look like a terrible Greek tragedy; both John Kennedy and Lyndon Johnson would have their Bays of Pigs—but one would last for several days and the other, for several years.

Normally this country supports its wars. They are not things to be sought after; but if unavoidable, and all other things being equal, the people will rally around—for a limited period of time, perhaps because this is a democracy —and give the administration the benefit of the doubt. But this war very quickly became different. Its historical roots were questionable; it was very far away and not noticeably connected to American security; it inflicted a particularly high price on noncombatants, something abhorrent to the American mind; and it had already been surrounded by a very considerable amount of disingenuousness. The more scrutiny the war received, the more the public would not like it. This was not because Americans were too soft and too unwilling to take on a difficult, complicated challenge, but because it was only with time that they would find the war not only untidy, but unworthy and unwinnable. And this, the long-range public distaste for the war, was, like the bogging down of American forces, entirely predictable.

Almost from the start the war was questioned. The major columnists of the country sensed that the more the country committed itself to Vietnam, the deeper it seemed to get, yet without getting any closer to victory. There was growing distrust of the President, who was, to use James Reston's phrase, escalating by stealth. Step by step the Americans were drawn in deeper and deeper. Now there were 500,000 in Vietnam, but even that many seemed to be sucked in by the lush countryside. The most powerful nation in the world, one which had brought tangible physical power to an awesome new degree, appeared to be using that power against a people who seemed, at best, to be mounted on water buffalo. Hawks and doves were named, and for a time it was fashionable to be a hawk. Hawks were tough and respectable; there was nothing queer about hawks. Doves were soft, dubious, perhaps unpatriotic; they might, under certain conditions, give away most of Southeast Asia. For a time doves would dress in hawks' clothing, keeping their dark secret as hidden as possible. But as the nation learned more and more about the war, the migration went in only one direction—from hawk to dove. The more that was perceived, the more respectable it became to be a dove. The real opposition began on the campuses. A new generation with a vast untapped political potential of its own felt particularly strongly about the war, and felt itself basically unrepresented in America. It had felt itself represented when Kennedy was alive; Johnson it regarded as much older, both because of years and because of style. As for the House of Representatives, it wrote it off as a citadel of old men in their fifties and sixties. This generation was a potent political force; for a politician in his late thirties or early forties not to deal with it, not to sense its moods and priorities, would have been like a politician in the late 1930s not taking into account the preferences of blue-collar workers. Twelve and a half million Americans had come of voting age since the 1964 election, and while they would not be a lifetime political force for the Lyndon Johnsons of America, they would for the Robert Kennedys and John Lindsays—a politician who neglected them on the war might never get them back. Political authorities noting these statistics have always pointed out that traditionally the young do not vote; but, as Kennedy aide Fred Dutton pointed out, the poor never voted either, until Roosevelt came along, and then they had a reason; and perhaps, in 1968, this would also be true of the young. (Not all politicians sensed this. Much later in the year a former Kennedy man was called in by Humphrey to discuss ways in which he might attract the youth. "Young people," said Humphrey, "they don't vote." Yes, said his assistant Bill Connell, "all they do is smoke pot.") To the young the war was regarded as *their* work, the work of old men wallowing in the past, repeating the old mistakes of American life. The college students felt the war intensely; it was not a vague issue, but indeed one that might take their lives. In home after home, their influence on their parents would be spectacular—this was to be one reason why the upper-middle class suburbs would be so dovish in 1968.

There developed a certain rhythm to the opposition to the war; it increased in multiples. The longer the war went on, the more people learned about it, and the more they were driven into opposition, thus encouraging others to dissent. The longer the war went on, the more it was not just a little war, but rather a war which began to dominate

American life. Men who had formerly kept their doubts private were now moved to express them. Now it was affecting not just the automatic doves, the people whose opposition was easily predictable, but more conservative establishment figures—men who watched carefully and were worried not so much about the war itself but about what it was doing to America. Gradually they came in; and as establishment figures came in, the opposition became more respectable, and thus even more doves surfaced. By 1967 the opposition to the war was at least as respectable as that in support of it, and it was growing all the time. The war was now backfiring; all the promises of Johnson and Westmoreland were being undermined daily. The doubters were beginning to look increasingly prophetic. Day by day, starting in late 1966, opposition to the war was becoming increasingly centralized; it was hard to gauge electorally, but it was there and growing.

The American public thinks of Lyndon Johnson as being too much of a politician. Poll after poll shows this, and as such the myth has grown that Johnson, whatever else, is a master politician. Curiously, Johnson is not a particularly good politician at all. He understands the Senate, how to maneuver and how to manipulate and overpower men there—how to deal with their weaknesses and strengths at close quarters—but he does not understand national politics, the delicate and complex balance of a country, particularly well. He tried to play Senate politics at the Democratic Convention in 1960, and was destroyed. Now in the White House he proved himself a bad politician again. He was unwilling to trust the public, but tried instead to outsmart it—in doing so, becoming increasingly a prisoner of his massive vanity. He was unable to confess error to a population remarkably tolerant of error, particularly if it is self-confessed. Of course a man who confesses to error is ipso facto not a politician; he is an honest man. The more opposition mounted, the more Johnson responded to it; but he responded with temporary measures: tricks, gimmicks, peace feelers, flying trips to Hawaii, trips to Vietnam, the bringing home of Westmoreland. Of course every time he did something, every time there was a trip or a gimmick, there would be a positive response—the nation would be pleased, the polls would show an increase in his popularity, and the doves would be on the defensive. But the war was not just a temporary thing. Though it was pleasant and colloquial to talk about bringing back coonskins, the war was, in reality, a cruel hopeless conflict which could not be won, which would not go away, and in which the balance had not been altered. Very powerful forces were at work there, and they would not be gimmicked. What Lyndon Johnson was doing all those years, starting in 1965, was buying time for his war; but again, he was doing so at the price of his own credibility, and again, it was a very high price indeed. Each time the cry against the war rose, he would fend off the critics, but he would use up a little more of his credibility. Thus he was buying temporary success but creating long-term problems. A smart politician doesn't do that. Instead, he suffers immediate problems and takes the long-range gain—he is willing to let the polls be low early in the administration if he is accruing gains which will help him at election time.

Moreover Lyndon Johnson was mistaken in his ideas about consensus opinion and his own position within the Democratic party. The consensus he was after was a national one, half Republican and half Democratic, but the dissent happened to be in the Democratic party which might block his chance to run again. One had only to look at the Senate Foreign Relations Committee, where almost all of the Democrats dissented and many of the Republicans assented, to understand the curious political split. Johnson was taking his own normal constituency for granted, counting on the traditional mythology, and concentrating instead on taking over what he believed was the middle. This might seem like a smart strategy, but in the process his natural base, the liberal wing of his own party—a faction of great influence and vocal power in this country—had almost completely turned on him. Thus the people who should have normally been most devotedly for him, willing to work for him, to contribute to his campaign, to publicize his many virtues, were most devotedly and passionately against him.

In this period of growing social and political dissatisfaction, the role of Robert Kennedy was crucial. He was at the exact median point of American idealism and American power. He understood the potency of America's idealism, as a domestic if not an international force, and yet he had also exercised American power. The correlation was such that his speeches could be written by young radicals like Adam Walinsky and Peter Edelman, and yet his children named after Douglas Dillon and Maxwell Taylor. Though Kennedy was part of the politics of the past, and had dealt skillfully, if at times somewhat roughly, with the old bosses, he understood the mandate of the new politics and the importance of keeping up with the kids. If he had been a partner, and for a long time an enthusiastic one, to early decisions in Vietnam, by the end of

his brother's presidency he had been one of the first to
sense that things were not working out. In 1968 reporters
traveling with him, or with one of his aides, like Kenny
O'Donnell, would hear again and again the lament about
those days: They kept promising us, they kept misleading
us. From the start Kennedy had doubted the validity of the
American commitment of combat troops, sensing that the
war was unwinnable. He went out of his way to keep himself
informed on Vietnam, talking to all the dissenters, to people
who had visited Hanoi. At a time when the administration
was carefully screening itself from any informed doubter,
making sure that no criticism reached the President's ears,
Kennedy was talking to all the people who were voicing
their private and public doubts about the war. He knew
also what the war was doing to the country, that it was
sharpening the existing divisions, making the thin fabric
which bound American life that much thinner.

Yet his position was particularly vulnerable. In a sense
there were not just two political parties in America in the
late sixties, but really three—the Democrats headed by
Johnson, the Republicans, and the Kennedys, almost a party
unto themselves. It was a government in exile with its own
shadow cabinet and with Robert Kennedy as the titular
head. Everything he did was viewed as part of his own
candidacy—every move, every motive was doubted; nothing
could be innocent. If he spoke out on Vietnam it would not
be judged as a statement by a concerned politician on a
crucial issue, but as an instance of petty political maneuver-
ing. Yet the other half of that coin was his power: dissent
by Robert Kennedy on the war was not idle dissent, it was
dissent by so powerful a political figure on so important an
issue as to represent a frontal challenge to the administration. With Robert Kennedy on their side the doves would

become that much more respectable. The Kennedys are not soft, they are tough; they are Irish; they are formidable practicing politicians, and one is not ashamed to have them as colleagues. Had any other politician in America spoken, as Robert Kennedy almost innocently had, of giving blood to the Vietcong, his career as a serious political figure would have been over; for Kennedy it was a temporary slip. If Robert Kennedy became a dove, a lot of other people, senators, writers and plain citizens, would feel more at ease in joining them; and those tenuously critical of the administration would be encouraged and strengthened, and they would become more sharply critical. The entire rhythm of protest would be accelerated that much more.

In early 1966 Robert Kennedy broke with the administration over Vietnam. There was no single clear point of demarcation, rather it was more a matter of tone and emphasis. He did not really attack the war or the President, he simply said that the emphasis of the war was wrong, that the administration was placing too much emphasis on military solutions as opposed to political solutions, perhaps a coalition, perhaps a bombing halt. It was not so much criticism as implied criticism; it was not so much an attack upon the administration as it was implied support of the dissenters. But both the administration and the dissenters knew where Kennedy was headed. If Lyndon Johnson had escalated the war by stealth, Robert Kennedy was becoming a dove by stealth—but his course was clear. In November 1966, right after the congressional elections, at a time when American political conversation turns inevitably to the next presidential election, a group of *Time* magazine writers assembled at dinner. One reporter, just back from Vietnam and knowledgeable about the war and the coming frustration there, predicted that Kennedy would run for the presidency in 1968—not because he wanted to, not because he intended to, but because forces outside his control would demand that he do so. The war could only get worse, and as the war became worse the public malaise would grow, and by March 1968, the crucial time—the time of the primaries —the pressure on Kennedy as the leader of the opposition would be unbearable. He would have to either run or surrender leadership. For that position was not just his alone, the party at this particular time inevitably would have a bright young man who would represent fresher ideas and a rallying point. The Kennedy phenomenon had made the Kennedys the controllers of that particular position, and after the assassination it had fallen by succession to Robert Kennedy. With their power and their ability to attract intellectuals the Kennedys so dominated the young leadership of the party that anyone else virtually had to fall into their orbit, clear it with them whether or not he ran. But that slot which Robert Kennedy held as the youthful attractive figure challenging the old order was one which would exist without him, it was a natural vacancy, not a man-made one— and his control of it might be only temporary.

His dissent grew, and with it, the opposition to the war. The White House predictions about imminent victory came and went, developing a rhythm of their own. Optimism about imminent victory was followed by a call for more troops, which was followed by more optimism for a more imminent victory. The ghettos became increasingly restless; city after city burned. The unique ghetto was the one which did not burn. As these forces mounted, Kennedy himself became increasingly radical and listened more and more to radical *social* voices. By early 1967 he was preparing to make a major address on Vietnam—a real and serious break with the administration which would become a watershed of opposition. He traveled through Europe meeting heads of state. In Paris he might even have been the recipient of a peace feeler, though one never knew (peace feelers are where you find them, if you want to find them; there was a time in 1966 when the mayor of every city in every neutral country proclaimed that he had just received a peace feeler). Then he returned to Washington to meet with Johnson for a final break.

All the bitterness and acrimony between these two powerful men, perhaps the two most powerful men in the country—one with actual power, the other with potential power—surfaced at the meeting. Kennedy had never been generous with the President after his brother's assassination. He felt that Johnson was a usurper of his brother's office, and a destroyer of his brother's dream, the dream of all the fine young men. Now that dream was being betrayed, being dragged into a hopeless war. Johnson, proud and vain, nursed long-held antagonism for Robert Kennedy. Kennedy had not wanted him on the ticket in 1960; he had treated him with disdain for three years in office, and had then wanted to be Johnson's vice-president. Johnson felt that Kennedy had never forgiven him for his ascension, that he had behaved ungenerously to him—"All that boy has done since I became President," he told one friend, "is snipe at me. He's been running for office since I was sworn in." His feelings were sharpened by the ease with which Kennedy handled public relations, by the glamour which was attached to Kennedy and which eluded him, and he was particularly bitter about Vietnam. He felt he was carrying out the Kennedy mandate, using the Kennedy people, and now he was being politically attacked by the young man who started it. Robert Kennedy himself had said in 1962, in Saigon, "We are going to win and we are going to stay here until we win." The President was angry and bitter. He began the meeting by denouncing Kennedy for having made alleged peace-talk leaks.

Kennedy immediately replied that he had not leaked anything. "That came from your state department," he said.

"It's your state department," Johnson said angrily.

Then they began to argue bitterly. Kennedy, according to some reports, called the President a son of a bitch. Then Johnson began to talk about the war, to criticize Kennedy for running down his own country. He told Kennedy that he would soon be in serious political difficulty. "We are going to win this war, and in six months all of you doves will be politically dead." The President continued, in a line of argument he frequently used; the anger showed in his voice. Criticism by Kennedy and others encouraged Hanoi to hold on. Hanoi was tired and losing, but the doves kept alive their false hopes and kept the war from ending. The doves were prolonging the war. If you persist, he said, "the blood of American boys will be on your hands." He looked at Kennedy and told him, "I could attack you in exactly those words and if I do, you will be finished."

"I don't have to sit here and listen to this kind of talk," Kennedy said. The meeting broke up.

Less than a month later, after an enormous amount of advance build-up, Kennedy made his major Vietnam speech. The build-up had been immense, and for days reporters had been clamoring for leaks. Would he be hawk or would he be dove? "We'll send up puffs of white smoke if it's dovish, gray if it's hawkish," said Frank Mankiewicz, his press secretary. The decision, when it came, was a clear break with the administration. While admitting his own responsibility for past mistakes, he finally came out and attacked the war itself and U.S. responsibility for it. "It is *we* who live in abundance and send our young men to die. It is our chemicals that scorch children and our bombs which level villages. . . ." He called for a bombing pause and a coalition settlement supervised by the United Nations. Johnson was not amused. He gave two speeches that same day, and also announced that Russia had agreed to discuss the limiting of the missile race.

Thus Robert Kennedy broke with the administration and acceded to the titular leadership of not only the Kennedy party, but also of those who were now leading the dissent on Vietnam and were looking for strong political leadership. (Many of them had been formerly anti-Kennedy; barely reconstructed Stevensonians.) It was perhaps smart politics, but it was done, ironically, without any political stratagem in mind. In early 1967 it was quite clear that Kennedy had no intention of running for office—he did it because he could not do otherwise. Yet in accepting the leadership of the opposition, he accepted certain obligations too. He was leading on an issue of such gravity that it would not easily be postponed; it held that quality of moral imperative. But he had thought, in accepting this leadership, that though it might be distasteful he could wait five years, until 1972. Yet his troops were rallying to him, not just because he was a Kennedy or because they wanted a restoration, but because he looked like the only Democrat capable of beating Johnson in 1968.

But he was really thinking in terms of 1972; he was not planning on 1968. The long-range forces he had counted on, the young people voting in large numbers, the dominance of television, the liberation from the bosses, would come with the new politics in 1972. But because of Vietnam, 1968— the transitional year from new politics to old politics— beckoned; and he was there.

Robert Kennedy was in many ways the most interesting figure in American politics, not only because he was a

Kennedy, not only because so much of his education had taken place in the public eye—it could be traced by putting together film clips of this decade—but primarily because he was a transitional figure in a transitional year. At a time of great flux in American life and politics, with old laws on the way out and new laws on the way in, Robert Kennedy was at exactly the halfway mark between the old and new. His career spanned the old politics of the past, he had worked successfully in it, electing his brother President; and he now planned on success in the coming politics of the future, to elect himself President. Thus there was a constant struggle, for his body, his soul and his campaign, between the traditionalists, the veterans of 1960—most often John Kennedy men: Larry O'Brien, Ted Sorensen and others—and the new breed, most often young men, more radical, and less professional in the pure sense. They were Bob Kennedy men first and foremost, prophets of the new politics—men like Adam Walinsky, the young speech writer, and Frank Mankiewicz, the press secretary. Though in part a struggle in tactics, it was more: it reflected a collision of forces in America just as much as a decade ago a debate between liberals and conservatives in the Senate had reflected a similar collision. The result was that Robert Kennedy, just as he was caught in the great contradictions between the thrusts of American power and American idealism, was also caught in the contradictory thrusts of the new and the old politics. But he would be too tied to the past, surrounded by men who knew more of the past than of the future, and this would force him into a fatal mistake.

This year was a long way from 1960 and, for the first time since the New Deal, American politics were reflecting the major changes in American life. As such, the battle around Kennedy reflected shifts in the society. The old machine-based, party-centered, economics-oriented traditionalist politics were shifting, in our affluence, to new styles. New issues were surfacing, old alliances were breaking up, and new forces were coming into our politics. The party machinery, once the dominant force in the Democratic party, was steadily being weakened. There was a new middle class which was moving to the suburbs; if a family was already making $10,000, how could the machine offer a better job? There was also the onslaught of television which was wiping out the middleman, the power broker who, in return for certain promises and controls, could offer the candidate exposure. Now someone with money, or the ability to attract money, and the right personality, someone who could bear exposure, could go directly to the people. Political power, which once rested with party officials and labor unions, was shifting to the suburbs. Labor unions, threatened by the rise of the Negro, particularly in housing and employment, were fast becoming a conservative force. The easy old coalition between labor and Negroes was no longer so easy; it barely existed. The two were among the American forces most in conflict. Yet other groups, traditionally Republican, might now, in suburbia, be wooed to the cause.

Yet if part of the new politics worked, so did some of the old. The mix varied greatly from state to state and region to region, depending on the affluence of the area, on the population shifts, and on how much the area represented the business and style of the old America and how much it represented the drives and technology of the new. The electronics industry with its all-engineer suburbs was new America; the textile mills, old America. Some states, like California, were almost totally new politics; others, like Indiana, were curiously old politics, strikingly unchanged from their voter profile in 1960 or 1956, albeit a bit more affluent.

Thus the new politics was the sum of many changes.

Labor and labor districts though more affluent were not very affluent, and their hold in the society was a somewhat marginal and insecure one. They no longer responded automatically to machine or union control. They feared the Negroes, and this undermined one part of the party's traditional base. Similarly however, in the suburbs a large portion of middle-class America, nominally Republican, had been freed from some of its economic fears. It had become materially successful, and now had time on its hands to worry about the course of American life. Most often it is bothered by moral issues. Its feeling on race is ambivalent. It does not feel the thrust of the Negro and his anger the way the blue-collar whites do. It would like to be for the Negro, and yet it is uneasy about the new anger of American blacks; it does not like anger or sweatiness on the part of anyone. In a sense labor now resembles the middle-class Republican America of thirty years ago. In the thirties, white-Protestant small-town America was the heartland of America. It had its share of the pie, but was worried about the upward push of labor in the Democratic party: Would that diminish the pie? Labor was the radical, on the outside trying to get in. Now, those sons of businessmen, well trained in the new technocratic America, have moved up. Very secure in their jobs, they have learned that labor is no threat. But labor, finally getting its share of the pie, is now uneasy about the upward drive of the Negro. Is it a threat? Will it diminish the piece of pie? Labor is on the inside these days, but without much security or generosity. George Wallace discovered this in the early sixties. He had sensed the anger and frustration of the blue-collar people and the new class division in American life; that the middle class was for the Negro but had fled to the suburbs leaving behind an angry blue-collar class to live next door to the Negroes. (In late July, 1968, Wallace turned to a reporter and said, "You reporters are for McCarthy, aren't you; and your editors are for Humphrey; *but your pressmen are for me.*") The new middle class had moved to the suburbs; it now had the time and energy to work in American politics. It was far removed from blind party loyalty, indeed it regarded party loyalty as just a little bit unsavory and almost dishonest; rather, it voted for the better man (as seen on television). Who got the suburbs, and could continually understand its needs, would most likely dominate the new politics.

Even the kids were different. They were largely middle class, affluent, not worried about their jobs—the jobs would always be there. They were a politically charged up generation, a product of stepped-up American education. They were in high school during the John Kennedy years; the civil-rights revolution was part of their times, it was a moral issue to them, and they were touched deeply by Vietnam. It was likely to be the most politically active generation in our history.

Technically, and Robert Kennedy understood this better than most people, the first year for the Democrats to operate under the new politics would be 1972. (Indeed his friend Fred Dutton had written a book on the new politics. It was to come out during the campaign and would warn Kennedy not to run until 1972; Dutton would have to revise the book under combat conditions.) The Republicans, less tied to the machine, would have a quicker shot at it if they chose the right candidate. If Kennedy himself was in a dilemma about his own decision, he seemed to view the opportunities of others much more clearly. Lindsay, he told one friend in January, was crazy not to go for it. It was wide open for him, and this was his year—just as 1960 had been Jack Kennedy's year. All it would take would be organization and audacity; the money and the talent would find the candidate once he announced. But the friend protested:

Lindsay was locked in by Rockefeller who had prior claim
to the same constituency. "If I were Lindsay," Kennedy said,
"I'd go to Rockefeller and I'd say, 'Governor, I admire you
and your record, and I think you're the man to lead the
liberals to victory this year. And we need the leadership,
and I want to be for you. But it's important that this time
we not be divided as before and that the liberals take the
leadership early. So I hope you'll announce. But if you don't
announce in three weeks, I'm going to announce myself.' He
could have gone all the way this year." By a hard-nosed
look, the thing for Robert Kennedy to do was to wait until
1972. But life was not like that; the forces brought to bear
by Vietnam were forcing him to make 1972 decisions at a
time when the structure was still old politics. Mayor Daley
of Chicago was still a powerful figure and there were other,
lesser, unsympathetic bosses to deal with. The moral forces
of the new politics were sweeping across the country in advance of the political realities of the new politics. Thus, a
terrible struggle for Kennedy.

It was a struggle which had begun as early as 1965,
when Kennedy was shaping his new direction and his own
staff—a surprisingly radical staff. He was gathering the
kind of men he would now listen to, and thus to a large
degree he was charting his own increasingly independent
course in politics. It was a struggle which would reach its
height, over whether or not Kennedy should run, in the late
fall of 1967, and winter of 1967 and 1968. It was a classic
struggle between the new politics people and the old pros.
On the one side there were the young radicals (of one very
young speech writer an older Kennedy aide said: "That kid
gets his draft notice and we're the only campaign in
town with a speech writer in Canada"), also people like

Mankiewicz who had come to Robert Kennedy rather than
Jack Kennedy, and a few of the older eggheads, like
Schlesinger and Galbraith. On the other side were the old
pros, the 1960 veterans, including Larry O'Brien who held,
at the time, that most radical of seats, Postmaster General
under Lyndon Johnson.

As early as the fall of 1966, two of Kennedy's legislative
aides had sensed the new currents, that the war would drag
on and that the only new thing in the political equation of
the war would be the growing national malaise. They saw
Lyndon Johnson increasingly a prisoner of the war, and
they believed that by 1968 the country would be ripe for a
new, modern and *moral* candidacy. There would be new
issues and a rejection of old foreign-policy clichés. More,
they felt it should be a Kennedy candidacy. They felt a
delicate and fragile balance would work for him in 1968.
It would bloom once, and if he did not rise to it, it might
never bloom again: for moral leadership once offered could
not be easily postponed, it might pass to someone else.
Walinsky and the others sensed that a Republican, Lindsay
most likely, might easily move in and become the hero, if
not winning, at least becoming the odds-on favorite for
1972. They did not figure on Eugene McCarthy.

Kennedy's staff was an interesting assortment. They
were by and large Robert Kennedy men first, more than Jack
Kennedy's, and attracted by what they saw as Robert Kennedy's instinct for radicalism. They would see the bumper
stickers saying "Bobby Ain't Jack," and they would say to reporters: yes, that's true, but not in the way these people
think. Jeff Greenfield kept copies of college editorials he had
written attacking Jack Kennedy's Vietnam policies. There
was a feeling among them that the early Kennedy years and
the early Kennedy people were too cold-war oriented. Walinsky had joined Robert Kennedy after the State Department

had tried to block pacifist A. J. Muste's peace march from Quebec to Guantanamo and Walinsky, a very young justice department attorney, had prepared a memo denying State's authority. Kennedy had backed Walinsky saying, "If an eighty year old man wants to walk eight hundred miles I don't think it endangers the country. . . ." Mankiewicz, a peace corps official, had been drawn to Kennedy during a briefing in late 1965. The Senator was about to embark on a major trip through Latin America and he met with high State Department officials. Kennedy had asked what he should say about the Dominican Republic intervention, and Jack Hood Vaughn, then Assistant Secretary of State for Latin American affairs, had said, "You could tell them what your brother said at the time of Cuba." The ice began to form and Kennedy said, "I hope you're not going around quoting President Kennedy to defend the Dominican Republic." It got worse from then on, Vaughn telling Kennedy not to worry because no one in Latin America cared about the Dominican events anyway. Kennedy asked what he should say in Brazil, and Vaughn suggested he say nothing, that's what the Latins usually do. They discussed problems of American oil companies in Peru—the government had moved against these companies and this had triggered a cutback in aid. Finally Kennedy looked at Vaughn and said, "Well Mr. Vaughn, the way you state it, the Alliance for Progress has come down to this: you can suspend the constitution and dissolve your political parties and exile your opposition and you'll continue to get all the aid you want, but if you play around with an oil company, it's cut off." There was no reply; it was very tense. At the meeting Mankiewicz, bitter about American policy in Latin America, had been the only official to speak out critically on American policies. The next day he breakfasted with Kennedy, and a few months later, faced with the prospect of leaving Washington, he went to work for Kennedy as a press secretary. These men pushed hard for a race, along with others such as Lowenstein who intended to have a candidate come hell or high water.

But the traditionalists had argued against it, men like Ted Sorensen, O'Brien. Amateurs willing to take risks in 1960, they had become professionals, establishment figures, by 1967 (witness Sorensen representing General Motors against Ralph Nader). The 1960 John Kennedy campaign had never been run outside the political establishment: it had been run to prove to the Democratic political apparatus, much of it Catholic and thus terribly sensitive on the issue, that a handsome young Catholic could win. However, they were now, in 1967, passing on the same clichés of American politics. The same men who had scoffed in 1960 when someone said a Catholic could not win, not yet anyway, were now saying yes, but you can't unseat a sitting president. They were wealthy and successful men now. They had important jobs which placed them in contact with powerful, wealthy men, and simultaneously removed them from the new forces now being generated in American politics. Sorensen seemed symbolic: heralded in the press as a great liberal who had taught Jack Kennedy his liberalism, and had masterminded the great victory, he had gained an insider's reputation, during the White House years, of being the most pragmatic politician of all, far removed from his liberalism. Following the assassination he did not plunge himself into the social issues with which the administration had been so concerned, but rather became just one more wealthy lawyer. Had he spent those post-assassination years working in ghettos or with Negroes, he might have felt the moral intensity of the times and he might have been more in touch with the country. Later in 1967 and 1968 his various public statements on the campaign sounded, ideologically, like those of someone from the Hubert Humphrey camp who had wandered into the Kennedy camp by mistake. (After the assassination he would talk publicly as though he had the right to barter the Kennedy mantle to Humphrey in exchange for some concessions on Vietnam.) His was in all a curious performance; and he had vigorously opposed Kennedy's making the race. Symbolically, of all the old Kennedy people who got together at a Kennedy meeting in December, 1967, the one most sympathetic to the race was Kenny O'Donnell. He was not yet for Kennedy's making it, but very close to it ("I'm almost there now," he said at the time). He was in Massachusetts and could feel directly the first pressure of the college kids going for McCarthy; feel the potency of the new force, and feel it slip away from the Kennedys.

The traditionalists passed on the myth that the country was more hawkish than you thought, which was not true. The country was less hawkish than you thought. The move was from hawk to dove and fast, and the polls which they carried to the meeting and quoted were wrong for two reasons: first because people do not tell pollsters the truth about how they feel if somehow they think it might mark them as unpatriotic, so that there is a very considerable built-in error; and secondly, and perhaps more important, because the questions were badly posed, and certainly not posed the way they would be in a vigorous and intelligent political campaign. Do you favor the war, are you against it, do you want to win, do you want to lose, do you want to escalate, or de-escalate. (Do you want to take a free trip around the world, all expenses paid, with a week with Brigitte Bardot in Paris. Do you want to take the same free trip around the world, all expenses paid, with the same week in Paris and the same week with Brigitte if it is going to give you terminal cancer?)

Another reason why the traditionalists counseled the conventional wisdom was that they had served in the presidency and seen the wide and extraordinary range of its powers. (Indeed they were not the only people who believed that you could not unseat a sitting president. The airlines thought so too. American Airlines which, like TWA, wanted domestic routes, would offer a 727 to the Kennedys at the start of the campaign for a rough rental of about $130,000 a month; after Johnson withdrew the price suddenly came down to about $30,000. The price for an Electra, roughly $70,000 a month while Johnson was still a candidate, dropped to $18,000. It was a quick study in presidential power.) These 1960 men had become traditional professional politicians, and to challenge the traditional laws was to challenge their own being. They had, after all, a candidate who might easily become president of the United States if he waited, and as such they felt they had something to lose. They had become conservative low-risk politicians. Some of them, like Pierre Salinger, a little lazy, a little arrogant, had said too many silly things about Vietnam. (After Kennedy finally went in he ran into Salinger and teased him about this. "Are you a hawk or a dove now, Pierre?" he asked. Salinger answered, quickly and seriously, "Oh-I'm-a-dove-now-I'm-a-dove-now.") Also, and this was crucial, there were basically differing views of Vietnam and the nation. After Kennedy made his major speech on Vietnam, in early 1967, he turned to Edelman, one of the young radicals, and asked, "Am I a big enough dove for you now, Peter?" No, said Edelman. "Good," said the Senator, "that makes me feel a little better." But of that same speech Sorensen would tell Jimmy Breslin that it was a mistake "because Bob Kennedy is the only hope in this country for your children and my children. And we can't afford to have him in controversies this early."

Kennedy's own instincts were probably to run. His

wife Ethel badly wanted him to. She sensed his moral commitment, and she sensed that he would be miserable and
never forgive himself if he didn't go. Kennedy sensed the
changes. But if he had the advantages of the past, the name,
the ability to assemble bright young men, the ability to
make headlines, he also had the liabilities of the past. He
was surrounded by advisers who had aged, and he was
particularly vulnerable to them. They had been advisers,
intellectual advisers, to Jack Kennedy, and that was part
of his blind spot. That meant they were automatically superior, perhaps more intellectual than he was. He had not
realized that in the restless chase of the last four years he
had gone beyond them; he now knew more about the country
and its mood than they did. He did not trust his instincts,
and it was a crucial mistake.

Gene McCarthy, not tied to the past, able to accept the
issue on its moral value alone, went in. It seemed at the
beginning a particularly frail candidacy. As late as February 3, the Gallup poll would show President Johnson's national margin over McCarthy to be 71 percent to 18, with 11
undecided. McCarthy's campaign seemed to lack the
glamour, the drive, *charisma*, one expected in a national
campaign. (Everyone expected a candidate to have charisma. Even Pat Paulsen, the Smothers Brothers' presidential
candidate, was once asked: "Mr. Paulsen, do you have charisma?" "No," he answered, "I had it once in the Marine
Corps but I haven't had any since.") McCarthy was seen,
after having announced for the presidency, eating alone in
restaurants in Washington and New York. His scheduling
was bad. Hours and hours of his prime time seemed to be
wasted. His meetings were often only half filled. The campaign was run on a low key from the start, and, as it turned

out later, a deliberately low key. Some of his closest aides and backers were worried from the start. They thought low key was all right, but there was a point where it bordered on laziness, and they sometimes wondered whether there was something physically ailing the candidate, something he had not told them about.

Sometimes McCarthy seemed to mock the entire process—laughing at the system, laughing at the traditional rites of vote-seeking, even mocking himself. If he had to give good lines, if he couldn't help being witty, then at least he could throw them away. Mary McGrory, a columnist who loved McCarthy, wrote that he was trying to run for the presidency without raising his voice. There was something unbending in him, a furious pride, and so at a time when he was doing something which genuinely dazzled the entire American intellectual establishment, when he probably could have had the best advisers and speech writers in the country, he had very few. His staff was often shockingly weak. He could not bear to solicit their aid, they had to volunteer it. And even then, when they did, it did not work well. He did not take well to other men's advice, nor did he use their ideas. This was a sharp contrast to the Kennedys who have always had an extraordinary ability to attract intellectuals and to retain them; to use just enough of their material to keep them committed, to make them feel they are making the breakthrough, winning the candidate to their view. McCarthy was also unlike Humphrey who has always been weak with intellectuals, unable to hold onto them because with all his energy he seemed anxious to prove that he didn't need them, he could do it all himself, thus leaving them unfulfilled.

McCarthy did not go through the usual pretensions either. He did not like the press and would not do the little things which made the daily life of reporters easier and endeared a candidate to them. He did not give them fire and, worst of all, he did not seem like a man running for the presidency. It all seemed terribly small-time. I remember trying to call Blair Clark, McCarthy's campaign manager, in early December after he announced. There was no campaign manager home; no answering service; it was only after many tries that a Negro maid answered. I gave my name, sensing, even as I did, that it would never reach Clark (it did not). One recalled McCarthy early in December at a meeting before a temple in Great Neck, Long Island. A long day for McCarthy: first a speech, then a press conference, the candidate patiently answering question after question for the television people. Finally he thought he was finished. "Now can we have a press conference for the writing reporters?" someone asked.

"I thought we just had one," McCarthy said.

"No you've had two conferences and both were for television. Now we can get serious?" the reporter asked.

McCarthy protested again: Look, he pointed to some reporters, they had asked questions and he had answered them, ergo a press conference. "I thought it was a press conference," he repeated.

"You've got a lot to learn," said the reporter.

"Yes," said McCarthy, "I have a lot to learn."

It was to get worse. The press would consistently underestimate his chances and, in McCarthy's view, underplay his activities; and he would grow embittered and occasionally petulant. He knew what they wanted him to do and say; he just as obstinately refused to do it. If they wanted anger, he would give them calmness. He would deliberately keep them waiting, often argue with them. A well-known columnist once asked for a copy of his speech. "What do you care?" McCarthy asked back, "You've never accurately reported my speeches before." Once he let the reporters sit around waiting in a lobby for hours. When they finally sent an aide up to see him, to express their displeasure, he snapped, "Why don't you go down there and play them some music." To the mighty Walter Cronkite, interviewing him, he would point out that young David Schoumacher, the regular CBS man and a favorite of his, asked better questions. He was bitter toward the press. One sensed that many of the frustrations he felt about American society were symbolized by his dislike for the press; he felt he wasn't demagogic enough for the American press. He felt they did not give him credit for his intellectual superiority, they wanted showmanship and they did not understand how he was handling this particular issue. The press did underestimate him. Reporters would see him ambling through his schedule in New Hampshire, giving what were predominantly bad speeches. The first three times I heard him he was simply terrible, giving his regular lecture-circuit $1,000-special on the History of Humanitarian Thought in the West. Stevenson without Stevenson, I decided. The reporters did not believe his own explanation—that the issue was already too emotional; it was there, deep in the people themselves, and all they needed was a political outlet for it and that was what he was providing. He was playing it very well, the quiet man. He had felt the mood; he had decided that the people felt there was already too much divisiveness in the country. His style was not to be divisive. He came across well in some of those small meetings. They listened and decided that yes, Gene McCarthy is a gentleman.

More, he had a cool analytical eye and he realized, himself, that American politics were changing and changing quickly. Sometimes it seemed he could analyze better than he could campaign. He sensed very early the new power of the kids, the massive influence of television (whose reporters he treated better than writing reporters) and, more important, he sensed that simply by running he would get his share of television time. He saw early that the old liberalism was increasingly irrelevant, and that the old coalition was fractured and by and large meaningless. The old liberals, he said, would speak with pride on how hard they had fought and were still fighting to pass civil-rights legislation, but that much of this was now viewed as irrelevant. "Johnson," he told me in December while campaigning, "is going out with a list of achievements, the laundry list, all these bills he's passed, all these things he's done. What he doesn't realize is that the people he's trying to convince don't care: he hasn't answered the questions that bother them. It's become a moral question, a question of values. He hasn't got their answers." He was articulating new issues and new priorities for an affluent America, shifting the issues of the Democratic party from the old economic orientation to new moral ones, asking what the quality of American life would be and what the thrust of American life would be. He was saying, in effect, that the more traditional liberalism of the last decade had failed because, though liberal legislation had been passed, the immense burden of America's military budget and foreign aid commitments had made the victories meaningless and left social programs more bankrupt than the nation realized. He was in this sense setting forth and clarifying the issues, not just for this campaign but for the next decade.

The New Hampshire campaign in early December was pieced together almost against McCarthy's will. His advisers tried to tell him that running for president was different from running for the Senate, that it was not a small, closed operation, that he needed the national press, and most of all that he had to enter New Hampshire. McCarthy did not want to enter. On that particular trip he wanted to tell all those nice, sincere, decent doves that he liked them and shared their idealism, but that he did not like their state; it had too many mountains, too few Democrats and too many hawks for his taste. One sensed that he was thinking about it—the long campaign ahead, all the snow, all the sore throats he would get. Just twenty-one days was all it would take, his New Hampshire people pleaded, just twenty-one days. They were the best people he had, and their quality of backbiting was surprisingly low for such good liberals; but he shook his head. All right they said, just fourteen days. Give us fourteen days in New Hampshire. Advisers like Lowenstein were arguing that if he went after the presidency, he had to go after each primary, he could not afford to be frightened away. A victory in a so-called dovish state such as Wisconsin would not be a victory unless he had also done well in so-called hawkish states. So he ambled, almost bumbling, through New Hampshire, appearing at meetings which were sometimes painfully small, talking about the need for changes in American life in a typically McCarthy style: "In the past, when a country won a war the successful leaders always stayed on one generation too long, but now, after World War II, with the invention of penicillin they have stayed on two generations too long, and that's the trouble with most of the world."

But the army of students was there too. It had been organized for more than a year, primarily by Lowenstein and a few sub-Lowensteins who traveled all over the country, telling the students that their dissent was not unique and that there would be an outlet this year. Lowenstein had alternated between the Reform Democratic clubs and the students—mixing in both, always late, always disorganized, and yet touching thousands of people. I remember one evening late in the spring of 1967 at Lowenstein's apartment. What, you've never met Norman Thomas? You've got to come by the house tomorrow night. And so I went, the next evening, to meet Norman Thomas. It was an extraordinary evening: Norman Thomas, almost blind now, Frank Graham, the former Senator from North Carolina who was successfully red-baited years ago, Mrs. Lowenstein, quite pregnant and quite confused—wondering who all these people were—and about twenty students, but no Lowenstein—he was circling above LaGuardia, in from another college visit. Some of the students were New Left, some of them very angry and bitter about the country and the war. Three very radical ones were arguing furiously with Thomas, saying that the war was racial and genocidal, white men deliberately killing yellow men. Thomas, turning with the sound, barely able to see, argued patiently that no, it wasn't a racial war, this country made a mistake. There was just too much American vanity and it was getting us in deeper. This was the radical Norman Thomas, my father's hero? Many of the people in charge, he was saying, feel about Negroes the same way you do. Those generals, a girl shrieked, those generals feel anything about Negroes? Yes, said Mr. Thomas. Vintage stuff. Eventually Lowenstein arrived and packed everyone off to a West Side reform club meeting where he spent half the night attacking Johnson and the war, saying Johnson will be beaten, the politicians are wrong, it is in the air. Volunteers were asked for, and a few appeared.

These were bad days for Robert Kennedy. He was playing Hamlet—thinking about the race constantly, wanting to make it, being led there by his emotions again and again, only to be brought back from the brink by the cold words of his closest advisers. His position was terribly ambivalent. He had chartered an entire political course only to halt at its most crucial moment. He was still telling people that he would support Johnson for the presidency. He had failed to come out for McCarthy (if he were going to come out for McCarthy, he might as well come out for himself). Columnist Murray Kempton who had frequently penned love notes to Kennedy in the past, and who felt deeply for him, was writing bitterly in early January: "As of now I prefer Eugene McCarthy as a candidate for President of the United States. An obvious reason is that McCarthy has the guts to go. A less obvious but more significant reason is that I was not at all surprised that he would, and I'm not the least surprised that Kennedy wouldn't."

But it was the cartoonist Jules Feiffer with his fine eye for our contemporary foibles who caught the failure of Kennedy the best. In a cartoon strip entitled "The Bobby Twins," Feiffer portrayed a television debate between the Good Bobby and the Bad Bobby:

The Good Bobby: We're going in there and we're killing South Vietnamese. We're killing children, we're killing women. . . .

The Good Bobby: We're killing innocent people because we don't want to have the war fought on American soil.

The Good Bobby: Do we have that right, here in the United States, to perform these acts because we want to protect ourselves?

The Good Bobby: I very seriously question whether we have that right.

The Good Bobby: All of us should examine our own consciences on what we are doing in South Vietnam.

The Bad Bobby: I will back the Democratic candidate in 1968. I expect that will be President Johnson.

The Good Bobby: I think we're going to have a difficult
time explaining this to ourselves.

But by late January it was no longer just a trickle of
volunteers. In Cambridge, where feeling runs particularly
strongly against the war, it was the minority which was *not*
opposed and which was not activist. And so now, gathering
from every state, the army marched on New Hampshire.
Not everyone, it seemed, had completely turned off the system. These kids were quite obviously the best of a generation. Kennedy would later note ruefully that he had the B
and B-minus kids and McCarthy had the A kids. Most of
them were upper-middle class. Many of them were the sons
and daughters of those who voted for Richard Nixon in
1960, who felt more at ease with Nelson Rockefeller than
anyone else. The kids were at ease convincing the Hampshiremen that the war was an immoral cause; they had all
practiced on their parents before.

Among the Jewish students there is something striking,
the new security of American life. They are the sons of the
affluent Jews in the suburbs, but they look more like their
immigrant grandfathers, those radical Socialists from the
old world with their beards. They were men who never felt
shame about their political feelings, not at all like the next
generation which wanted so desperately to be Americanized,
which shaved its beards and out-WASP-ed the WASPs
politically. No, these kids are much more secure in American life, and they seem almost to have their grandfathers'
political views in a contemporary setting. They are all part
of an affluent new society with jobs secure and waiting after
college. Material security is part of their birthright. Their
worries are different than their parents' were. They now
worry about what kind of a country they live in, and they
worry about the morality of American life and its affluence.

These volunteers are not interested in the great battles of their parents' day, the Depression and How It Was Solved by Franklin Roosevelt and Us. They are more interested in the moral thrust of America. They see not so much what has been done, as what has not been done. They do not doubt that capitalism, as a material system, works much better than communism, but they wonder openly about the use of its affluence. They are bored with the anti-communism of their parents and of most of the national journals, so bored, in fact, that any new youth-oriented publication, like *Ramparts*, gets the benefit of the doubt (just as the Communists get the benefit of the doubt), precisely because it is anti-Establishment, precisely because it is different; thus it is theirs. But in New Hampshire these kids were on their best behavior. They had found a tangible cause into which they could channel all that energy and frustration, and they did. They were intense, believing in their cause with a ferocity unmatched in contemporary politics. Many of the young men had been drawn from the brink of draft-card burning. Dan Dodd, a young student up from the Union Theological Seminary, told a reporter, "I was thinking of turning in my draft card but then the campaign began. We're not going to build grass-roots politics in time to end the war by November, but if we can end the present President's career, maybe we can do it by then." They were even willing to use a little cosmetology in order to help McCarthy; the girls' skirts became a little longer, beards were shaved off or, if not, were confined to manning the phones at headquarters. A note stuck on one of the bulletin boards there, just before the primary, read: "Over 40 percent we go on to Wisconsin; 30 percent back to school; 20 percent we burn our draft cards; 10 percent we leave the country."

They were carefully rehearsed in how not to offend the Hampshiremen; just how hard to push the issues;

and how to test for the extent of hawkishness, to sense whether it is fragile and can be turned around, or whether it is deep and hard-core and not worth the effort. The volunteers became overnight a very effective force; young, intelligent, very attractive, and surprisingly well-organized. They made a formidable impression in New Hampshire. They had intense devotion to cause and intense belief in themselves, and watching them, I realized something about the McCarthy campaign which was to recur again and again in the months to come: when people cheered McCarthy, they were cheering themselves.

Now too, in early January, there was money available. The big New York money, which traditionally has supported reform candidates—Kefauver, Stevenson, Humphrey, Javits—was beginning to go for McCarthy. But slowly, not in one great outpouring. These people were worried about the war, worried about the ghettos, and worried about the gold outflow, yet they were a little wary. They were tough-minded, and they weren't sure that their tiger was a real tiger; he looked a little soft. But Galbraith and others would argue their doubts away, and gradually the money came in. If it was coming in to McCarthy, then it was also not coming in to Lyndon Johnson. This was one more sign that he was in serious trouble—sitting President or not, he would need money and he would need active volunteers, and his chances of getting them were diminishing every day. Politically too, he was paying a price for the increasing isolation of the White House. If the country had paid a price in the exodus of talented men from the White House because of Vietnam, so had the administration. Now, strikingly without talent, it faced a national election.

Johnson has always had a problem with talented people, he has always had a reputation for mishandling and abusing staff, almost trying to humiliate and destroy the men around him. With Vietnam, the situation was worse than ever. Moyers, the brightest of Johnson's own people, was gone, and to a degree, Johnson was unprepared for national elections. In 1964 he had been aided by a number of Kennedy people whose loyalty in that year was not in doubt. But now it was different. He had Larry O'Brien, a highly knowledgeable technician whom he had carefully weaned away from the Kennedys. He had prevented him from resigning along with all the other Irish Mafia by an offer of the postmaster generalship. Robert Kennedy understood this; he told a friend he knew what it meant for a boy who had been as poor as Larry O'Brien to sit in the Cabinet of the United States. Kenny O'Donnell in particular was bitter about O'Brien because they had agreed, together with Dave Powers, to resign ensemble, and then O'Brien had stayed on. In 1968, when O'Brien came back to the fold, he and O'Donnell would, in a friend's words, "communicate but not speak to each other." But Kennedy had been too understanding of the dilemma. O'Brien had never broken ties with him, though the ties were strained at times, and now, in early 1968, Johnson was uneasy. He did not trust O'Brien and this proved costly, for O'Brien had an unusual knowledge of New Hampshire and the technology of its politics. He had run Jack Kennedy's campaign there in 1960, and he knew its balance. He could have helped, if nothing else, to minimize mistakes. And there were incredible mistakes. The Johnson operatives, for reasons known only to themselves, allowed forty-five candidates to run in the President's name for twenty-four convention slots, thereby splitting up the vote and allowing McCarthy to get twenty of the delegates. But Johnson was never sure of O'Brien; he did not entirely trust him, and so he used Marvin Watson.

Marvin Watson symbolized in many ways the White House at its lowest ebb in 1968; he was the loyalty officer of the administration at a time when loyalty was becoming the transcending quality. Marvin Watson was known best to America as the man who wanted to monitor all the calls going in and out of the White House, and now he was the White House's political man. The campaign was disastrously run. McCarthy was smeared repeatedly as the agent of Hanoi. Governor John King said that any vote for McCarthy would be greeted "with cheers in Hanoi." Senator Thomas McIntyre said McCarthy would honor "draft dodgers and deserters." Radio spots attacked the "peace-at-any-price fuzzy thinkers who say 'Give up the goal, burn your draft card and surrender!'" But McCarthy, running quietly with his own special dignity, did not look like the candidate of Hanoi. The Johnson people were too dependent on the state machine. They had nearly all the local politicians, which made them look, particularly in their own eyes, unbeatable. They would be able to gather all the politicians at the top —men who were seemingly reflectors of what was going on underneath—and believed this meant they would carry the workers and small farmers. The White House felt, looking at these politicians, that there was no coercion in their support, though of course it was not overt, it was covert: McCarthy had looked like a long shot and the President, a sure shot. Besides, the role of a state organization is almost always overemphasized by politicians themselves, and political reporters. Because the machine dominates politics in the off season, it becomes the initial point of reference; politicians make their living at it, therefore they are presumed to know what is going on. The truth is that in a statewide gubernatorial election, a moderately well-run machine can function, can effect a certain limited percentage of votes, because it is dealing with jobs and the families of job holders; but the very same machine trying for a Senate race often blunders badly because patronage is not at stake and because there are other more important issues. And in New Hampshire, in 1968, there was a very basic issue: the war.

In January 1968, General Vo Nguyen Giap changed his strategy. Up until then the Vietnamese Communists, fighting their particular guerrilla war, had never made their challenge in the cities. It had always been in the rural areas, where the guerrillas could slip away using the natural resources of the land. As such, the toughness and resiliency of the enemy had never come across clearly to the American public. By the time television cameramen arrived the enemy would be gone; besides, the places were almost always nameless spots. But in January, General Giap launched the Tet offensive. Suddenly, it became painfully clear to the American public that the war was not going well; that the enemy was resilient and very tough; that most of the pacification work had been shattered; that we could barely protect Saigon; and that the predictions of the American leadership had been totally false. Up until then Lyndon Johnson had believed that the war was going well; perhaps not as well as some of the generals said, but well nonetheless. He believed that dissent was largely the work of a few east-coast intellectuals and professors, and that it would be rejected by the rest of the country, which was soundly patriotic. Now, day by day, as the nation watched the endless battles on its television sets, and read the discouraging accounts from Saigon, Johnson was becoming more and more a hollow man. He had staked his entire political future on the war. He had slowly used up his credibility; now it was gone. Now it was too late to bring General Westmoreland home again to address joint session. And for Lyndon Johnson it was worse than for most leaders, for he was not a lovable man. He did not generate charisma, had no popularity; he was the kind of man who needed tangible success to hold his troops in line, and now even that success eluded him.

When Robert Kennedy decided in December to stay out, the debate within his circle had not ended. If anything it had accelerated. Walinsky, the house radical (when on the road, during the campaign, friends would put signs on his office door: "Gone To Peking, back in two weeks." or "In Hanoi"), wanted to quit. It took great effort on the part of his friends to keep him on the staff, to keep him from resigning. Now he and others were warning the Senator of something Kennedy knew himself, that Robert Kennedy was becoming an old politician overnight, long hair or no. If it were true that in the new politics with the old broker out, a candidate could be created overnight, then it was also true that it was a fragile thing and could fade just as quickly.

He became restless again and he wanted to run. Two weeks before the New Hampshire primary he began to call friends regularly, asking their advice, hoping, said one friend, to hear them change their minds and tell him to go for it. He went regularly to colleges, knowing that he would be harassed and booed, that the disparity between what he had pledged to America and what he was doing would be challenged. It was almost a form of masochism; he sought their anger. Indeed when it was not there, when they did not challenge him, he was angry at their complacency and he would challenge them: how can you be so complacent when there is a war on and your contemporaries are dying?

He felt it all slipping away from him, and felt himself caught in the particular bind of 1968. Lowenstein remembers calling him about ten days before the New Hampshire primary, jubilant because it had begun to turn; it was all falling into place. "We're going to do it! We're going to do it!

It's the beginning of the end for Johnson," he said excitedly into the phone. "I expected the same enthusiasm at the other end, I was so carried away by what we were doing. But he was very cool, very restrained, and he said 'You don't think you're being too optimistic?' and then I realized how painful it must have been for him." Other friends called and told him that New Hampshire was going to break it open. They pleaded with him to make a tentative announcement; to say that he was thinking of entering, so that he could share in the vote, and so that he would not be accused of moving in on McCarthy's triumph after the primary. And in the last few days he began to move. Jesse Unruh, one of the powers in the Democratic party who had previously told him not to run, flew in from California with a poll which showed Kennedy beating Johnson roughly two to one, with McCarthy a distant third. This was crucial, for Unruh was the first of the Democratic party powers to favor the race. Up until then it had been nothing but eggheads and moralists, and when they would outline all the reasons for making the race, a Kennedy aide would say, "yes, I agree with all that, but how many delegates do you yourself have?" The Sunday before the primary Kennedy called his wife from the west coast and asked her to call Schlesinger and Galbraith and have them tell McCarthy that he was going in, a task that neither relished. Similarly Teddy Kennedy contacted Dick Goodwin, a Kennedy man now working for McCarthy in New Hampshire, and Goodwin passed along the word that Kennedy was considering coming in.

Then came the New Hampshire results; they were staggering to the outside world. As late as early March, a sampling made for *Time* magazine by Roper Associates gave Johnson 62 percent and McCarthy 11 percent. But McCarthy had polled a startling 42.2 percent of the Democratic vote to Johnson's 49.4. In addition, and this was to become a consistent factor, McCarthy ran very well among Republicans; with nothing but write-ins, he ran third on the Republican ticket, and he trailed the President by only 230 in overall votes; 29,021 to 28,791. It was a staggering victory for a country which was unprepared for it and yet delighted by it. There was one last meeting of all the Kennedy brass. Steve Smith, his brother-in-law, had formerly opposed the race, but was now for it: if it's in your blood, do it, he told the Senator. Most of the others were for it now. Burke Marshall, a trusted aide, was also for it, though cold logic was still against it. Two men still opposed it. One was Edward Kennedy, a traditionalist, highly structured, very good at working with delegates, reassuring them; a different kind of man from Robert, less committed to lost causes, and more at ease in the camaraderie of the Senate. The other, Ted Sorensen, still conservative and cautious, still waiting for 1972; arguing not the new politics but the old mathematics, pointing out that even if Robert won all the primaries he would still need three-quarters of all the delegates outside the South. Others, such as Schlesinger, who had earlier argued for the race, now told Kennedy to wait a little, not to rob McCarthy of his hour of glory, not to re-create the old fears and suspicions in the process. Some argued that he let McCarthy do the primaries and then move in; others argued that he wait, create an artificial draft by having people troop in to see him daily, pleading with him to run, and having the pleas carefully leaked to the papers, until finally, against all his better judgment, for love of country he would run. But Kennedy was a curiously unsubtle man, not given to political pantomime. And he blundered right in, gracelessly, unable to wait, seeming to deprive McCarthy of his sweetest hour. "He didn't even give us 24 hours so we could raise the money to pay our bills," one McCarthy kid told Mary McGrory. New issues were made, the old Bobby was temporarily re-created, and McCarthy, who had privately acted ungenerously to Kennedy in the weeks before and who was very chilly about the news that Kennedy was coming in, was handed the white-knight issue. He became Clean Gene. "Kennedy thinks that American youth belongs to him at the bequest of his brother," wrote Mary McGrory. "Seeing the romance flower between them and McCarthy, he moved with the ruthlessness of a Victorian father whose daughter has fallen in love with a dustman." But he was in nonetheless, and alive; pleased to be liberated from the indecision, pleased to be back out campaigning again. In the same Senate caucus room where John Kennedy had made his announcement eight years earlier, Robert Kennedy made his entry statement. Many of the old guard were there. Men like Pierre Salinger who wandered about patting people on the back and saying "just like old times." But he was wrong, it was not like old times. The candidate was different and, most important, the country was different.

II

Suddenly then, in the early spring, Robert Kennedy was running. A shy, abrupt and sometimes passionate man ("He's unassimilated, isn't he?" Robert Lowell once said, after watching him at a party), he was more at ease running his brother for president than running himself. Now devoid of his privacy, forcibly shorn of his shyness, he was trying to control some of his passion. The spot was hardly ideal. In the normally alien state of Indiana, he was campaigning in cities and villages, trying even the tiny hamlets; stopping at little crossroads where no candidate for president had ever been because it was part of the American ethic that the rich may run for office so long as they campaign harder and longer than the poor. He was campaigning among the black and white, though rarely among the black and white together, not in the America of the sixties. These were uneasy days in an uneasy territory, for he was marked, this Irish son of an Irish millionaire, as being not just the friend of the black (indeed practically the black candidate) but Catholic as well. This was hostile soil, a land which had given Richard Nixon, though in 1968 it was hard to believe, 225,000 more votes; and there to remind him of both the past and the present were the bumper stickers, "Nixon Is Safer." When they said safer, they meant, and everyone knew it, Kennedy is Unsafe. (Nixon memorabilia amused Kennedy, particularly a signboard which showed Nixon, trustworthy, healthy, sober, carrying a briefcase, and doing something sound and practical for his country, and said: "Nixon is the One." He would tease with the crowd. "Nixon's the one *what?* . . . Look at that briefcase. . . . I've been wondering all this time what's in that briefcase. . . . Do you think he's a briefcase salesman?")

Robert Kennedy's aides were masters at bringing him to the right places, big cities for big Democratic votes, so that over the television screens that night there would be flashed photographs of huge crowds mauling Robert Kennedy, and a message to be read by the bosses of the Democratic party. But now the aides tuned primarily to Indiana, sought ever smaller villages where hopefully they might avoid some of the shrieking teenagers who had so lovingly pursued Kennedy throughout the campaign and who showed up again and again on television. It was, they knew, counterproductive to their parents, and their parents could vote, and were not likely to vote for their daughter's singing idol or that ilk. Yet even in the little towns the campaign rhythm remained one of constant, concentric circles formed by age and passion. The inner circle was very very young, too young but passionate, "Who cares if his hair is a silly millimeter longer?" said the sign. The voters of 1972 and *1976.* The second ring was a mixed bag, still young, but of voting age; a few signs pro, a few signs against: "Defoliate Bobby," "Give Your Blood to American Troops Not the Vietcong." Then finally on the outer ring, quietly coming and listening and watching; neither jumping nor cheering nor stealing his cuff links, nor untying his tie, the good citizens of Indiana. They were often outside hearing range, for the sound equipment was uniformly terrible. There was no portable bull horn; it had been suggested but Ethel Kennedy had vetoed it. A bull horn, she said, looked too coarse on television, too much like Lyndon Johnson. They had come, the good Hoosiers, to see another one of those Kennedys.

They wondered if he were ready, and whether he was as good and as nice as Jack. "He isn't as handsome as Jack," said the woman in Peru, Indiana. "No," said the woman with her, "but he's still handsome just the same." They tried to measure him to sense whether or not he could be trusted. They would come and hear the shouting kids and wonder what it was all coming to anyway, and where it was all going to. The same question sometimes bothered the candidate.

There was already a ritual and an almost narcotic rhythm to the campaign, though it was still very early. The plane would land and, even if it was a smooth landing, everyone would clap; if it was rough, there would be enormous cheering. Everyone would then spill out of the plane. The aides would curse the local advanceman for not bunching up the crowd at the airport; instead it had been spilled all around the airport fence and would not show up on television ("always get a hall which is a little too small," said the same aide.) The band would play the Kennedy fight song, "This Man is Your Man," to the tune of "This Land is Your Land." Music by W. Guthrie; lyrics by T. Sorensen. There were the inevitable dogged McCarthy fans to heckle. One sensed that if Kennedy landed in a blizzard in Alaska at 3 A.M. in 1976 there would be five McCarthy people with homemade signs saying "Why Did You Wait Bobby?" or "McCarthy, Our Profile in Courage." "The McCarthy people always look like they're either going to or coming from a Quaker meeting," said a reporter.

Then a brief airport speech: I think we can do better in America, I think we can turn America around. Much cheering though the sound system does not work. Into bus and down into the heart of town; reporters screaming at bus driver not to lose contact with the lead car, not to let sightseers slip in the motorcade (A reminder of Dallas. For another Dallas was always in the back of everyone's mind and in Logansport, one day, Kennedy was speaking when we happened to look up to the roof of a building. There was a cop up there, poised with a telescopic rifle. It was a frightening sight. Someone asked the police chief what the cop was doing. "We want this man to leave our town the same way he entered it," he said.) Same speech in town, closing with the words (as Kennedy gave them) of George Bernard Shaw; "Some people see things as they are and ask why; I dream of things that never were and ask why not?" Shaw was basic to the campaign; he was the signal for reporters, making their phone calls or grabbing coffee, to run for the bus. Indeed, on occasion Kennedy closed a speech saying, "as George Bernard Shaw used to say, 'run for the bus.' "

We'd land in the next town and Dick Tuck, the wagonmaster, would look at the crowd and say that at least 50,000 people were waiting for us and had been waiting for six hours. Tuck looks, and there is no other word to describe him, bawdy. He is the surviving humorist of American politics; Tuck, the man who put the girl spy on the Goldwater train; who once hired a stewardess on Goldwater's plane to ask him whether he wanted coffee, tea or hemlock. He ran for state senator in California, making the Los Angeles river, which is dry, his major issue. "Either fill it up or paint it blue."

The great Tuck specialty, however, was the haunting of Richard Nixon. Tuck prepared a sign in Chinese for a Nixon visit to Chinatown which said, when translated in the newspapers the next day, "What About the Hughes Tool Loan?" Tuck hired a sweet little old lady to greet Nixon after the first Kennedy-Nixon television debate: "Don't worry, son. Kennedy beat you last night, but I'm sure you'll do better next time." (Later in 1968 Tuck worked at the

Republican convention for Nelson Rockefeller, where, among other things, he hired a group of pregnant women to carry signs reading: "Nixon is the One.")

Now Tuck was vaguely in charge of the press. As we drove into town he'd note that the bus driver estimates the crowd at the airport between 7,800 and 78,000. Though it was a clear day he'd add that "this crowd is much larger than the crowd Richard Nixon drew ten days ago on a day when it was not raining nearly as hard as it is today." He'd also quote several unidentified local officials at the airport saying they have just switched over from McCarthy. "You didn't talk to them?" he'd ask, surprised. Earlier in the day a reporter had complained that the candidate deviated from the prepared text. "Robert Kennedy is not a text deviate," Tuck snapped.

These were tough, exhausting days, beginning early in the morning, fifteen, sixteen speeches, endless trips, bumps in the sky, private interviews in the back of the plane for those that demanded them. "Senator, there's a Danish reporter who's come all the way over to see your campaign." There was trouble with one Dutch reporter who turned out not to be a reporter but a Dutch politician come aboard to study American politics and the Kennedy style so that he might try the same thing out on the Dutch. Then there'd be strategy conferences between the air pockets, and at stop after stop the same speech: I'm not satisfied with America the way it is; I think that we can do better; I think the violence and the divisions are unacceptable, and so I ask for your hand. And the humor to blunt the ruthless image which pursued him relentlessly. I talked to my brother Edward (great laughs because of the family), and asked him for some campaign buttons, and they arrived, 15,000 of them (small laughs of anticipation), and they all had his picture on them (big laugh now), and I told him he couldn't do that, I was the candidate (small laugh), and it was too late to enter the race, and besides, people would say he was ruthless (big laugh).

The campaign began in Indiana, and it was the search for a domino. Most campaigns begin in New Hampshire, a land of journalist overkill, with television reporters outnumbering Hampshiremen. New Hampshire is usually bigger than life; candidates die there and are born there, and it would have been a nice piece of turf for Robert Kennedy. New England, friendly, compact; a state where they still had all the old voter cards, and no kickback against the blacks there, not with that fine Protestant ethic. Even the hard core of Johnson's strength against McCarthy, those blue-collar workers who had voted for the President, were largely Catholic and would have gone to Kennedy, a more ethnically Catholic candidate than McCarthy. But they had let New Hampshire slip away. They had entered too late and Indiana was the first available primary. They came charging in, hoping that somehow Indiana would come around and then topple Nebraska; and then they would topple Oregon which would topple California, which would topple Mayor Daley, the fifty-first state. So the Kennedys were running hard but a little late. Three days after the announcement they had flown to Alabama and Tennessee, taking a regular flight to Atlanta, and chartering small planes over to Tuscaloosa. The charter man in Atlanta wanted some kind of proof of credit, having apparently read somewhere that the rich are the slowest in the world to part with their money, and so Fred Dutton, Kennedy's traveling aide, whipped out his Carte Blanche card and $1,800 worth of charter was charged to it. This was all fine, except that the rich *are* slow paying, and by June an angry Carte Blanche was threatening to suspend credit to Attorney Dutton unless he quickly paid his bill. It was symbolic of the entire campaign. In 1960 the Kennedys had planned everything long in advance, the preliminary trips had started in 1957 and 1958, the early scouting; then the candidate showed himself visually to the delegates and Ted Sorensen, carrying a little notebook, checked out the delegates. By 1960, when Jack Kennedy announced, the basic organization and strategy was already laid out; responsibility already carefully delegated. Now in 1968 they were instinct-shooting. The events were running ahead of the men; until the very day that Robert Kennedy announced, most of them thought they would be sitting it out until 1972. He entered on March 16, and Teddy called Gerard Doherty, one of Teddy's men: Look Gerry, you take Indiana. On March 22, he arrived there, with a week to get 5,500 signatures for the filing. Everywhere panicked phone calls were going out, and people were told to get down to Indiana. Why? asked one woman, a dedicated political worker in 1960 but now a mother of two. Because we need you, they said. Need me to do what? she asked. We don't know yet. But get down here by Friday; and off she went. So if they were running a little late they were also running very hard, with almost desperate energy; a campaign pieced together at the last minute. Two students from Fordham were put in charge of forty from Ohio State because they arrived at volunteer headquarters four hours ahead of the larger group, and pulled their assignments first. They were all, in the flurry of activity, sent to a white working-class neighborhood where they were less than welcome. If these blue-collar whites wanted to hear about Robert Kennedy, they did not want to hear about him from some smart-aleck college kids who should have been off at college studying a little harder, and who had probably burned their draft cards anyway. Eventually the kids were moved to a black ward where they were warmly welcomed and made common cause. Much of it was like this, and in many ways the Kennedys were curiously unsure of themselves despite their reputation for slickness and for being a part of the well-oiled Kennedy machine. ("Does the powerful Kennedy machine have any more typewriter paper?" asked a secretary on the plane one day.) Indeed they were so unsure of themselves that they had carefully and gratefully listened to the advice of one Gordon St. Angelo, the Indiana state chairman. The nice Mr. St. Angelo had given them all kinds of friendly advice, such as, "Stay out of Indiana." They had liked him, had thought of him as Their Mr. St. Angelo, only to discover once in Indiana, having disregarded his advice, that he was no friend at all, that he wished dark days for them, and had indeed devoted most of his working hours to calling press conferences where he discussed how much the Kennedys were spending in Indiana, buying all those votes, a tactic which, he confided to a reporter, was by far the most effective way to attack the Kennedys. They did not like Mr. St. Angelo and somehow, later, one sensed Mr. St. Angelo would get his.

The staff was briefed everywhere on what was obvious about Indiana: a conservative state, strong Ku Klux Klan in the old days, more like Kentucky and Tennessee than anything else; go easy on the race. So they were running a somewhat muted campaign, fearing both fore-lash and backlash. The problem was part religious and part racial. Southern Indiana was part of a great religious belt which began in the Midwest, heading southwest through Tennessee and Kentucky into Oklahoma (Oklahoma, traditional Democratic territory, had given Richard Nixon one of the largest percentages of victory in 1960), and in some of these areas the more fundamentalist churches were militantly anti-Catholic: preacher after preacher had taken the pulpit to campaign if not for Richard Nixon then against Jack Kennedy. The issue had burned like a brush fire, costing Jack immense numbers of votes. He had eased the religious issue some; he was young and handsome and did not look like a Catholic, and television had helped to break down some of the older prejudices. But if prejudices die, they die slowly, particularly in an area undergoing some economic difficulty, and in 1968 some of it was still there. (Larry O'Brien, one of the architects of the 1960 strategy which had been so dependent upon winning every single primary, proving that a handsome young Catholic could win, could still offer small and fervent prayers to Stuart Symington who, for reasons known only to God, had chosen not to enter Indiana in 1960.) And there was prejudice against Negroes too, and Robert Kennedy entered Indiana in the minds of white Indianans as the man most identified with the upward and now unruly thrust of the Negro. He was *their* candidate; he would go into their areas and be mobbed, much more so than Gene McCarthy, whose voting record was basically similar on race, but who seemed curiously dispassionate about that most passionate question. One looked at McCarthy on television and did not think of Negroes. McCarthy, like Nixon, seemed safer.

Kennedy faced many problems in Indiana and he had barely been in the race a week when the entire campaign changed. One night, with a minimum of fanfare, Lyndon Johnson withdrew as a candidate for reelection. Historians and reporters will speculate for years as to why Johnson did it, what his motives were. The most likely explanation is that he found himself tied to a hopelessly unpopular war and likely to be ravaged in the primaries by two critics and beaten by Kennedy, the politician he hated the most. As such he decided to withdraw as a candidate; and hope for one last chance to find peace. That destroyed Kennedy's most important issue, the war, and more important, removed his favorite opponent, for it was Johnson who made him look good, made him a necessity. Many liberals, uneasy about Kennedy, could now, with Johnson departed, relax and smile at McCarthy again. Gene McCarthy, who often seemed to be a more incisive analyst than candidate, had said with considerable prophecy the day Johnson withdrew that it would hurt Bobby the most because until then Bobby had played the role of Jack Kennedy campaigning against Lyndon Johnson. Now it was going to be much more difficult, it was going to have to be Robert Kennedy campaigning against Jack. Kennedy's opponents in Indiana were clean Gene McCarthy, a tough-minded candidate of considerable subtlety who was running on a similar platform (How do you attack McCarthy when you want his army? If you offend him, you offend his army), and Roger Branigin, the pleasant folksy governor. But these men were not his real opponents, the real opponent was Robert Kennedy himself. Finally he was the issue, and he was campaigning against himself, against the old fears and the old suspicions, though they might be different in different parts of the country. In the spring of this crucial year he had managed, because of his delayed entrance, to be at once too ruthless and too gutless for the liberals and the students, too radical for the middle class, too much the party man for some of the intellectuals, and too little the party man for most of the machines. He had, then, the look of a man who intended to rock the boat, and rock it he probably would. He was in that mood, he sensed the country needed a little rocking.

The suspicions of the good Hoosiers did not surprise him. Indeed he had anticipated and welcomed them. He had assumed they would have doubts about him for he knew who he was, and what he had come to champion in America, and he knew something about them and thus he assumed their doubts (indeed at times he would campaign hard, perhaps a little too hard, to ease their fears and suspicions), but the liberal suspicions, and the depth and intensity of them, had hurt and surprised him. He knew his own mistakes and he was willing to live with them, but now the animosity of the liberals shocked him. The liberal suspicions were not exactly new; they came and bloomed seasonally about the Kennedys. They existed about John Kennedy on his way to the White House, for Adlai Stevenson was their candidate then, and faded when Kennedy attained it. Indeed by the time of his death they had almost forgotten about Stevenson—so much so when one of the high priestesses of New York liberalism was asked to contribute to the Adlai Stevenson Institute in Chicago, she said no darling, *live* politicians were her hobby. They existed about Robert Kennedy, especially because he looked and acted more Irish than his brother and had that McCarthy committee in his background. They faded upon his performance as Attorney General, bloomed again when he became an instant New Yorker on his way to the Senate, when he challenged Ken Keating, a man with a reasonably liberal record and who had identified himself regularly with Israel ("Keating," the sign said in 1964, "Nasser's Number One Enemy, Israel's Number One Friend"). The suspicions faded even more in the late sixties, upon his performance as a Senator, and with the real fear of the war and the backdrop of The Man. They who had once feared him, and even perhaps voted for Ken Keating, had spent October and November depressed about the prospect of the forthcoming Johnson-Nixon-

Wallace race. They had loved him in the fall; they thought of him often and remembered what was good in his brother's administration and in his own record. Jack Kennedy would never have sent combat troops to Vietnam, they decided. Kennedy had thought of them often in this crucial time; he had played brinkmanship with the race, and had then entered gracelessly, rudely, and it now had all come back. But he was in, nonetheless, joining in this extraordinary campaign which had seen one after another of the traditional maxims fall.

Kennedy's own presence had helped transform the campaign; he had done what McCarthy might not have been able to do alone: he had driven Lyndon Johnson out and probably turned American policy on Vietnam around. A grateful liberal community, freed from its fear of the war and its fear of Lyndon Johnson, liberated momentarily from the attacks of the New Left, was celebrating its new freedom amid its old suspicions and dislikes of Robert Kennedy. It was symbolic of the fresh breezes suddenly flowing in American politics in the spring that the liberals once more had the luxury of disliking Robert Kennedy. He had helped slay the dragon only to become the dragon.

It was the race issue, not Vietnam, which hung over the campaign in Indiana. This was due in part to Johnson's withdrawal and the Paris peace talks which had so suddenly begun; with that Vietnam ebbed as an issue. (Abner Mikva, an attractive reform candidate in a liberal Chicago district, had said that up until March 31, you could not say hello to anyone in his district without their saying, "Hello-how-are-you-where-do-you-stand-on-Vietnam." "But after March 31, people looked away whenever you mentioned Vietnam; they did not want to hear about it, wanted to believe it had gone away. They only wanted to hear what you were going to do about *them*, and all this rioting.") For this was a far different time from 1960 when John Kennedy could easily put together the blacks and the blue-collar whites. Now both the whites and the blacks were restless, and it was indicative of the situation that in Gary, one of Indiana's few big industrial cities, a mayoralty primary had broken down almost fifty-fifty between the black wards and the blue-collar white wards; Robert Kennedy had been with the blacks on that one. In 1968 one sensed everywhere the new movement toward racial polarization, an ever spiraling hostility and a breakdown in communications. The racial gap seemed wider than ever, and seemed to be getting yet wider. The gap was not being narrowed, as good liberal Americans had assumed, and as it had for the Jews and the Italians and everyone before. The rich were getting richer in America, and the poor were getting poorer, and by and large the rich were white and the black were poor. The public schools which had allowed previous classes of American underprivileged to break out of their ghettos were now simply one more enforcer of the existing conditions. Schools confirmed existing inequities, graduating functional illiterates, showing the brighter black kids that it was really hopeless.

They seemed angrier daily, as the promise of America failed to come through for them, and sensed acutely their own poverty in an affluent nation. Their moderate leaders were now being seriously undermined. They had told their people to keep working, keep praying, and somehow it all would be arranged; the heart of America was good and Christian. But there had been too few victories. The awakening which had begun with the outlawing of school segregation in 1954 and had continued with the various street protests was now out of control; the taste glands had been whetted, awakened and accelerated. More radical leaders were springing up, thanks to television. As in white politics, television was diminishing the old established order. Formerly the Negro leadership had been tightly structured and perhaps a little compromised because their organizations were somewhat dependent on white support, but now radical leaders were springing up without traditional structured organizations. With the aid of television, they were now being catapulted headlong into living rooms, those of black and white alike, on the basis of their looks, their anger, their ability to speak. There was a heightening of consciousness, and a sharpening of the sense of anger, for now the expectations were far ahead of the white society's ability to deliver.

Worse, the white society, so deeply involved in the war in Vietnam, seemed not to realize that it was failing to deliver. The young were threatened by the draft, were forced to go to hopeless schools which would prepare them for guaranteed third-class jobs. Watching their televisions, they saw the anger in other cities. The mood became increasingly angry and violent. Those who had been the followers of nonviolence in the early sixties had turned off; they let their hair grow out into the new Afro style; racial pride was now emphasized; Malcolm X, who had been largely a joke to much of black America in 1960, seemed the prophet now with his black pride and black consciousness and his view that the core of the problem was not black inferiority but white immorality. (Feiffer caught some of the mood in a cartoon strip which showed an angry young black with a beard and dark glasses, saying: "As a matter of racial pride we want to be called 'blacks' . . . which has replaced the term 'Afro-American' . . . which replaced 'Negroes' . . . which replaced 'colored people' . . . which replaced 'darkies' . . . which replaced 'blacks.' ")

The nation seemed headed toward a kind of modified economic apartheid. It was moving very quickly toward it: whites leaving the cities for the suburbs, taking the good jobs and the favorable tax structure from the cities; white collars around poor, rotting black cores; the Negroes frustrated, living in slum conditions and unable to find decent jobs. If they found decent jobs, then they were unable to find decent housing and decent schools. Now the young blacks were totally outside the system, it meant nothing to them, held no promise. They would as soon destroy it as try and grope their way up it, and so they began to riot, tearing and burning down their black slums, their faces contorted with rage. It was the rage, not the causes of it, which showed up on white television sets; the whites, seeing that anger and that hatred, were now more frightened than ever. They decided, well, the hell with them, if that's the way they want to be, after all we've done for them; I always thought they were like that, and now the politicians are giving in to them too easily. Thus more whites moved to the suburbs, leaving behind only the blacks and those very poor whites who hated the blacks the most. So in early 1968 America was facing a social crisis of spectacular proportions, and it was ill-prepared. The country was hardly united. The last time there was a comparable crisis was the Great Depression, but then everyone was poor. The Congress of the United States and the president of the United States represented the poor. Now the poor were largely invisible; they had precious little representation; and they were on the outside of a society which was affluent, a society which looked around and saw the visible Negro, the middle-class Negro who had benefited from the progress of the last fourteen years, who was now super-visible. White America felt, Let the rest of them be like that; after all, we worked our way up (when a young Irish nun who worked in Chicago's west side, which is a jungle not even a ghetto, pleaded with Mayor Daley to come out there to *see* the conditions, the Mayor said, "Look, Sister, you and I came from the same place. We knew how tough it was. But we lifted ourselves up by the bootstraps . . ."). It was increasingly prepared to answer the Negro's anger by building bigger walls around the ghetto and sending more police in. Lyndon Johnson was imprisoned by the war in Vietnam and the complexities of the ghettos seemed far beyond his comprehension. Perhaps it was a generational thing, but he was still talking about the civil rights bills he had passed. Besides, those people who were protesting the ghettos most vigorously were also those who were protesting the war in Vietnam most vigorously, and that did not help their cause very much. So the polarization intensified.

But the polarization posed serious problems for any serious politician, white or black. It was difficult to talk to both societies at once, the poor angry black America and the affluent smug white one, which wanted black progress on *its* terms. If Martin Luther King, a moderate in 1964, talked as a moderate in 1967–68, he would lose his black constituency because he would seem too conservative, too much a Tom; yet if he talked radical, which would retain his black constituency and which he was now doing, he was in danger of losing the white semi-establishment following which was so basic to his cause. Similarly, if Robert Kennedy made the extra effort, as he did for three years, to walk in the ghettos, and talk to the leaders and represent their views on a national scale, then he immediately endangered himself among the whites as looking too radical, too identified with the blacks; perhaps he was even causing some of that restlessness, encouraging them to riot. It was becoming increasingly difficult in America, in 1968, to have any meaning in the black community and any credibility in the white. It was a simple fact of political life that there was a certain amount of happenstance in Kennedy's attempt to do it; anyone else as identified with blacks (and the view of Kennedy was that you had to make that identification, the country desperately needed someone who had some meaning for the Negro populace, otherwise they would turn off the country completely) would nominally have lost the whites. But he as a Kennedy, with that residue of glamour, and also as a Catholic (who moved the Slavs and the blue-collar working class), might be able to do it. Lindsay, as strong with the blacks, had a good deal more trouble with the blue-collar voters. So now, in 1968, Robert Kennedy was trying to put all the odd pieces back together. He was trying to keep the Negroes, who loved him with an intensity that was special in such a rich country, to bring back the kids and the liberals, and to hold on to the blue-collar whites as well. Perhaps a Kennedy could do what no one else in America could do, could walk that particular narrow path. He was doing reasonably well in the early days of April, talking about the divisions in the country; the need to be generous; saying we must end this divisiveness, we must work together; these problems can be handled, America has the capacity and the generosity to deal with them. On April 4, he went before a huge audience at Ball State University in Muncie, Indiana, and he spoke of this hope for a generous America, and during the question and answer period a young Negro asked him:

"You are placing great faith in white America. Is this faith justified?"

Kennedy answered, simply. Yes. And then added: "I think the vast majority of white people want to do the decent thing." And that was what he believed. He felt that most white people simply did not know what it was like to be a black man in their own country, what the schools and the housing were like; they did not understand the historical conditions which had created the black man's dilemma.

Then he boarded his plane to fly to Indianapolis and, as he did, an aide told him that Martin Luther King had been shot, was seriously wounded, and was probably dying in Memphis. He seemed staggered and for a while he did not mention Dr. King. When he finally began to talk he said, "To think that I just finished saying that white America wants to do the right thing, and even while I was talking this happened." It gets worse and worse, he said, "all this divisiveness, all this hate. We have to do something about the divisions and the hate."

He landed in Indianapolis and learned that yes, it was true, and Dr. King was dead. Then he went on to a previously scheduled rally in the ghetto area; he had not wanted to go, but others convinced him he must honor this obligation. He spoke to an audience which was primarily black and he told them the news about Dr. King. In the background you could hear the gasps and the wails, and then he gave, extemporaneously, perhaps the best speech of the campaign, perhaps the best speech of his life:

> Martin Luther King dedicated his life to love and to justice for his fellow human beings, and he died because of that effort. In this difficult day, in this difficult time for the United States, it is perhaps well to ask what kind of a nation we are and what direction we want to move in. For those of you who are black—considering the evidence there evidently is that they were white people who were responsible—you can be filled with bitterness, with hatred and a desire for revenge. We can move in that direction as a country in great polarization—black people among black, white people among white, filled with hatred toward one another.
>
> Or we can make an effort, as Martin Luther King did, to understand and to comprehend and to replace that

violence, that strain of bloodshed that has spread across our land, with an effort to understand and love.

For those of you who are black and are tempted to be filled with hatred and distrust, at the injustice of such an act, against all white people, I can only say I feel in my heart the same kind of feeling. I had a member of my family killed, but he was killed by a white man. But we have to make an effort in the United States, we have to make an effort to understand, to go beyond these rather difficult times. My favorite poet was Aeschylus. He wrote: "Even in our sleep, pain which cannot forget falls drop by drop upon the heart until in our own despair against our will, comes wisdom through the awful grace of God."

What we need in the United States is not division, what we need in the United States is not hatred, what we need in the United States is not violence or lawlessness, but love and wisdom and compassion toward one another, and a feeling of justice toward those who still suffer within our country, whether they be white or whether they be black. So I shall ask you tonight to return home to say a prayer for the family of Martin Luther King, that's true, but more important to say a prayer for our own country, which all of us love—a prayer for understanding and that compassion of which I spoke. We can do well in this country, we will have difficult times, we've had difficult times in the past. We will have difficult times in the future. It is not the end of violence. It is not the end of lawlessness. It is not the end of disorder. But the vast majority of white people and the vast majority of black people in this country want to live together, want to improve the quality of our life, and want justice for all human beings who abide in our land. Let us dedicate ourselves to what the Greeks wrote so many years ago: to tame the savageness of man and make gentle the life of this world. Let us dedicate ourselves to that, and say a prayer for our country and for our people.

It was a sign of the changing new and angry times that Kennedy's very appearance in the ghetto was considered more important by the press than his speech. He was one of the rare American political figures who could, on a night of such anger and vengeance, go safely into the black quarters of the cities; others would go that night, and in the nights to follow, in unmarked cars or fly quickly over in helicopters as city after city burned.

They had been tied together, King and Kennedy, in what was essentially the same cause: working within the system to bring white and black together. They had both worked, for the last eight years, to make America more tolerable for the black. It was Robert Kennedy's phone call to a Georgia judge which had sprung King from jail in 1960, and which had probably won Jack Kennedy not only the election, but the affection of King's father, Martin King Sr.—a hard Baptist preacher with no love for white men and particularly for Catholics. (He later told reporters that he had planned to vote for Nixon because he did not trust Catholics, but would now vote enthusiastically for Kennedy. "Imagine Martin Luther King having a father who's a bigot," Jack Kennedy said later. "Well, we all have our fathers. . . .") The relationship after John Kennedy's election had been guarded, King and the Kennedys were not of the same style, and they were mutually suspicious at first. King felt that the Kennedys were dragging their feet on civil rights, which was correct—they simply did not understand how far there was to go and how slowly they were moving; and the Kennedys found King's brand of moralism somewhat heavy in the fast pragmatic world in which they operated, where idealism was carefully masked with cynicism. Nonetheless the justice department under Robert Kennedy was drawn increasingly into civil rights, not particularly because it wanted to be, but because the action was there and because the Kennedy administration, drawn in by events, had to come down on one side or the other, and finally there was only one side. By the end of the administration, the justice department virtually served as a coordinator for The Movement. It quietly lent its organizational skills to King and his people; organization had never been their strong point. They would choose an idea, more likely a target, jump in, and await the Lord to hand down the organizational plan, said one admiring follower. At the time of Jack Kennedy's assassination, Martin Luther King was holding higher hopes for Lyndon Johnson than he did for the late President (though Robert Kennedy was another matter, King had high hopes for him). He had seen in Johnson a son of the South trying to cleanse his past, had thought him deeply committed on civil rights, and anxious to prove his liberation. (This might have been a double miscalculation on King's part; he was from the South and Johnson was from the South, and perhaps both of them had thought the battle front would remain in the South. It was an area and a set of problems which Johnson understood far better than the problems of the ghettos.) Then the war came along, dominating the Johnson years and destroying the Great Society. Those years particularly undermined moderate leaders like King, who preached non-violence, love and reconciliation, hoping that the moral conscience of America would turn. It was a plea which did not particularly offend white America, but in the late sixties it fell on deaf ears among the alienated young blacks of the North. These young men were in the North because they had forsaken their past; the Protestant religion of their parents had failed, their god was dead; King was hot and they were cool. In the past year King had been pushed by events into increasing radicalism. His doubts about American society mounting, his criticism of the society sharpening, his white following diminishing, he was no longer so beloved by the white establishment. At the time of his death he had been organizing the Poor People's March on Washington. Had that failed, it was feared that it would have been one failure too many, and that the more radical leaders would take over his following, particularly among younger blacks. But now he was dead, the victim of one more assassin, and the campaign was breaking off. The Kennedys sent a plane to Memphis to bring King's body back to Atlanta, and all the great figures of America went to Atlanta.

In Atlanta there were additional dilemmas. The rioting had started throughout the country, and Chicago and Washington and Pittsburgh were burning. Lindsay's walk had helped ease tension in New York but the nation seemed to be just short of revolt. Kennedy wanted to go on national television and discuss what was happening, and why the Negroes were rioting, and there was discussion among a very few friends as to whether he should. His point was strong: most of white America would see only the rioting and the anger; Kennedy knew why this rioting was taking place and he thought people would listen to him, and besides, he felt the country needed some leadership at that moment. But he was warned that anything he might do would be misinterpreted, would be attributed to political motive. The rednecks would say, look at that damn nigger-lover, and the liberals would say, he'll exploit anything. Reluctantly he decided against it. Later that night an informal meeting between Kennedy and a number of black leaders took place. Though some of the men, such as the Reverend Ralph Abernathy and John Lewis, the former head of Snick, were sympathetic, almost all the black anger in America seemed to be unleashed on Kennedy in that room, one constant outpouring of bitterness. Why should we support a white man? Why should we bother with America's election? You people kill our leaders. Kennedy painfully tried to talk with them, not to answer them, saying "If you think I'm going to give you a campaign speech, you're mistaken. I'm not here to campaign. I'm sorry. I'm here to pay my respects to a friend and a leader. I can't campaign. I know how you feel and I know your anger, but I can't make a speech to you, I'm sorry."

The King funeral: a dark, somber affair, a broiling hot sun. Every important black man in the country was there. White leaders were everywhere. The little church was so crowded that the group of Senators which had flown down had to stay outside. There was only room for presidential candidates inside. King's people were wearing their poor people's uniforms as badges of honor. One of King's people was trying to move the enormous crowd in front of the church so that the mule-drawn wagon would be able to start. The crowd refused to move. He was begging them now, "Make it easier for the family, this is a way to honor Martin," but they refused to move. They have moved too often at the requests of officials all their lives, and they will not be moved. Then the march from the church to Morehouse College. More than five miles under the grueling sun. It was a strange assemblage of the mighty and the poor. It went through Atlanta; stores all closed, in honor of Dr. King, and in honor of keeping them from being destroyed (Rich's, the famous store, closed its downtown store, but left its suburban store open. Perhaps there is no honor in the suburbs). Along the way some of the older Negroes began to lead in singing; the walk had become a shuffle, slow, hot, burdened. Someone tried "We Shall Overcome," but it seemed tainted. Rather, they moved back to some of the older ones.

> *I'm on my way to Freedom*
> *We shall Not be Moved*
> *I'm on my way to Freedom*

We shall not be moved
Just like a tree that's planted near the water
We shall not be moved.

Martin's gone ahead
But we shall not be moved
Martin's gone ahead
But we shall not be moved
Just like a tree that's planted near the water
We shall not be moved.

"I'm coming Martin," someone wailed, "I'm coming now," and the rest said, yes, yes, we're coming.

Along the route Kennedy became the star. As we got closer to Morehouse there were crowds of Negroes standing in front of their houses, handing out cool water to marchers. When Kennedy came along, slight, almost hard to find in the crowd, they began to clap, *Yes, Bobby, Bobby,* and more clapping. "It's as if they're anointing him," a friend of mine said. Someone else complained later that even here he was campaigning. Perhaps, but it seems American, in 1968, that a funeral should be part of the campaign.

Several days later we were talking during a break in the campaign; Kennedy started discussing the fabric of America. I said that it seemed very thin, stretched far too thin; there has been so much violence that any quality of doubt or buffer has been used up, now everyone believes the worst. There were 50,000 people or more at the funeral, many of them the best people in the country, all having come to make a witness, all this passion, and yet, all it would have taken was one nut, pulling one trigger or throwing one bomb, to have set off the entire country. Yes, said Kennedy with a touch of bitterness, the richest country in the world. White people living better than they ever did before; no matter who they are, having it better: if they had rented, now they own. If they had ridden buses or walked, now they own one or two cars. If they had sweated, now they have a summer place. Now they go out to dinner once or twice a week. But all they think about is how much they have to pay in taxes, and how much more they pay in taxes than five or ten years ago. It is extraordinary how ungenerous they have become, he said. They don't see the poor and they don't want to.

All this distrust, he said, everyone in America distrusting everyone else. Then he became very critical of President Johnson: he never went into a ghetto. He knew he had the Negroes and decided they had nowhere else to go, and he didn't care about the ghettos. He was going to run on crime in the streets, and they knew this, knew that he felt he didn't have to go after their votes. Look at Dr. King, he couldn't get through to the White House, the administration wouldn't see him. They thought he was an enemy because of Vietnam. So the Negroes felt more and more isolated politically.

I nodded, yes, but how much of it could really be blamed on the President? Wasn't it a little too easy to blame it all on Johnson? How much of it was the diverse pull of the country; perhaps we had become too rich, and as such, less dependent on each other, allowing the selfish rather than the dependent tendencies to become dominant. So that now the things which divided us were stronger than the things which united us. We were not bound together tightly, but were permitted the luxury of divergent pulls. People behaved best in adversity, worst in luxury. His face darkened for a minute; after all, what I was saying was that if he became president he would end up as beaten by the system as Johnson had been. Then, rather coldly, the informality of the last ten minutes gone, he said, "I don't think so at all. I think the country wants to be led and needs to be led. I think it wants to do the right thing." And then he was off campaigning and moving again.

From the funeral he flew back to Indiana, ending up in Terre Haute in Southern Indiana. It has the look of a depressed city. (One develops a fine eye for poverty in America after campaigning. One can sense where the money has departed and where the money and the jobs have arrived.) In the downtown area, store fronts were closed. Terre Haute was cool to the candidate. It was the day after the King funeral, and white America, by and large, was not mourning Dr. King, rather it was frightened by the violence which took place in the wake of the assassination, and it felt that the politicians were too permissive. As he rode into town several people shouted coon-catcher, coon-catcher, at him. His speech was weak and edgy and somewhat defensive on civil rights; with a new emphasis on the fact that the violence is unacceptable. The audience was almost entirely white, only a couple of Negroes there. I asked one what he thought was happening. "Oh he's my man. He's my man all right." What about the rest of Terre Haute? "These people? These people?" and he laughed. That night several of the reporters claimed that in the last day Kennedy had been trimming on civil rights. His staff denied it, but the reporters insisted. The talk was pleasantly abrasive, and everyone was in a reasonably good mood because the schedule had eased off a bit, for a day, and there was time to eat for a change. One of the reporters kept telling one of the young speech writers, "What I can't stand about your guy, what I find hard to stomach, is that back right after the war, when I came home, and I led an open housing drive on the campus, and it was a lonely fight, your guy was on the McCarthy committee. That's what I can't stand. And now he's a big liberal." One of the speech writers, who was approximately eight years old when this transpired, was enjoying it all, saying, "You should have had a richer father that's all. That was your first mistake." It was all reasonably good natured, but it could have gone sour at any minute. The staff was restless; there was too much time and they were not used to it. We had checked into the hotel in the early afternoon and there was nothing scheduled until the next morning. "Four colleges in the area and all of them on vacation when we got here. Best scheduling of the trip."

The next morning Kennedy breakfasted with a group of 150 women in Terre Haute and gave a pedestrian speech. He was not a particularly good speaker, and here he was ill at ease. But then in the question-and-answer period, and this is equally typical, he was very good. He fielded their questions and he had decided that while they were all good Democrats, they were *complacent,* and so he got carried away on the subject of the poor in America. "They are hidden in our society. No one sees them any more. They're invisible. A small minority in a rich country. Yet I am stunned by the lack of awareness of the rest of us toward them and their problems. We don't see them. We pay all these taxes and pass all these programs to help them, and yet the programs don't reach them and the taxes go for other things, and every year their lives are more helpless than ever and yet we wonder what's wrong with them, after all we did for them." It went on like that, very good stuff, not exactly what the good ladies of Terre Haute had set out to hear, but it was very effective. There were almost no reporters present.

We got off to Gary which is a very tough town, perhaps the most polarized city in America. On the plane Kennedy talked about his problem in the state. Since the King funeral he had had two days of cold receptions. "So far in Indiana

they seem to want to see me as a member of the black race
—I don't think I can win if that happens. If it keeps up
I'm lost. That breakfast was very good and you could feel
them coming around, but how many people in Indiana
will get that much exposure, how many chances will you
have to talk at that length?" He stopped for a moment.
"These people never ask me, 'What are you going to do
about the Negro problem, or what can we do for the Negro?'
They always ask: 'What are you going to do about the
violence.' " Then he continued with a private and highly
informed analysis of varying Negro groups in the country.
He saw the Southern Christian Leadership Conference
splitting apart inevitably with Dr. King dead. There are
too many conflicting ambitions and conflicting pulls which
have been kept submerged only because of the sheer power
and prestige of King himself. Now with him gone, they will
begin to surface. Besides, there is no one person who has
all the qualities of Dr. King: one is his intellectual equal,
another has his ability to speak, another has his instinct for
the moral position and how to dramatize it, but no one had
all the pieces like Dr. King. What about Stokely and Rap?
someone asked. Beyond bringing in, he said, it's all gone
too far. They're too bitter, been hit on the head, harassed
and arrested too many times. As far as America goes, you
can forget about them; your only hope is the other young
Negroes. Keep them in, and give them alternatives, and
make it possible for them to stay inside the system. It can be
done, but you have to move quickly and you have to be
willing to take some heat in the process. I mean, they're not
going to tell you how grateful they are.

Kennedy had been making a major part of his pitch on the
ghettos an attempt to get private industry involved. He had
decided that there had been too much reliance in the past

upon government action, and that nothing could be done in the ghettos until there were jobs available. This put him in a different group from most of the older Democrats who, from the New Deal days, had an instinctive reliance on the government's ability to handle any problem; but it did put him in the rough category of younger men, like Chuck Percy of Illinois, who felt that government's encouraging business to operate in the ghetto would have more long-term results than overdependence on government programs. It also put him at odds with some of his allies.

Michael Harrington, the young socialist who had articulated the plight of the poor in America, had switched from McCarthy to Kennedy despite the reliance on the private sector, and in Indiana Dick Goodwin brought Harrington in to meet the candidate. "I guess you don't like all the things I say about free enterprise," Kennedy said.

"I guess you don't like all the things I say about socialism," Harrington answered.

Goodwin interjected: "Mike told the television people he couldn't support Rockefeller because Rockefeller wouldn't really spend 150 billion dollars for the cities."

Kennedy looked at Harrington, "My God, you didn't say I would, did you?"

Gary. A very tough town; it is black and white and not together; it is steel mills. The kind of city America's poets once wrote so lyrically about, *Oh I hear the blast of your furnaces, Oh America, the flame of your furnaces, the might of your steely strength*. Well, that was a long time ago. Now Gary seems to reek of all of America's urban ills, its drabness, *Oh I taste the sweet pollution of your air, Oh America, I see the blast of your furnaces covering the linen on my wash line*. Gary is depressing, one sees it and senses the revolt against the industrial revolution which is going on in America. Yes, the city brought them all here, the Negroes and the poor whites and the Slavs, and offered them jobs. They won their great battles, got their unions, kept their jobs, made good wages and yet now the quality of life often seems terrible. The reception for the candidate was mixed—unadulterated enthusiasm from the blacks, more cautious from the whites, who were interested but worried (a few "Bobby Ain't Jack" bumper stickers).

Much of the black reception appeared to be for Dick Tuck; he is something of a hero in Gary. He was dispatched there last fall, by Kennedy, to keep the Democratic machine of John Krupa from stealing the election from Dick Hatcher, the black candidate. Tuck, who knew exactly how a machine operates, kept the Krupa machine from voting the dead and the imaginary (and also kept about 5,000 Negroes on the register). He had heard of a plot to have all the voting machines in the black wards break down at the height of the voting, and so he sent off to nearby Chicago for ten Negro pinball machine repairmen, whose credentials he faked, and whom he tutored on a model of the voting machine. At one point Tuck warned them sternly when they began experimenting on how to run the totals a little higher so they registered too quickly. On election day, sure enough, when the machines started breaking down, always in the black wards, Tuck's men fixed them in minutes instead of hours. Tuck also beat the machine on another ploy traditional with machines which want to discourage Negro voting. The machine had been sending out registered letters to Negroes which said that there was some evidence that the individual was not properly registered. Naturally a registered letter terrifies people in ghettos since it usually means someone wants to reclaim something, wants money or plans an arrest. So the Negroes would not open the letters, and they would come back unopened and the machine could strike the blacks off the rolls. Tuck got hold of the lists and proved the letters were only going to blacks. When Hatcher was elected, Tuck became something of a folk hero in Gary, though he ran up a bill of $130 at Gary's Steel Club, which is where the local establishment meets and eats. As soon as the election was over he disappeared and there were great efforts to find him. The bill eventually ended up in Chicago with some Kennedy people there. After a few months, when Tuck arrived in town, someone presented him with the bill. He scanned it for a minute, and then said: "That's outrageous. I wouldn't pay it if I were you."

In Gary the whites remained edgy; there were few of them along the streets as the motorcade pulled through. Yet there were some around and some of them cheered, and considering the racial division in the city, even that was a hopeful sign. "They should really be hating him here," said one of his press people. "But maybe the magic still works." The audience in a Gary hall was about two to one black. The speech was good, mainly on the different vision of America that whites and Negroes have, and what America has promised and delivered or failed to deliver to each; how each sees a different thing. "Then the whites say, 'Why don't the Negroes come up and work hard and earn it like the Poles and the Italians?' But it's more difficult. The jobs have gone to the suburbs, or been taken over by machines, and are beyond the reach of them as they were not before with people of limited background."

But the Gary trip had gone reasonably well, and a week later, when the entourage made a trip on the famed Wabash Cannonball, the reporters, restless on the train ride, composed a song to the tune of "The Wabash Cannonball," called "The Ruthless Cannonball." One verse went:

He has the Poles in Gary
The blacks will fill his hall,
There are no ethnic problems
On the Ruthless Cannonball.

Then it was back to Indianapolis. The suspicion that Kennedy had been trimming persisted. That night Mankiewicz was asked: "Will he place greater emphasis on reconciliation rather than divisiveness?"

It had been a long day for Mankiewicz and he answered, "Well, I think you can say he will not urge divisiveness."

One day out to go to West Virginia for a day of campaigning. Why West Virginia? someone asked Tuck. "That's the only way you can get news coverage," said Tuck. "You get it by going in and out as many times as possible. Candidate arrives, news, candidate leaves, news, candidate arrives again. Television cameramen everywhere." The day in West Virginia was a long nostalgic one: Robert retracing the footsteps of his brother, telling the people how much the Kennedy family owed to West Virginia. The crowds were good in tiny town after tiny town. Kennedy talked about economic progress, of bringing in industry, and yet it had a hollow sound. One looked at the mountains, the gaps, and the population, and one sensed the hopelessness of it, that no new industry would come in here, and that the talented young people would almost certainly have to leave. Some of the stops were infinitesimally small. Oceana: so small that no one seemed to want to give the population. Finally, it was given as 3,000. Oceana is not even a crossroads, it is barely a stop. The candidate stopped, and kids spilled all over him and the car. "I want to be introduced in Oceana," he said, "where's the Mayor?" Mayor. Where's the Mayor?

Someone was dispatched to find the Mayor. Eventually the Mayor, a balding man, materialized from the back of the crowd. "Mayor, say something nice about me. Introduce me." The Mayor looked at him; they had never met before. Then he got up on the car with Kennedy and said, "I give you the next President of the United States." It was the best and simplest introduction of the campaign. "Very good," says Kennedy, "We'll take you with us the rest of the way." A few words on America; that it must do better, and we departed from Oceana.

The day was long and hard and he ended it in Charlestown with what was billed as a major foreign-policy speech. This one was not about Vietnam, but rather about the Soviet Union and coexistence. It was absolutely appalling, perhaps the worst speech of the campaign. It read as though the first part of it was written in 1960, about showing the Russians our might, and the second part in 1968, about desperately searching for new ways of leaving the cold war behind. It seemed to alternate paragraphs in this manner, a truly bewildering piece of work. Kennedy himself seemed to understand the discrepancies, and became confused and embarrassed midway through. "You ought to introduce your speech writers to each other," one reporter later told him. Another added: "I thought you told those hawks where to get off." He paused. "Those doves, too." Kennedy laughed and took it well. He had been introduced that night by John D. (Jay) Rockefeller IV. Tall, thirty years old, a millionaire now serving in the West Virginia legislature and running, one knew, for Governor. And eventually, after that, for president (though perhaps he will be slowed down and have to run for vice-president first). The press knew all this and was annoyed. It was all too perfect; Rockefeller, tall, bespectacled, had sat up there with his wife, the former Sharon Percy of Illinois (he will cut into the Republican vote in Illinois), and what was worse and most galling, he had made a very intelligent and graceful introduction. Now in the back of the plane flying to Washington, Kennedy was praising him: hadn't young Jay Rockefeller given a fine speech, wasn't that good? The reporters were noticeably cool. They were annoyed by this instant celebrity and the fact that young Jay, unlike Uncle Nelson, had the good sense and the good fortune to join a party which might love him. One of them made a strongly anti-Young-Jay remark. You didn't like the speech, asked Kennedy, surprised. No, said the reporter, it isn't just the speech, it's the whole damn thing of him coming down here and practically buying a base, with all his money, and cashing in on his name. No, said Kennedy, he's better than that. He went to Japan and learned Japanese and did some good things there, and then he came back and he wanted to work in the poverty program and so he came down here, and he was very good at it. The people like him very much. Sure, sure, said one of the reporters, and what he was really saying was Must American politics be like this? Are we going to have only Kennedys and Rockefellers the rest of our lives? The atmosphere was getting a little tense. You guys are pretty rough, said Kennedy, what's your real objection? He's too ruthless, said a reporter, and everyone relaxed. Why did we spend the day in West Virginia? someone asked him. I don't know, he answered.

The campaign rested for one day in Washington; husbands met wives, children were reintroduced to fathers, there was a desperate search for clean socks, and then back to the plane early Monday morning. The plane was headed back to Indiana. On board, the candidate was in a good mood. "Are you ready for my speech?" he asked a reporter.

The reporter replied that he had memorized the Kennedy speech, had indeed amused many friends by giving it at cocktail parties on Sunday. "No, not *that* speech, my new speech about the four vice-presidents who came from Indiana. It's my best historical speech." I'm getting off the plane, the reporter replied. "Or my new speech on the Negroes," he said, mocking himself, mocking the clichés of American race, "how they're going too fast . . . how you can't expect people who have lived one way for more than 200 years to have everything overnight . . . and then my conclusion, that they have to earn their rights just like all the Americans did, all the other people who came to this country and worked hard and earned a place. Now it's their turn to make it on their own. . . ."

The plane started in the East, and it was filled with television teams, some working for the networks, some independent, some doing instant documentaries, some working for the candidate. Everywhere he went they followed. The candidate would come aboard, would stop to talk for a moment—How are you? How is your wife?—and all of television would move in, as if to inhale him. Your comments—wife has a headache—are recorded for posterity; every little word is gobbled up. It is the age of documented irrelevance. This sort of thing caused some anger among the working reporters, or writing press as they are affectionately known, the new minority in American journalism. ("Who's the pool TV man getting him when he shaves tomorrow?" asked one reporter.) The plane zipped across the sky, pushing through occasional turbulence. (Once when John Glenn, the astronaut, was traveling with him and the air was particularly bumpy, Kennedy turned to two reporters sitting behind him and said, "I have a small announcement to make: John Glenn is terrified.") Bloody Marys were broken out by the time the plane crossed the Appalachians; the drinks were there, they were free and there seemed to be no earthly reason not to drink them.

A campaign humor also began to emerge. Now when the reporters went to a restaurant and the food was late, they would say, the service is *unacceptable,* I think we can do better. Or on the genuinely terrible hotel rooms in Indianapolis: I think we can do better, I think we can turn the Indiana hotel industry around. Much of it, of course, fastened on Indiana. We had all been here too long; there was a constant laundry problem, and a constant food problem. Indiana, someone said, is where they say French dressing on your salad, and it's *orange.*

We landed in Indiana and everyone was relaxed. Mankiewicz was on the press bus and was now in particularly good form. We were off to Vincennes and other historical sights. "Vincennes, as you all know, was founded by George Rogers Clark. As you are all aware, Mr. Clark was credited with saying, 'don't trust anyone over thirty.' Now does anyone want to hear about William Henry Harrison?" Tell us about the pacification program, Frank, someone asked. "Well the pacification program is going reasonably well in Indiana," said Mankiewicz, picking up the Saigon language, "but you must remember that they are a proud people with a culture and a tradition all their own, and therefore these things take time. You can't expect things overnight. We Americans are too impatient, we expect too much." Someone asked how long Kennedy would stop in town. "I don't know," Mankiewicz answered. "First he'll make a speech. Then he'll answer some questions. Then he'll be besieged by a surging throng of mature adult voters."

Much of the humor was unfair, but Indiana was a state which had not changed, and much of it was rural and some of the reporters were bitter about being on an expense account in an area where there was so little opportunity to exploit it. But one did feel, in Indiana, that one had stepped back a bit in time. Later after the campaign, when Gene McCarthy was complaining about his defeat there, he would say of Indiana: "They kept talking about the poet out there. I asked if they were talking about Shakespeare, or even my friend Robert Lowell. But it was James Whitcomb Riley. You could hardly expect to win under those conditions."

This day had been given over to television. Kennedy was to campaign on several levels: the normal one which was to make an impact on the towns he visited, the secondary one which was to make an impact on the normal local, state and national coverage, and now a third one which was to create images which his own television teams could use for his television commercials. This last was perhaps the most vital part of the campaign; perhaps one percent of the voters might see him in the flesh, but through television almost all the voters would see him. So the day was devoted to television clips: Was he an outsider as Roger Branigin charged? A tourist? Part of the day was scheduled so that Robert Kennedy would visit and be filmed at every shrine in Indiana. He would come on the screen knowing Indiana's history and being reflected in it—the Lewis and Clark Memorial, the Lincoln Shrine. In addition, a major effort would be made to counter the ruthless image. Was he ruthless? The television clips would show him a little shy, wittier than people thought, a little slight, and he would not look ruthless but rather would look victimized by all that ruthless talk. Most important it would show him answering questions from the good people of Indiana. They would stumble a little in their questions, which would show the natural touch, though they wouldn't stumble too much. It would have a sense of real questions put by real people; the questioners must not look like they just came from doing a soap commercial, though they should not be too ugly either. Long leathered faces of farmers were very good because everybody trusts long leather-faced farmers. Everybody knows that they speak with eternal wisdom and that they are bothered by questions which bother everyone. As for students, they should not be too bearded. It would be better to have fairly clean-cut students.

Kennedy's advisers had learned long ago that he was far better at questions and answers, particularly tough questions, than he was at set speeches. At set speeches he tensed and went flat. In questions and answers he came alive; he felt challenged and felt a personal relationship with the questioner. In 1964, during his Senate race, the best television clips had come from a meeting with Columbia students; semi-hostile, they had poured it to him, tough ungenerous questions. The best part of him had responded; the intelligence, the candor and the humor had flashed through. Probably it had hurt Keating, for Keating had matched it with little of his own. The television clips for Kennedy had to be a little different than those for most candidates. For most candidates the job was simply to introduce him—here, this is what he looks like, and please get the good side of his face. With Kennedy it was different. Everyone knew what he looked like; along with Lyndon Johnson he was probably the best known public figure in America. The problem with Kennedy was the reaction to him. A lot of people recognized him and did not like what they recognized. When he was running for the Senate, he and his aides had discovered what they had already suspected—that he had a very high antipathy quotient, a polling measure developed by the firm of Bennett and Chaikin.

This test reflected the number of people who, when polled, registered a serious objection to a political figure. In 1964 Keating had what was to them an alarmingly low antipathy quotient of six. It surpassed even that of Dwight Eisenhower in 1956, which was seven. In 1964 when Lyndon Johnson's A.Q. was 17 (before the escalation), Robert Kennedy had a staggering A.Q. of 36, though many of the people who disliked him might vote for him. Now in Indiana the Kennedy people realized that they had a similar problem on their hands; and that while McCarthy might not be that well known, there were few people who felt strongly against him. All that particular day the advisers tried to get the candidate away from the crowds (which would reinforce the A.Q., showing the sweaty, unruly side of the candidate, or at least an image which projected as sweaty and unruly), and away from reporters. They tried to get him in an indigenous setting, with no teeny-boppers, this man is not discordant. They got him to tiny little crossroad stops, barred reporters, got him into general stores, and encouraged the people to ask questions: the quiet Kennedy in a quiet surrounding.

In addition, he did the usual twelve stops, his voice ragged at the end. The reporters were still claiming that he was cutting back on civil rights, which he was. (Someone had mentioned to Tuck that Kennedy was giving an Indiana speech, and Tuck became angry. "There is no Indiana speech. When are you guys going to learn that? The Indiana speech died in 1956. Anything you say here goes everywhere. These people here have seen the war just like everyone else, just like Chicago and New York. It's not 1930. If you ask the people in Indiana what concerns them it's not Indiana. The Governor is running around saying that the only issue is Indiana for Indianans and we're going to beat him on that; he's underestimating these people. There is no Indiana speech or a New York or Wisconsin speech. Learn that will you.") Late that night, after 11 P.M., Kennedy went to dinner with a few friends and magazine writers. It was very late and he was very tired; all the ideas about preserving the candidate, the conservation of the candidate's energy, were shot. There was just too much to do, and too little time, and besides, one of the problems of his campaign was that the candidate lacked a Robert Kennedy—someone who would do for him what he did for Jack Kennedy in 1960, who would handle all the endless details quickly and correctly and intelligently, and make sure the candidate himself was bothered with only a minimal amount of detail. That was hopeless now. These days he would campaign all day long and then go out very late at night to discuss the next day with aides—sometimes finishing dinner at 2 A.M.; drawing on his exceptional physical condition and energy. "You guys are always complaining about the fact that he doesn't go into detail on Vietnam and on civil rights in his short speeches," Dutton once said, "one reason is sheer fatigue. How much energy does a candidate have. Fourteen speeches a day and you want him to touch all the points on civil rights." That night he was talking about his main campaign poster. He did not like the photograph which was both boyish and surly boyish—"like the guitar player in a high school rock-and-roll band," he said.

"Like a bad guitar player in a bad high school band," Warren Rogers of *Look* corrected. Kennedy agreed.

The food was late, and he and John Glenn were both frequently interrupted by autograph hunters. Finally he turned to a friend and asked whether it was worth it, couldn't it just be done on television, couldn't you sit back and do it from the studios as some of his younger assistants were insisting. (Again the new politics/old politics split; the younger people thought most of the traditional campaigning was a waste of time and money, television could do it all. They wanted him to do less street campaigning, to pay less attention to newspapers.)

No, said Dick Goodwin, "You have to go out there and do it all and you have to show that you don't have contempt for them, that you value who they are."

"You could afford to do more by television if you weren't so rich," someone else said. "You're too rich not to get out there and mix. McCarthy ought to run a television campaign."

Someone else said that it was all insane, that it didn't matter any more. Visiting people was a thing of the past (though election results would consistently show that Kennedy ran better where he campaigned personally). The newspapers were a thing of the past. You didn't get any space from Pulliam (Eugene Pulliam was the arch-conservative owner of the two Indianapolis newspapers whose treatment of Kennedy and his campaign was scandalous). Forget it—it probably makes you a little bit of an underdog. Papers have less influence than anything else in this campaign.

But this too was quickly challenged. Newspapers, another aide said, were still important, in a limited sense. Not so much the reporters, except inasmuch as they can influence the columnists, and the columnists in turn influence other reporters, and finally the columnists influence the television commentators who still lack confidence of their own judgments. So one columnist saying one thing can trigger an entire series of comments. (Eugene McCarthy, referring to the same characteristic and a little bit bitter over his coverage and bitter about the American press in general, once compared all reporters to blackbirds sitting on a telephone wire. One flies off and they all fly off. One flies back and they all fly back.) Thus James Reston was very important and a campaign should consider his influence on other writers. Kennedy asked why Reston didn't like him, and one of his staff people said it wasn't dislike, it was just that he wasn't at ease with Kennedy.

He likes you, I said, turning to John Glenn. He thinks you represent the traditional American values as much as anyone these days. At a dinner party, in 1964, right after Glenn had announced for the Senate, Tom Wicker and I had complained bitterly about him and about the entire glamour syndrome of American politics. So Glenn had walked in space, what did he know about the earth. Was he just one more Kennedy satellite, like Salinger who was now running in California? We were quite strong willed but Reston had defended him. Reston liked the way he talked and what he believed; more, when he landed that day after the space flight and saw his wife for the first time, Reston had caught him "looking first at his Annie, and I liked the look in his eye."

I know, Glenn nodded, I'm having lunch with him in ten days.

The television commentators, Kennedy said, they're the ones. He mentioned a young correspondent covering McCarthy. "Boy, what I wouldn't give to have someone like that on my side." Another aide said yes, and named two other reporters covering McCarthy who were allegedly sympathetic to the McCarthy cause. "They're all doves you know, and because of that they give McCarthy a free ride. Is that fair?" I told Kennedy there were a number of reporters covering him who were sympathetic to him because of his positions on race and Vietnam, and who were treating him a little gently. "You don't expect me to be fair, do you?" he said.

The dinner moved on to a quick discussion of what television would do to politics. There was a general assumption that it would throw the rascals out. "What about the new rascals it throws in?" someone asked, and mentioned Ronald Reagan. A sore point. Kennedy and Reagan had debated the question of Vietnam on international television a year before, and the general consensus was that Reagan had destroyed Kennedy. Part of the trouble had been the setting; they had answered questions on Vietnam posed by foreign students, militantly anti-American, and the questions were shrill, angry and hostile. Reagan became the cool defender of the country, while Kennedy, if he tried to discuss the substance, looked like he was supporting the kids. He had been placed in a clearly embarrassing position; he was off balance and edgy. "Next time you debate him, get a panel of right-wing kids to ask the questions," someone said. I dissented: Reagan seemed to me to have memorized his cards and nothing more, while Kennedy, in contrast, had tried to answer each question with his own spontaneous responses, essentially the kind of intelligence and self-dependence which shows up very well over a long tough campaign, where automatic cards are not enough. Reagan had bobbled one question rather badly; a student had asked him something concerning the Geneva accords. He had answered smoothly and glibly but had misquoted and misrepresented the accords, and the kid caught him dead to rights. He had a copy of the accords right there and had read it out. It was the kind of mistake which, in a tough campaign, might be a fatal flaw. A misstep here and the intense pressure and fatigue of the campaign would magnify it, and the candidate would try and cover up and make yet another mistake, and soon he would be off balance, off his natural rhythm. Today an American campaign is a ruthlessly cruel and searching business; those television cameras look at you and look back, in Dylan Thomas' words, "to the bed you were born on." Anyway, I had thought there were fatal flaws in Reagan. Kennedy agreed and said that I could judge any future debates between them.

The campaign was a curious, almost contradictory affair. There was no doubt that it was, technically, beginning to go well, that McCarthy was not exactly catching fire though he was running, as usual, a clever campaign that was easily underestimated. (His television was quite good, particularly a last-minute half-hour paid interview with Garry Moore, a real live Hoosier, a local boy, doing the interviewing. It was a slick piece of work, Moore taking the low road, and McCarthy the high road: Senator, isn't it just terrible the way some candidates are spending money? Well Garry, I don't want to comment on that, let's talk about *my* campaign.) As for Branigin, they were sure he'd inevitably diminish as a candidate. Their first polls taken before they entered, the Kennedys always take polls before they enter anything, had shown them tied with Branigin 33–33. But they were convinced that, as the campaign intensified, Branigin, who was playing only to local chauvinism, would fade, the issues in 1968 were simply too great for an Indiana-for-Indianans pitch. They were, of course, building up the Branigin threat, casting themselves as underdogs, a favorite Kennedy trick since the West Virginia primary in 1960 where they poor-mouthed, and poor-mouthed the better to magnify the victory once it was in. The trick, of course, was highly suspect, and when the Kennedys were genuinely pessimistic, as in the last few days of Oregon, the reporters thought they were being put-on.

The problem in Indiana was not so much whether it would be a victory, that looked better and better in late April (though the size was always a question, they wanted fifty percent as a means of ending McCarthy right then and there), but the tone and the balance of the campaign. It had become a curiously contradictory affair, reflecting the changing views of the candidate himself, the changing nature of the country, and the differences among his own advisers. In the beginning, when he had first challenged Johnson, the campaign had been by its very nature new politics and high-risk politics. It was defying the taboos, it was going outside the party establishment, indeed up against it. Its main issues were moral ones; it sharpened rather than muted the differences between Kennedy and the administration. Since the party apparatus was hostile, the campaign's only resource was shock—quick striking victories, fashioned on dramatization of the issues, in primary after primary until California, where a smashing victory would destroy the President. Though the race was mathematically impossible, it somehow seemed within reach. This was particularly so because one sensed that Johnson was a hollow man, and when he went, he would go down quickly. While this phase of the campaign was on, the younger more radical advisers were more in command. They were the shock troops and they believed in the moral issues and in the sharpening of them. They had always been the advocates of the race, because of the preemptive quality of the issues. They knew little about the delegates, and their strategy was simple; make the delegates come to you.

Then Johnson withdrew, and a more traditional campaign began. Vietnam disappeared, temporarily at least, as a viable issue. (In Indiana Kennedy had fumbled around with it. To raise it as a major issue was considered unpatriotic because of the Paris peace talks, and yet he doubted the seriousness of these peace talks; indeed the war was the issue which had forced him into the race.) At the same time, delegates once locked, even if uneasily, to the President of the United States, became unlocked. "Dick Daley's office was like a revolving door for Kennedy people for a few days," said one Chicago politician. The tone of the campaign had changed, had become muted; the role of the young radicals, and the other Robert Kennedy people, tempered, much to their annoyance.

Tonight, two weeks after Johnson's withdrawal, Kennedy was on a plane talking with a small group of reporters. The campaign seemed to have gone slack, to have lost its intensity since Johnson pulled out; the quality of spirit, of excitement, almost of a crusade, that had marked the first couple of weeks seemed to have gone. The crowds were noticeably less emotional, and the Kennedy people themselves seemed less spirited; indeed the campaign *was* more cautious. One of the reporters mentioned this and asked Kennedy whether he wished Johnson were back in the race. "No," he said, "it's much better now. It's not as dramatic, and you people [reporters] miss that. Not as exciting. But it's better now. All those delegates are unlocked. The other way was much more exciting but it was more uphill." I disagreed with him; it seemed to me that Johnson's withdrawal had reinstated McCarthy as an important candidate, and that it was going to be much tougher now.

Kennedy started talking about the party. He mentioned the dinner in Philadelphia right after the Johnson withdrawal, an occasion that shattered Walinsky and his colleagues because Kennedy had praised all the old hacks of the party. He said that had he entered New Hampshire against Johnson "there wouldn't be one Democrat in the entire country talking to me. I couldn't have gone to any party dinners at all. They would have booed me. They would all accuse me of dividing the party. Now [because of McCarthy] they know that the division was already there."

Someone mentioned the loyalty of the party people to Johnson, but Kennedy brushed that aside. They were never loyal to Johnson, he said, though they were loyal to the office.

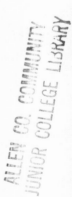

Johnson had been weak with the party, not tending to small party affairs, not going to party dinners ("nobody listens to what you say at them, but it's important to go, important to show that you care"), whereas Humphrey had been very good at tending to party functions. Hubert, he said, had more money in the bank with the pros than Lyndon did. Then he spoke warmly of Humphrey; Humphrey is getting a few breaks, "and if anyone ever deserved a break, he does."

That night, the discussion with several Kennedy aides was about Mayor Daley. (I was writing a piece about Daley when I switched off to cover Kennedy, and I would soon be switching back to the Mayor for a few weeks.) Daley's presence hovered over this entire campaign. Though big city bosses are generally on their way out, he is the last truly powerful one, and though his power is likely to ebb and be diluted nationally in the future, his strength at this convention was immense. He controlled the big Illinois delegation, and some of the smaller bosses with smaller delegations would key on Illinois. This campaign was a curious one, not so much a horse race as a horse show, parading in front of Daley, showing him how much class and style and power you've got, and hoping he agrees. Daley was the judge. Unless the showings in the primaries and the polls were very good, he would probably go to Humphrey, and the Kennedy people were aware of this, aware that Daley was more comfortable with Humphrey than with the more radical, abrasive Kennedy. "One of his other big mistakes in 1968," said Mankiewicz, referring to the failure to enter the race earlier, "is going to be that he thinks Dick Daley regards him in the same light that he regarded Jack Kennedy. It's a very different time now."

There was general agreement about this, for this was a group of the newer Kennedy people. Someone noted the enormous difference in styles and worlds of Daley and

Kennedy. When Kennedy was trying to decide whether or not to enter the race, he made one rather odd last-minute attempt to maneuver Johnson on the war; he proposed an objective panel on the war which would recommend ways of getting out with honor. The White House leaked word of this to reporters. Kennedy was enraged, and called Daley, asking him for advice about what to do. Daley's advice was immediate: Just deny it. "Can you imagine that," said the Kennedy man, "there's Bob with forty of the most important reporters in the country waiting outside his hotel door, and the White House has already leaked it—a pretty official damn leak—and Daley says, *deny it*. Cook County is a long way from modern politics."

There was a general assumption that Kennedy was to have a much tougher time ahead with Daley than he realized, that a coolness existed which the Senator had not realized. ("What hotel is Bob Kennedy taking over in Chicago?" a reporter asked a Daley aide in late April, and the Daley man answered, "Bobby Kennedy isn't taking over anything in this city.") The one thing working for Kennedy was that despite Daley's probable preference for Humphrey, he likes winners above all, that's why he had steadily expanded his power base, and the Kennedy people believed that they could prove that they had the winner and that Humphrey simply couldn't carry a weak ticket. One Kennedy man recalled being in Chicago with Jack Kennedy in 1960, at the time of the debates, when Daley was actively for Kennedy. "Jack arrived and was preparing for the debate and he kept asking us, 'Where's Daley? Where's Daley? Anybody heard from Daley?' And no Daley of course. So we had the debate, and the moment it was over, who's the first guy bursting into the television studios, surrounded by a phalanx of his yes-men? Why Daley of course. He knew for the first time he'd got a *winner*."

Kennedy became more dependent on the traditionalists who had opposed the race but were now more at ease with it. They knew delegates, they worked among the delegates, but they also were a tempering influence on the campaign. The delegates, many of whom were tied to the big city machines, were uneasy with Kennedy's radicalism and his ties to Negroes. In Chicago, for instance, the militant blacks Kennedy had touched were the sworn enemies of Daley and his machine. Daley was uneasy with Kennedy's appeals; if this young man were elected he might threaten the city machine. He might give federal money directly to these wild black men, and thus cut off the machine's power among the poor blacks through traditional patronage. He might just finance Dick Daley's opposition, and Daley was not happy about the course of it. And Daley might now be the most important single man in the party. And so the delegates were uneasy with the course of the campaign. A basic split soon developed between the radicals, the Robert Kennedy people, and the traditionalists or Jack Kennedy people, with someone like Fred Dutton serving vaguely in the middle as an interpreter to the generations. "The young people think the New Politics is already here and they want Bob to lead it in, or failing that, to be a martyr to it," said one staff man. "What they don't see is that Bob is a transitional figure with ties to both the new and the old, but that he also wants very much to win. They have too much conviction. They are too sure of themselves for the complexities and pluralism of American politics. Walinsky makes too many flat statements such as 'the country is against the war,' or 'the country is for the Negro.' The kind of thing they want Bob to do is the sort of thing you do from the pulpit or from the editorial page, but not necessarily in politics. They want something new, the sharpening of issues and differences. You could almost call it the politics of abrasiveness. The traditionalists want to soften the differences, ease them over, say something like there's no real difference here between you and me, but our guy is better and besides, he's a winner."

The young radicals for their part thought that the cutback on race ("I was the chief law enforcement of this country . . .") was a mistake, morally and politically. The entire country already knew where Kennedy stood on the race issue, particularly those who hated Negroes. There was no sense in 1968, with its instant communications, of trying to fool them. Those who hated Negroes would know where Robert Kennedy stood—either they would hate him too, or they would come aboard. But cutting back was harmful among the liberals with whom he was in already serious trouble. His image was blurred. If national reporters and television reflected his edginess on race, as they were bound to and as they did, then it would hurt him once more there. It would re-create the image of the too political Bobby, and this finally would backfire. (What is the difference between you and Barry Goldwater on some of these programs in the ghetto—about plans to involve the private sector more in the cities, he was once asked. "The difference is that I mean it," he answered.) The view, expressed by Walinsky, was "we should do our own thing, and win and then let the delegates come to us." The young men were still bitter about the failure to enter the race the previous fall ("We'd have the nomination by now," one said in late April), about the loss of their real base to McCarthy—the professors, liberals, intellectuals, kids. They thought that this had thrown Kennedy off balance in the campaign. Because he had come in late, McCarthy had picked up Kennedy's natural base and as a result Kennedy was forced to appeal to blue-collar people, which contradicted his appeal to blacks and liberals. Had he entered early he would have been right on balance, running from strength with Negroes, kids and liberals, and pitching to blue collar simply by his presence. He would have been able to go into working-class neighborhoods and instead of talking about law enforcement, he could talk from a stronger position, putting the emphasis on the need for generosity, and reconciliation in America.

There was an additional problem here; Robert Kennedy's course had been one of the traditional politician turning toward an increasingly radical position. In the process, men like Walinsky had played a considerable role. They always felt that it was an uphill one: softening your real advice on three out of four positions so that you did not look too much like a radical, and so that you looked like you had good common sense, were a professional, and then slipping in your advice on the fourth point. Now the young aides saw other men coming up and using what they considered to be self-serving conservatism: trimming on what they really felt in order to ingratiate themselves. "You-know-I'm-liberal-myself,-but-is-the-country-really-ready-for-this." The younger men regarded Sorensen as the arch enemy; they had looked to Richard Goodwin, though he had served in the earlier administration, as a soul brother. (Goodwin, was a swing figure politically. After having run some shabby errands for Johnson on the war, he had become deeply involved with the opposition to it. Of all the Kennedy people, he alone had gone to work for McCarthy—showing up in New Hampshire and telling Seymour Hersh, McCarthy's then press secretary, "Just you and me, Sy, and one typewriter, and we're going to bring down the President of the United States." When he finally came back to Kennedy, after Wisconsin, he called the candidate and made sure he realized that it was not Gene McCarthy or Bob Kennedy who had brought Lyndon Johnson down, but Dick Goodwin.

It was a call which delighted Kennedy with its egocentrism.) But Goodwin, after joining the Kennedy campaign, had busied himself becoming Kennedy's television expert, and had participated to a limited degree in ideological conflicts. Indeed some of the other staffers felt that Goodwin seemed a little unsure of himself in the Kennedy camp, as though he felt he might be a little distrusted for his prior service in the enemy camp. The radicals' best friend in court was the candidate himself, and they felt he had surrounded himself with too many men who were now viewed as professionals, whereas they were viewed only as amateurs.

Thus the uneven and at times contradictory tone of the campaign. The formal tone was constricted but then again and again the passion would break through, in question-and-answer sessions, where the candidate would react, more often than not, to the smugness and complacency of white America. It would jar him out of his own nervousness. One of the most poignant examples was at Purdue. It was a conservative audience, not with him at the beginning, during his dull speech. But then, during the question-and-answer period, he began to talk about the poor in America, about what it was like to grow up with rats in Bedford Stuyvesant, how the schools maim, what it was like to be in an Indian school and read only the white man's characterization of Indian life. Finally there was a deep and moving description of the disenfranchised in America: ". . . the almost impassable barriers between the poor and the rest of the country." It won a prolonged standing ovation from the audience, converted several otherwise critical reporters, and led one Washington columnist to say, "Scotty Reston always claimed that Jack Kennedy never educated the people on their country, but you've just seen as good an example of it as you'll see in American politics."

Probably the best example of the passion and the anger came in late April when Kennedy met with medical students at Indiana University. It is a fact of American life that the medical profession has become a hard core of American conservatism. In 1964, as I traveled with Goldwater, the hard core of the committee at those $100 a plate dinners was doctors, and here at Indianapolis they were in their embryo stage, the new young conservatives, Reagan country. (One looked at them and listened to their questions and recalled a great Goldwater rally in suburban Chicago in 1964, and the very posh teen-age children going around in their Madras sports jackets with huge signs saying "We Want Freedom.") The hall was packed and, for a Kennedy audience, markedly reserved. In the balcony, a Negro, obviously a maintenance man, shouted "We want Kennedy." Immediately about a dozen others, all students, shouted back "oh no we don't."

"Some of my people," he began, "have been trying to organize a committee of doctors for Kennedy in Indiana. And they're still trying." Mild applause. Then the speech, strong but not terribly well done, an indictment of U.S. medical programs. We are lagging behind other countries, and twelve other nations, "some of them Communist," have a higher life-expectancy rate than the U.S.; a call for the restructuring of American medical care, which included expanded programs and greater decentralization of decision making. When he finished, the applause was polite. Then a flood of questions, almost all conservative, almost all dubious and hostile. Where would the money come from, someone asked. "The federal govement will have to make some available," he said. "Money implies control," a student shouted. "Barry Goldwater lost that struggle four years ago," he said. It went on, and finally, angry now, angry at the smugness, he said, "The fact is there are people who suffer in this country and some of the rest of us have a responsibility. I look around me here and I don't see many black faces. Frankly, the poor have difficulty entering your profession. You can say that the federal government does this or fails here or doesn't do that, but it is really our society that is responsible. That there are more rats than people in New York is intolerable; after all, the poor are the ones who are doing most of the fighting in Vietnam, while white students sit here in medical school."

With that they began to hiss and boo, and they began to shout, "We're going, we're going, we've signed up."

"Oh yes," he said, "going there sometime in the future. It's not the same thing. The dying is going on now, *right now,* while we're talking." What about college deferments? someone shouted; he was against them. What about medical school deferments, are you against them? "Well, the way things are going here, I guess the answer is yes. I don't want to say anything you might approve of."

Later, on the plane, he kept shaking his head about the afternoon. "They were so comfortable," he said, "so comfortable. Didn't you think they were comfortable?"

Election night. The old excitement. The hotel filled with all the team: faces from the past, new faces, the good looking Kennedy women with their expensive coats (you can always recognize the rich women because they put money into their coats a non-political expert told me). A buoyant atmosphere, and the feeling that Kennedy will go to about forty-five percent and the hope that McCarthy will be disposed of, so that they can get on with the business at hand—Hubert. Early returns were very good. The Negroes were coming in just fine. One black precinct which John Kraft, the pollster, had told them to look for came in: Branigin 16, McCarthy 52, Kennedy 697. "I think that's my favorite precinct," said Mankiewicz. Winners' words, winners' smiles. The Poles in Gary came through, 2-to-1, despite the machine. More smiles. A Negro ward came in and it had Kennedy over Branigin by only 166 to 102. Someone complained about it. "There's nothing wrong with that total," said Larry O'Brien, "I would say that the regular organization is functioning effectively in that ward. They had the foresight to bring whiskey." Winners' words again. The lead seemed to be about 45-to-26-to-26. The television sets were all on that afternoon and one TV newscaster said that Kennedy's showing was disappointing. "Disappointing to who," said Tuck, "not to you, you sonofabitch, you never liked us anyway." (Later that night, a reporter, wandering through the crowd, picked up a TV broadcaster and pleaded with his home office. "Yes, yes I know the other networks have had him on, and have interviewed him, but Tuck refuses to let him go on with us until we pronounce him a winner. You declare him a winner and I'll get him on. It's that damn Tuck.") McCarthy, on the television, was saying that it wasn't a defeat. "Well, I don't know," Kennedy said, "I don't know whether people think it's so good to be second or third. That's not the way I was brought up. I always was taught that it's much better to win." He was laughing. "I learned that when I was about two." It was coming on, not exactly what they had wanted, they had wanted that fifty, but it was forty-two in a conservative state and with a rushed-up campaign, and they had those Slav wards, 2-to-1; a fine gift for the omnipresent Mayor Daley. Larry O'Brien was already on the television spreading the sweet syrup; how happy they were, how they had come into Indiana and run against such a fine popular governor like Roger Branigin, and they were pleased to do so well against such difficult odds. And it had been a fine campaign, a clean one, and Roger Branigin, well, he was a fine governor, imagine beating him here in Indiana. Adam Walinsky wanted to issue a statement calling the returns a victory for social justice. Someone told him, no Adam, not this time.

And the candidate? He was celebrating by having dinner with two intense young McCarthy workers whom he had found, dispirited, in the lobby. They were still a little bitter and they complained about the quality of Kennedy's young people, and the fact that when they went into the ghettos none of the Negroes would listen to them. Kennedy suggested that perhaps McCarthy hadn't worked hard enough in the ghettos.

"But you're a Kennedy," the girl said. "It sounds like a newspaper rehash, but it still is right. You have the name."

"Look," he said, "I agree I have a tremendous advantage with my last name. But let me ask you why can't McCarthy go into a ghetto? Why can't he go into a poor neighborhood? Can you tell me when he's been involved in those areas?"

"You've got a tremendous headstart in those areas," the girl insisted. "But he was there first on the war. He declared himself first."

And with that, Indiana was finished.

III

He was an odd and beguiling figure. Patrick Anderson had once written that Robert Kennedy was not a simple man, but many simple men; a good description. His reputation was for ruthlessness, yet in 1968, there was no major political figure whose image so contrasted with the reality. Part of it was simply the quality of change. He was a man of constant growth and change, and while journalistic stereotypes are, more often than not, accurate as long as the person involved stands still, they are likely to be several years out of date if he changes as much as Kennedy did. Most politicians seem somewhat attractive from a distance, but under closer examination they fade: the pettiness, the vanities, the little vulgarities come out. This was to hurt McCarthy as the campaign progressed, for some of the young people who worked most directly with him would find some of their enthusiasm dimmed by his lack of generosity, his cool, almost arrogant, introversion. Robert Kennedy was different. Under closer examination he was far more winning than most, with little bitterness or pettiness. For in those days, if one was a Kennedy there was little reason to feel embittered or cheated. There was little false vanity or false modesty because, as a Kennedy, the action swirled around him; he was automatically at the center of things. Even when a Kennedy is out of power his telephone still rings. He seemed like the other Kennedys, still a fresh figure in our politics, which in some measure was a benefit of his wealth. For it is true that having money as a national politician is not so important as *not* having money. There is a gradual erosion to a politician who lacks wealth—too many years attending too many dinners, asking too many rich men favors, listening to their inanities and then thanking them. Kennedys and Rockefellers are spared that. He was intelligent and knowledgeable about the world; indeed there was now no one in his entourage who knew more of the world. This too was indicative of the change of the past few years; for there were men who had once been major intellectual influences on his brother, who had taught the Kennedys about America and about the world. But Robert Kennedy had passed them by now. There might be people who knew more about one particular country, but none who knew as much about as many things. He had traveled too much, been briefed too often by very able people; he had access again and again to the most powerful and informed people in the world. His was the best education a rich family and a powerful nation could provide. He was quick to admit his own mistakes (the only major figure who had been involved in Vietnam to have done so; a fine index of the intellectual integrity of our times), and curiously fatalistic about himself, for if one is a Kennedy there is a sense that it can all be achieved, but also that it can all be snatched away.

Thus again and again, during the campaign, reporters would ask him what his long range plans were, and he would answer that you never really knew; you lived day to day; it was all like Russian roulette. He could talk with striking detachment about his own career (though not about John Kennedy's, that was still emotional. One could easily criticize anything Robert Kennedy had done in his lifetime, but one did not criticize aspects of Jack Kennedy's career without quickly and sharply changing the tone of the conversation; his voice getting a little icier, the eyes getting a little harder). He could sit one night and talk fatalistically about Indiana, on the eve of the primary, about the people, they had given him at least a fair chance, about the people who hated him in the state, the transplanted Kentuckians, and Tennesseans, out of place, scared for their jobs, scared by the Negroes, scared by Robert Kennedy. Sometimes, he had said that night, you could feel them hate straight at you. "I can understand that." As for the kids working for McCarthy who hated him, he understood that too. He probably would feel exactly the same if he were one of them; but they were good, weren't they? What he wouldn't give to have them on his side. McCarthy had the A kids, the best of them, and that was hard to take. They'll come back some day, someone said. He answered, Oh, perhaps eventually, but it will probably never be the same thing. They may never forgive themselves or me for making it happen.

His sense of humor was very good in small groups and he could be very funny. Yet he often seemed ill at ease in his public appearances, and he performed worst in a sterile television studio without any audience. He performed best under intense critical, indeed emotional, circumstances and under heckling. In public he would be cool toward a business group, unless they were so smug that he was angered, and he would spend long hours with a young people's group or with Negroes. (Nevertheless, he could, on occasion, flash moments of almost absent-minded rudeness for such a normally sensitive man. A reporter traveling in upstate New York in early 1968 would come across a pleasant congenial Democratic functionary who hated Robert Kennedy with a very special passion. The reason was simple. In 1964 he had driven Kennedy around his section of the state in his own car. Kennedy had sat in the front seat and said to him snappishly, "Turn off the heater!" The driver had done nothing, waited ten minutes, and then, "It's a little warm in here, would you like the heater turned down, Mister Kennedy?" Kennedy had answered, "Yes, please.") Conversation with him was never particularly easy, and he was often abrupt. A reporter did not really interview him; at best he talked his way through with him, not so much asking questions as proffering ideas and judging his reactions. "You have to learn to read the pauses," his former press secretary Ed Guthman once said of him. Young radicals uneasy and distrusting of him would find him interested in their ideas and willing to listen at great length. High ranking labor leaders expecting to tell him about their demands on minimum wage might find themselves questioned sharply, even rudely, on what they were doing to end discrimination in their unions. He lacked Jack Kennedy's absolute confidence in himself and his charm, and most important, his confidence that he could project that charm. "More than any man I ever knew," John Kenneth Galbraith once said of Jack Kennedy, he "liked being himself and was at ease with himself." The people around Robert Kennedy were regularly telling him to loosen up, but it did not come easily: his knuckles would be cracking away, his hands wrestling with each other—he was not a loose man. He was less graceful and more committed than his brother.

Kennedy had the dual advantage of being rich, which gave him one kind of asset, and of coming from a home where the Anglo-Saxon prejudice against the Irish had generated a rage to succeed and to excel, and which would prevent the squandering of money. The Kennedys would not let their money distort or soften them. They would dominate the money; the money would not dominate them. They understood, as few wealthy families in this country understood, its advantages and its liabilities. Joe Kennedy, said a contemporary, "is sort of like a caterpillar. He couldn't

quite become a butterfly, but his boys were going to fly, no
matter what." Robert came from way down the list of children, the seventh of nine ("When you come from that far
down you have to struggle to survive," he later said). He was
by far the smallest of the boys and in a family in which there
was a relentless success cult, his lack of size drove him
even harder. That, and the fact that he came along at the
tail end of World War II, and always felt a strong sense
of disappointment at not having seen combat, were frustrations which drove him even harder in the postwar years. He
did not learn much at college but he learned from his personal experience. As his life touched things in the outside
world, he would become interested in them. He had had, as
a young man, a special quality which would later set him
apart from most men in public life: that indignation, an
almost primitive and innocent anger—that things were
not what they should be or were supposed to be. Had he
not had the wealth and family position which springboarded
him into immediate public service, he might either have
lost this indignation through the erosion of a thousand
smaller deals and battles at a lower level, or his very intensity might have blocked out a public career, for men that intense are not always trusted by their peers; they are often
considered extremist, in the American vernacular. But because of his family he was able both to enter public life at a
very high level and retain that intensity.

In his public career, that outrage was turned at first
to relatively minor issues, indeed sometimes to the wrong
issues. But as he became a full-fledged public servant, he
turned it to the great and dark questions of American life.
This quality took him to stands and causes far beyond those
accepted by more traditional liberals who accepted the society at face value. At dinner late one night in Indiana, Kennedy and Bill Haddad, an ex-newspaperman who had also

served in the Peace Corps and the poverty program, and I were talking about the campaign. It seemed to me, I said, that as the campaign developed it was taking Kennedy further and further outside the establishment; that the more he saw of the country, the more he was turned off by the establishment and the existing representatives of existing institutions, and the more he was involved with the poor. (Indeed, Dick Harwood of *The Washington Post* would a month later write an incisive story pointing out that Kennedy had earlier said McCarthy faced the danger of being a one-issue man on Vietnam, but now Kennedy himself, tied to the poor, was sounding like a one-issue man.) Yes, Kennedy said, it was pointless to talk about the problem in America being black and white, it was really rich and poor, which was a much more complex subject. But if you keep going this way, I asked, won't you finally have to take on the establishment. Kennedy nodded. And what if you take over and find that the very institutions of government and the society are strangling the country and perpetuating the imbalance? Haddad asked him. "Then we will have to change the institutions," he answered quietly. Then he began to talk about the problems that would be involved in changing the institutions in this country non-violently. Haddad looked over at me as if this were a signal victory. Many months afterward he said that this was the first moment when he was convinced that Kennedy was different from other politicians and that he was the one major political figure who understood where everything was going and how serious it was. "He was willing to change the institutions. Even John Kennedy didn't go that far. John Kennedy's instinct, when he ran up against the institutions, was to try and challenge them, to elevate them. Which worked a little, but really didn't work. Before, when I was in the Peace Corps and things would go wrong, I'd go running over to the White House and scream at Kenny

O'Donnell. 'You think you run the country! You don't even run it from here to across the street!' and he would answer 'The trouble with you Haddad is that you think we don't know it.' And now here was Bob, seeing how deep it went, and how bad it was, and then suddenly breaking through— it was like finally seeing the blue sky. You had a sense he could go all the way and do something about it."

He could bring into American politics some of the very best people in the game: fresh, intelligent, even joyous men of a variety of views, and he could inspire them to an extraordinary degree. That was in part because he did not like sycophants, and because, more than most strong men who like power, he could listen to the quiet dissenting voices. Indeed one of the better epitaphs might have later read that, in a time of growing pessimism about American life among many of the best-informed young men, Robert Kennedy had nonetheless served as a rallying point for many of the most talented young men of the nation; men who were scarred by the events of the past decade, but still saw, through him, a hope of turning the country around. Yet he could also tolerate, on the fringes, self-serving and frivolous people; so that to the outsider, the Robert Kennedy people were blurred. Was it Fred Dutton, a rare practicing intellectual in American politics, or Mankiewicz, the thoughtful press secretary, who had decided to work for Kennedy when the Senator had denounced the government's refusal of burial privileges to Robert Thompson, a Distinguished Service Medal winner but also an ex-member of the Communist party? Or was it John Lewis, the former head of Snick, a poor Negro boy from Troy, Alabama, still hopeful that the American dream might work, or was it some silly socialite? I remember once being in a crowd of some of his young social friends and wondering how in God's name he could tolerate them, and deciding there must be some mean, perverse little Irish quirk in Kennedy which permitted him to accept the fawn-ing of these people: one more victory for his family.

He was visualized as a total politician, yet he fre-quently did things which were, technically at least, bad politics. His championing of the California grape pickers was, at best, high-risk politics and, by traditional standards, bad politics. One makes powerful enemies for marginally effective friends. His constant reiteration about the plight of the American Indians, their suicide rate, their hopeless-ness, had little impact on a crisis-belching American middle class which can accept no more than two causes at a given time.

He had become the chief spokesman of the dispossessed in this country and, God knows, the conservatives and reac-tionaries knew it. (In Texas, it was virtually impossible to get anyone to work for him in 1968. Someone finally asked Judge Woodrow Wilson Bean, one of the few men openly supporting Kennedy, why he was doing it, and Bean an-swered: "Because if he's elected, anyone from Texas will need a pass to get into Washington, and I'm going to be the man handing out the passes.") Yet, as he started his race, he was distrusted by liberals and intellectuals to a surprising degree. People who felt deeply about his brother regarded him with grave misgivings and deep suspicion, though in 1968 he had a far greater proven record than Jack Kennedy had in 1960.

Part of it was that he was a Kennedy, which meant that everything was bigger than life. He could not be judged like other men; more had been given to him, more was ex-pected of him, and more would be doubted about him. In Indiana, for example, he had attracted a much bigger press corps because he was a Kennedy, but similarly, when he won, a striking victory in a conservative state, he got sur-prisingly little credit for his victory. Only a landslide or a defeat would move the press. Indeed *The New York Times* and two of the networks called McCarthy the big winner in Indiana, because he had not been eliminated. The other part of it was the Kennedys' own fault. Like the rest of us, they wanted things both ways but unlike the rest of us, they more often than not had it both ways. They wanted to be able to complain about the lack of privacy given them by the press, and yet be able to summon photographers and reporters from important magazines to reveal all kinds of innermost thoughts at opportune moments and permit all kinds of spontaneous family photographs. They wanted to be able to get the full measure and mileage out of the power and unity of the family, to the degree that outsiders felt that the power thrust of the family came first and issues second, and yet they wanted, at the same time, to convince the uneasy, sophisticated dissenter that they were doing all these things because of the issues involved. Then there was Camelot. The country at times liked Kennedy for being part of Camelot, and then hated him because of course there was no Camelot. And why did the Kennedys pretend there was? Wasn't it nice to have an American royal family at last, but who were these Kennedys, did they think they were better than the rest of us?

Thus he could not be like other men and this feeling extended to all of us; we all had our ambivalent feelings about him. I remember the night of Martin Luther King's funeral. I sat with Jack Nelson of the *Los Angeles Times,* one of the most distinguished reporters in the country, a strong idealistic man, and perhaps as knowledgeable about race in the South as any man in the country, and a fan of Kennedy's. We were talking about the long, grueling march in the very hot weather from the church to Morehouse College. Kennedy had made the march and had evoked by far the most passionate response from Negroes along the way.

Yet he had taken off his jacket, as had some others, and I was complaining about this. I suppose I felt it was half youth-cult and half tough-cult, but Nelson was defending him. Others had taken their coats off; it was only normal; it was not demagogic. Why, he said, Martin Luther King would have taken off his coat at the funeral. No he wouldn't, I said, you just don't do that. No, said Nelson, King had even done it, at the funeral of Jimmie Lee Jackson, but when Kennedy does it, you all read too much into it. Case closed.

Yet finally when he was judged, he had to be judged not just on the past and the mythology of the past, but in his time, when America itself was changing so rapidly, and on his capacity for growth. They were not just the years before the White House, or even the three years in power, as the right hand of The Man, but also and equally important, those post-power years when he had stood outside the power establishment looking in, and had become consumed by the poor in America, and the inequities within the system. He had changed radically and he understood the rapid changes in America, and this did not always help him. Not only were many of the reporters describing the early Robert Kennedy, but they were also writing about their own version of America—vintage 1960. One man, Bill Wilson, a talented young television producer, an early Stevensonian, had worked with Jack Kennedy in 1960. He had not liked Robert Kennedy and had reluctantly come to work for him in 1968, but was startled by the change; "Now he is tough of mind and tough of spirit, not just tough of mouth."

Kennedy had begun his public career as a social illiterate. He worked for a time for the justice department, and then took a job with the McCarthy committee, a natural enough liaison worked out through his father, who admired Mc-

Carthy. (McCarthy and the elder Kennedy had become good friends; the elder Kennedy admired McCarthy for his enemies: liberals, members of the Eastern establishment, and the British.) Kennedy's role was not major, largely working out statistics on allies who were trading with the Communists during the Korean war, and he eventually ended up as a counsel for the Democrats on the committee. He admired McCarthy, did not dissent or even think to dissent from what he was doing. He did not see anything particularly destructive to it, and saw McCarthy being destroyed by Roy Cohn and David Schine who played to his desire for publicity. ("He was on a toboggan," he would later tell one interviewer. "It was so exciting and exhilarating as he went downhill that it didn't matter to him if he hit a tree at the bottom. Cohn and Schine took him up the mountain and showed him all those wonderful things. He destroyed himself for that—for publicity.") Kennedy broke with McCarthy more over Roy Cohn than anything else; a relationship which almost ended with a fistfight. He ended his tour of the McCarthy committee by serving as counsel for the Democrats, though he did remain loyal to McCarthy to the end, one of the few who did, as the Wisconsin Senator ravaged himself. At the end, Kennedy received an award as one of the Junior Chamber of Commerce's young men of the year but walked out during the main speech by Edward R. Murrow, who had distinguished himself to most of the nation by his battles with McCarthy.

After that he joined the Senate Rackets Committee, becoming a relentless chaser of hoods in general and Jimmy Hoffa in particular. Here the full force of his indignation was felt for the first time in this country. One reporter who covered the Teamster investigations was enormously impressed with Kennedy's determination, his single-mindedness, the way his anger exploded at Hoffa's operation and

Hoffa's belief that he was beyond American laws. "At once you admired what he was doing, the intensity of it all, and how well he did it, and at the same time you wondered a little about Kennedy and how he felt about labor in general," the reporter said. This was a feeling that much of labor's leadership was to retain; the leadership went for Jack Kennedy in 1960, but it always remained uneasy about Robert Kennedy. It felt that he had enjoyed the Hoffa prosecution a little too much, and this hurt him some in 1968. Kennedy's puritanism bloomed and flourished during the combat with the hoods and the toughs. Joe Gallo, one of the hoods investigated, later recalled that Kennedy had looked at him and said, " 'So you're Joe Gallo the Jukebox. You don't look so tough. I'd like to fight you myself.' So I hadda tell him I don't fight." Kennedy himself thought that the toughs, themselves, were overrated. He once told a friend that anyone who talked as much about being tough as Hoffa did, couldn't really be that tough. Yet a violent struggle emerged; they threatened each other, they swapped insults, they were ready to match each other in push-ups. Kennedy once drove home past midnight, the last person to leave the Senate office building, only to see the lights in Hoffa's Teamster office still on; he turned around and went back to his own office. Kennedy was in those days very much the prosecutor, not a great social-cause-and-effect man. He saw the American system working, and working well, and he simply saw Hoffa violating it. The Teamster years were not beneficial for him. Rather they benefitted Jack Kennedy, giving him needed national exposure, and hurt Robert Kennedy's standing with his future constituents, the liberals. He did, however, make some acquaintances among the extraordinary group of investigative reporters covering the Teamsters who were to become his most trusted friends: Wally Turner, John Seigenthaler, Ed Guthman. Yet Kennedy would retain, and find difficult to shake, the image of a prosecutor, and people in general, and liberals in particular, do not like prosecutors. Liberals do not like investigations of labor, even if it is corrupt. In those days it went against their instincts, it might be labor baiting, and yes, they would think, maybe Hoffa is abusive, but isn't he being singled out? In sum, Kennedy would lose more by the Hoffa investigation than he would gain. Hoffa would call him ruthless, and that would stick. Hoffa might be ruthless too, but he would not be running one day for the presidency of the United States.

He had never, of course, lost sight of the priority assignment in those days—to elect Jack Kennedy President. That ambition was the family ambition and it never dimmed. Was Seigenthaler a close friend through the Rackets Committee investigations? Well then, the Kennedys would later send Robert down to Nashville and use that connection as a base in searching for delegates, in meeting people. In 1956 they had an attractive young candidate, and they had come within a hair of the vice-presidency in the open convention. Beaten by Kefauver, Robert Kennedy, working the floor, had found that many delegates liked Jack Kennedy, thought him a real comer, but Estes, well old Estes had been to their homes, had sent them postcards. Between 1956 and 1960 a lot of postcards were sent out by the Kennedys and a lot of homes visited. (Jet travel has enormously changed political conventions. In the old days when travel was so slow, the proselytizing was done at the conventions and thus the delegates arrived more malleable. Now, with jets, they are visited, wined and dined locally and sought at their very doorsteps. By convention time one nominally knows whom they're for.) The interim years were thus crucial and the Kennedys became adept at all this; there were so many of them to go visiting and they always had the financial resources to do it. But the 1956 race proved valuable. Young Robert Kennedy traveled with the Stevenson campaign all over the country, sitting quietly, realizing that the election was lost, but that it was a fortuitous break that Kefauver rather than his brother was on the ticket (the onus would not go against the Catholics). He made endless notes on how badly the campaign was run, the poor timing, the waste of the candidate's time and energy, the failure to schedule well, the lack of press kits.

He was an excellent campaign manager for his brother in 1960. Though it was Jack Kennedy's campaign, an extraordinary number of the key men, the organizers, the drivers, were men brought in by Robert. It was as if Jack were in charge of the intellectual component, the speeches, the policies, the ideology, while Robert was in charge of organizing, of the talent, of the *loyalty*, picking and deciding which men could do it and which could not. Bobby would test the men; Jack would test the ideas. As campaign manager he had the total trust of his brother. He guarded Jack's interest zealously; Jack was a precious commodity and was not to be scratched, worn down or irritated. He understood Jack and his best interests. The brothers, different in style and in friends, had been brought much closer by politics; without the common link of Jack's destiny, they might have gone quite different ways, with different friends, different wives, different tastes. Now Jack Kennedy had a campaign manager who understood not only the candidate, but the family; someone who would not be too independent, or seek his own publicity, or get independent ideas, and someone who could take the heat. This latter is terribly important.

A campaign is a difficult thing and there are endless decisions to be made. Not only must the candidate be saved from making them in order to conserve his time, but more—

a lot of the decisions are cruel, they have an element of rejection in them, and they can make enemies. Thus a person whose campaign idea or campaign role is rejected must not be made to think that it was the candidate who had turned him down. He must think that it was unsympathetic underlings. In this case it was the illiberal Bobby who was blocking him out. It was also Bobby who had to separate the endless fights between the local reform groups and the local machines, while keeping both in the Kennedy camp. It must always be the Good Jack and the Bad Bobby. "I'm not running a popularity contest," he said at the time. "It doesn't matter if people like me or not. Jack can be nice to them. I don't try to antagonize people, but somebody has to be able to say No. If people are not getting off their behinds, how do you say that?" He was very good, always willing to take the heat, always willing to back up his people, and willing to try the unorthodox. (A young political science professor who bucked the organization in upstate New York, in 1960, got an enormous kickback from the machine, which went directly to Robert Kennedy: Was one young egghead worth five old professionals, even if Kennedy himself had given the go ahead on the strategy earlier? The professor, to his surprise, found that Kennedy backed him up. He became a lifelong and influential devotee.) Kennedy was at times rough and almost too devoted to his purpose. Anyone, in those simplistic days, who opposed Jack was a bad guy likely to be roughly treated; and even friends found their sensibilities trampled on. A lifetime of intelligent and dedicated service to certain principles meant nothing to Kennedy if the person was somehow blocking, or likely to help block, Jack Kennedy's presidential ambitions. Harsh words were spoken; and years later people would exonerate Jack Kennedy and remember Bobby Kennedy. It was at the convention that he told the unhappy Humphrey, wavering between Stevenson and Kennedy, "Hubert, we want your announcement and the pledge of the Minnesota delegation today or else." To which Humphrey replied: "Go to hell." But he ran an excellent campaign. They had enough delegates, and they kept them in line. If he was frequently and justifiably accused of twisting arms one notch too many, it was also true that on the first ballot their calculations were almost letter perfect. It was also true that the first ballot was vital. The bosses still had their doubts about Kennedy and the liberals still loved Stevenson, and any defection might start an outbound tide. If they missed on the first ballot, they might miss completely. But the convention was won, and so was the campaign. Jack became the handsome young President and Robert took the heat; he had won for his brother but lost for himself.

If it is not traditional to appoint the campaign manager Attorney General, it is not exactly unusual either. So the question very early became whether Jack would appoint Robert to the justice department. The President was reluctantly inclined toward it, he wanted Robert Kennedy around and he trusted his advice. Joseph Kennedy was enthusiastically for it; the cries of dynasty hardly frightened or embarrassed him. Nothing would have pleased him more than to have founded a dynasty. Robert himself was dubious. He remembered that when Nixon had visited South Carolina during the 1960 campaign, Bill Rogers, the Attorney General and one of the ablest members of the Eisenhower administration, had been forced to hide in the plane because of his unpopularity. (Eight years later Robert Kennedy, visiting Atlanta, would see a young girl named Kathy McGrath, a twenty-two-year-old secretary who had come to the airport to meet him. When she asked for his autograph he would write: "To Kathy. You are now in charge of my campaign in Georgia. Good luck. You'll need it. Bob Kennedy.") Besides, there were other things in the administration which he would have liked to try, perhaps in State or Defense, places where he could learn and could soften the intensity of feeling against him. Jack Kennedy, wanting his brother in this special role, finally decided to go ahead, though noting to a friend: "I'd like to open the door at about 3 A.M. and announce that Bobby is the Attorney General and then shut the door and run like hell." Jack Kennedy, witty, gracious, charming, had always been amused by his younger brother's ability to take the heat for him. In 1962 a group of congressmen dropped by the White House to pay the President a visit. It was a pleasant amiable session and finally one Southern congressman said, "Mister President, I'm afraid I'm going to have to attack you in a speech for all this civil-rights activity." The President laughed and said: "Why can't you just call Bobby a son of a bitch?"

The early days of the John Kennedy administration were marked by a certain arrogance of the hard-nosed— we're eggheads, but we're tough too—and Robert Kennedy was one of the leading offenders. It was a time when activist eggheads with muscles were in, and old soft eggheads, many of them Stevensonians, were out. The newer men were in their late thirties and early forties, more often than not combat veterans of the war, well-read, articulate, playing down their idealism; it was not something one talked about. Chester Bowles was almost symbolic of the old kind, though many of the administration's best ambassadorial appointments were made by him. He was too avowedly liberal, too quick to talk openly, in daily conversation, about idealism. Robert Kennedy was to finally emerge, in instance after instance, as the single most important liberal influence in the administration, but the very idea of this would have

appalled him. In those days he would have been embarrassed to go around spouting liberal ideology; his liberalism
was camouflaged under the tough-guy exterior. When
Bowles appeared ready to blab about having been against
the Bay of Pigs, Robert Kennedy's finger went into his
stomach: *you were for it, remember that.* (The story went
around the country and it wasn't the Bowles people who
put it out either.) Indeed part of the mystique of the administration was toughness—Floyd Patterson's photograph
hung in the Attorney General's office until Patterson lost
the heavyweight title. Shortly after the administration
started, with speaking invitations coming in from everywhere and very few being accepted, one came in from a
Polish group. Come on, he said, let's take that one. I like
the Poles, they're tough.

When Burke Marshall was being looked over for Assistant Attorney General, the early doubts about him were that
he wasn't tough enough; which was true. Marshall on the
outside is a mild, quiet man; his fingers do not go into people's stomachs, yet he proved in those years to be a man of as
much steel and fiber as anyone that administration produced. He became as close to Robert Kennedy as anyone,
and Kennedy, at the end, probably relied upon his basic
judgment more than that of anyone else. He also had a part
in teaching the young Attorney General that tough talk is
not always toughness; that steel does not necessarily come
from swaggering, boasting and hard talk (the New Frontier
had a lot of that), but from quiet inner conviction. Nonetheless, to the end, the word tough had a fascination for
Robert Kennedy. It was still a quality he admired, though
he might have given a much different description of it by
1968.

The years as Attorney General were very important for
him in a variety of ways. For one thing they gave him an

identifiable public record. Instead of being a shadowy figure slipping in and out of the back door, blamed for all that was bad, and credited with little that was good, he became a man with a record which could be checked. He was more than just an Attorney General, he was like a deputy president, particularly after the Bay of Pigs. He advised the President on almost every major issue, seeing the world from the eye of the storm. (The President quite accurately felt that the traditional advisers who came with the offices were more identified with their own particular agencies than with the Kennedy administration.) He was a good Attorney General, getting better. He made good, even excellent appointments. He gave people their head. Most important, on the great questions of the day, he was very good.

On civil rights both he and his brother entered with a nominal interest, and Robert Kennedy left with a growing sensitivity. They had both come from Massachusetts where the race question was for a long time a minor ethnic political issue. Had they been from Illinois or New York they might have been more immediately sensitive to the complexities and depth of black feelings. Rather they had run in 1960 as traditional liberal Democratic politicians: hold the old coalition together, be *for* (rather than against) the Negro, don't say anything against them, give whoever their anointed leaders are the minimal reward, usually one notch above what the previous administration gave. Besides, 1960 was the last year of the old order. The Negroes, given the 1954 Supreme Court ruling on segregation in the schools, had waited for six years for the courts to give them their share of the action. Now, in 1960, the young restless kids who had received no benefit from the legal change were taking the matter into their own hands. They began with sit-ins, demanding the right to eat bad overpriced hamburgers just like any other American. They radically changed the pace and tempo of the race question in America, and inevitably, the federal government would be involved in a growing number of moral decisions. The Kennedys did not realize this at first, they were still thinking in traditional terms. They had done a little more for the Negro than the previous administration and they had not yet realized that a revolution had started. They were like most important and influential Americans of that time; they were far more interested in foreign crises than the coming domestic storm. In addition, their hesitance to take the initiative on civil rights at the start of the administration reflected their nervousness after the narrow victory of 1960; one sensed that they planned to go slow in the first administration, then run again, in 1964, win by a landslide, and *then* move ahead on civil rights.

In 1963 Robert Kennedy decided to meet with a group of Negro intellectuals and artists. Just why was never clear, but the impression was strong that he wanted to hear what was on their minds, wanted to be praised a little, and wanted to create continuing ties of friendship—perhaps toward 1964. He asked James Baldwin, the peripatetic writer and protester, to arrange it. Many of the Negroes invited never exactly understood what it was they were being so impatiently summoned to, but arrived at Baldwin's desperate plea. The meeting was a disaster. Kennedy totally misjudged the temper of the Negroes who, meeting in a large group with a white man, all went to the more militant position. (Six years later I asked him what he learned from the meeting. He said, "Never meet with more than two or three Negroes at a time. Never with eighteen. With eighteen it's hopeless. Everyone has to be more militant. Now I realize what they were saying, and why, and why they were so angry, but what was hard to take at the time were the ones who let me take the roasting and then came over afterward to sympathize.") A young civil-rights worker who had been beaten on the head during one of the then-recent Freedom

Rides got up and said that it made him sick being there. He apparently meant that it made him sick having to sit there and ask for his rights which by constitutional right were already his. Kennedy, however, misunderstood and thought him to be saying that it made him sick to be with Robert Kennedy. Kennedy had been under the impression that the Kennedys were *for* the Negroes, and that, of course, the Negroes understood this, and so he pointed to administration accomplishments. They were stunned; to them Kennedy was talking about one drop in a very big bucket, and they had thought he had, at least, realized this, realized how little had been done for the Negroes. At the end of the meeting Baldwin told people that "Bobby Kennedy was a little surprised at the depth of Negro feeling. We were a little shocked at the extent of his naïveté."

But the momentum of American life was headed toward new and militant demands, and the protesters carried the administration with them. Again and again the administration was caught in civil-rights crises, inevitably to land on the side of the Negroes, and inevitably to bring greater affection for the Kennedys from the Negroes. Similarly, there developed in Robert Kennedy a growing sensitivity to the problem of black and white in America. The Kennedys became committed on civil rights in those years simply because there was nowhere else to go, except backward. Thus in 1968, in a black neighborhood, a handmade sign over a Kennedy storefront would read:

> *Kennedy white but alright.*
> *The one before, he opened the door.*

On foreign affairs he became a surprisingly cool and thoughtful influence. In an administration heavy with political scientists, Robert Kennedy's basic value to the President was that he had excellent common sense, judged people well, and often followed his own best instincts. (Following one's best instincts and common sense would have avoided both the Bay of Pigs and the ground war in Vietnam.) His role grew after the Bay of Pigs. The President needed him, and one sensed that the President set out to expand Robert's world, picking the Attorney General for foreign assignment as the President's representative and thus putting his younger brother into situations which might expand and broaden his view of the world. I went on his first major trip, in August 1961, when Kennedy represented the President at the independence ceremonies at the Ivory Coast. He was shy, uncertain of himself. (I remember him wrestling with both his French and his speech: "Your President, Houphouet-Boigny, is the George Washington of your country." Then he listed all the similarities between American and Ivorien history.) But even here, certain characteristics came through. He wanted a candid and thorough briefing before leaving and he was appalled by the lack of knowledge and interest of the first three men the State Department sent over. He kept sending them back until the Department sent over a young man named Brandon Grove who had just spent three years in the Ivory Coast, and who knew the background and the current political balance. Kennedy immediately drafted him for the trip, and later took him on his world tour in 1962. The other thing he demonstrated on arrival was his disdain for normal diplomatic procedures, many of which are hopelessly out of date in a contemporary world. The embassy there had scheduled a series of meetings with all the official people. Instead, he wanted to talk with students, labor leaders (as much as they had them), and of course he wanted to get out into the boondocks to see how the people lived. The embassy felt he ran roughshod over it, pushed its members around, made unnecessary and unfair demands, and insulted its good Ivorien friends. Almost everyone else loved it. This would not be the last embassy to feel this way.

He behaved particularly well during the Cuban missile-crisis in 1962. At the height of the crisis, when the two main choices were a naval blockade and a surprise air strike to eliminate the missile sites, most advisers appeared to favor the bombing. Robert Kennedy strongly opposed it. The air strike, he said, sounded like a Pearl Harbor in reverse. It would be hard to explain to the rest of the world—particularly after the Bay of Pigs—why a great nation was bombing such a small one, and most people would doubt that the missile sites really existed. He did not want his brother to become the Tojo of the sixties. Dean Acheson, a power man and a man with a considerable reputation, attempted to destroy the Attorney General's argument. The young man, he said, simply wasn't dealing with the realities of power and this was a situation where you used power. But Kennedy insisted: American tradition and ideals were completely against such a bombing raid and the world would never understand it. Douglas Dillon, originally for the air strikes, swung around on the basis of the Attorney General's argument. "What changed my mind," he later told Elie Abel, who chronicled the crisis, "was Bob's argument that we ought to be true to ourselves as Americans, that surprise attack was not in our tradition. Frankly these considerations had not occurred to me until Bob raised them. . . ." Later during the same crisis the Attorney General was useful again. Khrushchev had sent a Friday note which was conciliatory but then made a Saturday broadcast which seemed more threatening. It was Robert Kennedy's simple but sound idea to ignore the Saturday message and simply respond to the Friday one.

On Vietnam he was one of the principal authors of the counterinsurgency commitment. An early enthusiast, he forced everyone in Washington to go to special classes on counterinsurgency. Yet even then his judgment was helpful. During 1963 when I was in Vietnam and was not exactly the favorite reporter of the Kennedy administration, the administration saw that a major foreign-policy disaster was shaping up and wished that the crisis would go away or, failing that, that my colleagues and I would go away. Michael Forrestal, the White House man on Vietnam, saw, probably more than any other Washington official, what was coming. He saw it clearly and used his influence to change Washington policy. At the time he told me that if you wanted to get dissident ideas through to the President (which is a very important thing, given the constantly increasing power of the executive branch, the natural isolation of the Presidency, and the instinct of most men to tell powerful men what they want to hear), the single person most open to suggestion and to accepting bad news was Robert Kennedy.

Those were nevertheless good and heady days for the Kennedys, a confluence of power, intelligence, style and glamour perhaps never seen before in this country. Everyone, it seemed, was bright, handsome and tough and had a good-looking wife. They set a style which those of us on the outside might envy, for it was true that the Kennedys, with their wealth, could have free what money could not buy. They could get other immensely talented people to work for them who would not work for other politicians no matter how correct the politician's ideological position or voting record. Those who were simply wealthy found glamour; those who had glamour and wealth found power. It was, in

fact, too good a time. They inhaled people; thoughtful journalists and intellectuals who could not be bought in the
real sense were taken over by the Kennedys and the glamour.
They became too close, they went regularly to Hickory Hill,
saw only what they wanted to see, and finally in the eyes of
their colleagues they became Kennedy satellites, Kennedy
insiders. Their gossip would be listened to, their presence
at a dinner party sought, their post-administration books
bought, but finally they would be seen as Kennedy men, and
this would come back to haunt Robert Kennedy. Years later,
when his own candidacy was advanced, many of the people
who now spoke for him were a little tarnished, their independence questioned, their intellectual judgment no longer
so valued. There was, in some places, a Camelot backlash.
Robert Kennedy would be in a position where his enemies
would be armed and his supporters disarmed. Other younger
men coming along, viewing his candidacy, would deliberately stand a little further back: no one was going to inhale
them. He was not going to get the benefit of the doubt.

It would always be a point of dispute: whether the
dominant force was Kennedyism, the Kennedys first, right
or wrong, or whether it was issues, those particular causes
he came to articulate, which formed the real pull. To some
journalists and critics resisting the pull and the glamour,
there was a feeling that the Kennedys, starting back before
1960, had always practiced manipulation with issues; that
the basic inner ideology was simply The Family, right or
wrong; and that many in the inner circle were motivated
not so much by causes and social issues, as simply by the
fact that this team was a winning one—it had won once
before and now there would be a restoration. Thus there was
a feeling among many reporters, particularly in the early
and mid-sixties, that it was not enough to like the Kennedys
part way, to be partially sympathetic but still to write about

their warts (though they had fewer warts). One had to go all the way with them. (Laura Bergquist of *Look*, a sympathetic journalist-friend of the family, recalled asking the then Attorney General a tough question about bombings in the South at a magazine writer's luncheon. Kennedy, unhappy with the subject, fumbled the question. Later an angry Ethel Kennedy grabbed Miss Bergquist in the ladies' room and said to her fiercely, "I thought you were a friend of my husband's.") This all led to a feeling that the Kennedys were overzealously policing up their image, and finally a belief that the Manchester affair, messy and demeaning as it was, was exactly what they had long deserved. (Even though Manchester did violate his contract, and Robert Kennedy, caught between his sister-in-law and his own political career, behaved honorably, if perhaps unwisely from a political point of view.)

My own feeling was that this sense of Kennedyism had begun to ebb in the last two years of Robert Kennedy's life; that it was one more reflection of the change in his viewpoint; that in the post-assassination period, issues and human grievances began to consume him and that he judged people not so much on how they related to the Kennedys, but on how they related to issues. Hence some of the differences between the old Kennedy advisers and journalistic friends, and the newer more issue-oriented Kennedy friends and journalistic friends: George Smathers, the Florida Senator who led the fight against minimum wage for migrant workers, was an old Kennedy friend; Cesar Chavez was a new Kennedy friend.

But the symbol of the conflict between the Kennedys and their critics was the uneasy relationship between the candidate and *The New York Times*. Kennedy got on reasonably well with the reporters, but the editors were another thing; there was a tension going back to the early Jack Kennedy days when John Oakes, the editor of the editorial page, had once implied that Sorensen, not Jack Kennedy, was primarily responsible for the writing of *Profiles in Courage*. Jack Kennedy went to considerable length to point out that this was false. That tension had never eased. The great strength of *The Times* is that it will stand alone; it can and does resist fad, idol, and even president of the United States. Hence an almost inevitable clash between two powerful contemporary institutions—*The New York Times* and the Kennedys. The Kennedys, because they were liberals, assumed *The Times* would be in their hip pocket, or at least sympathetic, which it clearly was not. It was as if this very assumption of the Kennedys brought out a stronger sense of *The Times'* independence, a conscious desire not to be swept away. (Thus Kennedy would be annoyed with what he felt was *The Times'* instinct for publishing photographs of the handsome young Mayor of New York, John Lindsay, playing tennis or riding a bike, rather than of the handsome young Senator from New York. He once asked Mankiewicz to call *The Times* to suggest that the paper photograph Kennedy playing handball in the Senate gym. Mankiewicz did. *The Times* was not amused.) *The Times* editors, for their part, felt the Kennedys were manipulative on issues and manipulative of the press. I remember being with the young publisher of *The Times*. Arthur Ochs Sulzberger, in early 1966 when his wife criticized him sharply for the abundance of Bobby stories in his paper; she insisted that he was going to be responsible for making Kennedy president. At the end, during his last campaign, there seemed finally to be a certain justification to the Kennedy complaints that there was a double standard against them, that *The Times* was viewing Robert Kennedy more on the past than on the present, and lent credence to the old attacks on Kennedy for ruthlessness and spending too much money. (The

Oregon campaign, *The Times* wrote, was "too relentless and too aggressive in its single-minded pursuit of power.") There was some bitterness later in the year when Nelson Rockefeller, running belatedly for the Republican nomination, began spending money, in the words of one Kennedy aide, "like a drunken sailor"—with the enthusiastic support of *The Times*.

That time of excitement ended with the assassination. In those post-assassination days, Robert Kennedy was like a man in shock. He had devoted everything to his older brother, had thought little of himself, and now it was all gone, insanely destroyed. He was also without a political base, for Lyndon Johnson was now President and Robert Kennedy and Johnson had always been opponents. The sharp things Johnson had said about Jack in 1960 rolled off Jack's back, but not off Robert's; and Robert Kennedy had reciprocated by ignoring Johnson during the years in office. There was deep hostility and suspicion. Robert Kennedy offered himself as ambassador to South Vietnam and was rejected by the President who thought it too dangerous. He wanted the vice-presidency. Some of his advisers, like Kenny O'Donnell, suggested a frontal attack—putting so much pressure on through the party organization, which was at that time still more pro-Kennedy than pro-Johnson, that the President would have to yield. But he turned this down and started to campaign.

He went to Poland where he was greeted by tumultuous crowds. He broke all kinds of protocol and enraged the American Embassy by disregarding its instructions, showing up late for official dinners, barnstorming all over the country. At one point, standing on top of a car, he began to speak to a group crowding around. Inside the car was the patrician ambassador John Moors Cabot who told a Kennedy aide, "Would you mind telling the Attorney General the roof is falling in on us." This delighted the aides; they took the words and inscribed them on a silver tray which they gave to the Attorney General. Polish officials were furious with his conduct. "Do you know who you shook hands with this morning in the market?" asked an indignant deputy minister of foreign affairs. "My maid." The trip seemed to rejuvenate him.

But Lyndon Johnson was unmoved. He did not want Robert Kennedy as his vice-president. Kennedy of course knew this would happen, that he would be the last person Johnson wanted ". . . because my name is Kennedy, because he wants a Johnson administration with no Kennedys in it, because we travel different paths, because I suppose some businessmen would object and I'd cost them a few votes in the South." Eventually the President called Kennedy in to break the news. It was a relatively pleasant meeting, Johnson praised Kennedy's past service, said he had a bright future, wanted him to run the campaign, but did not want him on the ticket. As the Attorney General left he turned and said almost wistfully, "I could have helped you a lot." But it did not end well; a few days later Johnson called in three reporters and over a very long lunch regaled them with the story of how he had broken the news to Kennedy. He told how Kennedy had gulped when he heard it. Kennedy was furious when he learned of this; the already bad feelings between the two became even worse. At the convention Johnson was still nervous about his own hold on the party, and the Kennedy electricity. A film on John F. Kennedy had been carefully censored and just as carefully scheduled by the President. There was no mention of Robert Kennedy in it, and it was not shown until after the vice-presidential nomination was completed. Robert Kennedy introduced the film and it was the most dramatic and emotional moment of the entire convention, fifteen minutes of wild cheering. Finally he spoke, quoting from *Romeo and Juliet:*

When he shall die
Take him and cut him out in little stars,
And he will make the face of heaven so fine
That all the world will be in love with night
And pay no worship to the garish sun.

Without a base, anxious to keep his career alive and continue the restoration ("And if anything happens to me Bobby will take my place, and if anything happens to him it will be Teddy," Jack Kennedy had once said describing how he had taken Joe Jr.'s place as the family politician), Robert Kennedy turned to New York for the Senate seat. It was not something which appealed to him; there was already one Kennedy in the Senate, and besides Robert Kennedy was an activist, a doer, he did not particularly want to be a junior member of a deliberative body. But there was nowhere else to go, and he came to New York to run against Kenneth Keating. To a degree this would undermine even more his credentials with liberals, for Keating was a man who, though leading the league in anti-Communist, anti-Nasser and anti-Sukarno speeches, had an enviable record for domestic legislation. Many liberals would finally vote for Kennedy, but they would do it grudgingly, feeling somehow that they were deserting Keating who had a right to their loyalty. It was a fairly banal campaign. Each ran around the state courting the ethnic vote, particularly the Jewish vote which was regarded as a swing factor. They made every temple breakfast in town; they wore their yarmulkes all over the city. Keating recounted his many speeches against Nasser and said he would make Israel a member of NATO; Kennedy imported Abe Ribicoff to talk to Jews. "The things you are saying against Bob Kennedy are exactly the same things you said four years ago against Jack Kennedy," Ribicoff told Jewish groups.

The main issue against Kennedy was that he was a carpetbagger; that plus the fact that no one was angry with

Keating. He was white-haired, he was nice, he looked like
a Senator and he was virtuous on the Goldwater issue (his
virtue consisted of failing to endorse Goldwater; an endorse-
ment, of course, would have been suicidal). He was not,
however, a particularly good target for a young man, a
carpetbagger, and a man around whom a good deal of suspicion still swirled. Yet Kennedy was the heir of the great
family, and a nation still mourned an assassinated President. "I am for Robert Kennedy," wrote Murray Kempton
who reflected some of the emotion of the times but was to
become a bitter critic in 1968, "because he is a decent and
talented young man terribly wounded whom I do not want
to look upon wounded further. This is like being for Bonnie
Prince Charlie; it has to do with commitment to a divine
right and there are no reasonable arguments for a divine
right." Two things finally sealed Kennedy's victory. One
was his use of television which was far better than Keating's. Kennedy's television spots were fresh and modern;
Keating always seemed to be backed by an American flag.
The Kennedy radio spots were well done too. Over and over
the voice would come: "Think about it for a minute: which
of the candidates running for United States Senator has the
better chance of becoming a great U.S. Senator . . . a *great*
U.S. Senator. . . . On November 3, vote for Robert Kennedy."
It was effective, slick stuff; it caught just the right implica-
tion for the Kennedy camp, that though Keating was a very
nice old man, perhaps he was not really as good as his
voting record, maybe he wasn't a really strong figure. The
other asset was Goldwater. In New York State Goldwater
was the kiss of death. Johnson would carry New York by
2.6 million votes. Kennedy was aware of this as the campaign progressed. He put greater emphasis on supporting
not just Bob Kennedy, but the Johnson-Humphrey-Kennedy
ticket; he emphasized that he was the only candidate who

was *for* Lyndon Johnson. In the final days Hubert Humphrey came in to campaign for him. Thus he won, but with the galling fact that he had come in on Lyndon Johnson's coattails. It annoyed him. The rest of the country might not pay attention to it, but it was something that he and Lyndon Johnson both knew, and that was two people too many.

Nominally a Senate seat from New York is a weak power base. The Senate bestows power by seniority and by security so that the most important and powerful members come from small states with one-party electorates and one-crop economies. They were the men who survived, who worked their way up in the Washington jungle. They would return home briefly to make the pro-sheep farmer speech and then return to Washington where they gained seniority; they played the game and eventually dominated the Washington scene. This was the direct opposite of Kennedy politics, the provocative politics of youth and energy, injecting themselves into issues, speaking out, having immediate media impact on the world outside Washington rather than the world inside. The Kennedys are not known for waiting.

Under normal conditions a junior senate seat, particularly from New York where one must speak for the polyglot of ethnic, business, industrial and labor groups, might have led him to quick obscurity, especially with his party in the White House, or might have saddled him with endless speeches promoting all of New York's vast and conflicting groups. The Ukrainian speech one day, the Jewish speech the next, then the pro-cop speech and then the pro-parking violator speech. But the Johnson presidency soon became dominated by Vietnam, and the Democratic party became at once the party of power and the party of dissent. Kennedy was thus pushed more and more into a special role; because he was a Kennedy, his constituency was not just

New York, his constituency was national. On issue after issue, as Johnson became imprisoned by the war, people looked to Kennedy for leadership. Gradually, through the hearings he held on urban problems in the Senate, through trips to Mississippi and to the grape pickers in California and to the Indians in New Mexico, he became the spokesman for the poor and the restless and the dissatisfied in America. Thus when America suddenly began to go through great social change, all of this heightened by the war in Vietnam (which drained off money and sharpened existing divisions), Kennedy was, by chance and not especially desire, on the outside looking in. He was outside the power establishment and he could feel, himself, some of the futility which the dispossessed felt. His course became one of increased radicalism. "The difference between him and Humphrey," said one of his friends midway through the campaign, "is that Humphrey started out, in 1948, outside the establishment and slowly and steadily was incorporated into it, step by step until, in 1968, he was an official establishment figure. When the columnists talk about Humphrey being the man of reconciliation because he can bring together the labor unions and the Southern governors, they're really talking about him reconciling two different parts of the establishment—they may have made it by quite different roads, but they're both there nevertheless. Now Kennedy began in power, but because of events was thrown out of the establishment and thus has looked at American society from the outside. There is one other difference; one was out in 1948 and the other was out in 1967, and that means a very great deal of difference in outlook."

IV ────────────

Nebraska came and went quickly. It was a triumph of imported organization and style. Indiana had taken all the time and effort, but the Kennedys, it was one of their great assets, had the resources to send yet another team into Nebraska to schedule the candidate properly, to save his time, and to get him the proper exposure. McCarthy was already stretched too thin in Indiana. His eye was on Oregon and California. He lacked sufficient organizational structure; he had virtually forgotten about Nebraska until too late. Then his campaign was a disaster; a hodgepodge of misscheduling, wasted time and effort, and long hours trying to get to the wrong town. His frustration built as he sensed that the Kennedys were moving around smoothly, seeing more people, getting in and out of towns quickly, and choosing the right towns. There is occasionally a moment when a candidate finds himself *lost* in an area, and that happened to McCarthy in Nebraska. Nebraska is a difficult state for a Democrat to campaign in anyway; its population is stretched thin and far. At the outset the Kennedys had been more worried about Nebraska than any other state. It had treated John Kennedy roughly, and it seemed to distrust Easterners; Easterners were different and had too long imposed their ideas, their taste, their accents, and worse, their government on the Midwest. In particular, the Kennedys, Eastern, rich and patrician, had seemed out of place in Nebraska. Jack Kennedy had hated

the idea of farm issues. He had once appointed John Kenneth Galbraith, a former agricultural economist, his chief
farm expert, saying, "Ken, I don't want to hear about farm
policy from anyone but you—and I don't want to hear about
it from you either." Orville Freeman, named Secretary of
Agriculture under Kennedy, had explained his appointment
at the time: "I think it has something to do with the fact
that they don't have a school of agriculture at Harvard."
Now Robert Kennedy would mock that cultural gap between
east and west in town after town in Nebraska: "Don't you
just feel it when you're looking at a fellow farmer? I come
from New York, a great farming state," he would say, laughing at their skeptical looks. "What? You don't accept that?
Well we're first in the production of sour cherries. . . ."

The scheduling had been good. They had been aided
by Phil Sorensen, Ted's brother and a former lieutenant
governor, and they managed to hit all the towns larger than
10,000. The Kennedys rented a train and used it to tie together many of the otherwise isolated towns—towns which
had been formed in the first place because of their proximity
to the Union Pacific. The Kennedys had reinvented trains
as a means of campaigning in Indiana. Trains now had
made the complete cycle in American politics, from the only
means of transportation to gimmick transportation scheduled by a candidate to give the television crews something
extra to cover; remembrances of an America Past. And it
had worked. When Robert Kennedy had boarded the Wabash
Cannonball he had no less a fellow traveler than David
Brinkley himself, there to cover Americana for NBC. That
particular ride had gone very well. Indeed when the Kennedy
canvassers checked with the public about which of the
candidate's television commercials they liked the best, a
majority cited the one about the Wabash Cannonball. This
irritated Goodwin and the advertising people a good deal,

and delighted Mankiewicz and the press staff. The train was cheap, colorful, and easy on the candidate. "We never realized how easy those old-style politicians had it," Dutton said one day after a train ride. "The trains are very easy. The candidate gets on, and he can rest. He has a whole car in which he can work with his advisers. There's no bumping around in the clouds, no jumping on and off the plane, no fighting your way through crowd after crowd. The crowds assemble for you; if there's any shoving, it's not you who gets shoved. You talk for a few minutes, you quote George Bernard Shaw so you don't leave any reporters behind, and then you can rest again."

In Nebraska the train touched tiny towns which had not seen an American presidential candidate since William Jennings Bryan. It was a tour which a lesser candidate, or a less well-known celebrity, might not have been able to make. Had McCarthy made the trip, the crowds simply might not have come. But this was a Kennedy and for days before there had been signs saying, "Yes, Robert Kennedy Is Coming to Ogallala," or "Meet Robert Kennedy Saturday in Downtown North Platte." Aboard the train the national reporters could hear the incredibly excited voices of the local radio reporters: "It's due any minute now, due in a minute. . . . Yes, there it is ladies and gentlemen, I see the light, I see the light of the train, it's coming down Main Street, people are running toward it, the train is *slowing down.* The children are pushing toward it. The police are fighting to keep the crowd back. Now the train is stopping. I see the press getting off. . . . *Television* crews are getting off. The crowd is surging forward, and *Yes,* Robert *Kennedy* is coming back on the platform. He's waving to the crowd. He looks smaller than you expect. . . ." He was in a good mood aboard the train. Earlier the train had gone through Julesburg, Colorado, the birthplace of Fred Dutton (a fact discovered at the last minute), and Ethel Kennedy, not telling anyone, had spent several hours making up posters. When the train stopped, she and friends rushed out and started a Dutton demonstration. "Sock it to 'em Freddy," "Fred Dutton's Brother for Attorney General," "Make Fred, Not War," read the signs. They demanded a speech and the candidate, now joining in, shouted: "Tell us about George Bernard Shaw, Fred."

The crowds were good all along the way. The candidate was relaxed, telling the crowds: "Richard Nixon is speaking up in front of the train. We thought that was only fair. He has no crowd at all." Then he would talk low key, a fairly conservative pitch: that the local people knew more about their business than some bureaucrat in Washington (which went over well; even in Washington no one loves faceless Washington bureaucrats), and a little bit on law and order and the divisions in the country, and then fairly hard on the war. Frank Morrison, the former governor and one of the few Democrats with real statewide appeal, had noted that the war was very simply *the* issue in Nebraska, the gut issue. People wouldn't talk about it much, he said, because they think it's unpatriotic to talk a lot about it, but it's there. The farmers were angry too, restless in a time of rising costs and low prices, and aware that most of the other whites in America had never had it so good. They were restless and angry and Kennedy told them they were being cheated, that he favored collective bargaining for them, a popular stand.

But there were still problems, and in some ways the campaign was not jelling the way they had hoped. The crowds were still coming, that part of the magic still worked, but the politicians were not. The bosses, and the leaders of the

Democratic party apparatus, were still suspicious and unreceptive, and this was being demonstrated by a marked
migration to Hubert Humphrey. It was becoming clearer
and clearer that Robert Kennedy's problem with the machines was very deep and serious, and that the apparatus
was almost as hostile to him as it was to McCarthy. For the
first time in many years, the party machinery, which had
traditionally been reasonably sympathetic to the pressures
and whims of the party eggheads and liberals, was un-
responsive to two candidates representing the intellectual
element.

The relationship between the Kennedys and the party
machinery had always been a tenuous one; they were not
of it, and yet they had never fought it, even in their earlier
years. In Massachusetts, where local politics are particularly
venal, they had simply by-passed the apparatus. They had
developed their own breathtaking popularity and that meant
that the party machinery would not make a frontal challenge. They were able to control the state delegation at
conventions, but in return they never really used any of
their power, popularity, or resources to clean up Massachusetts politics. Reformers in Massachusetts tend to be
somewhat cooler to the Kennedys than reformers in other
states; they have seen more of their cool indifferent side.
Massachusetts was a quagmire which the Kennedys tol-
erated and were careful not to step into. In 1960 their relationship with the machinery was guarded, but improved
steadily. Mayor Daley of Chicago, the most important and
most sophisticated of the traditional politicians, had been
for Jack Kennedy, first because of his friendship with Joe
Kennedy but also, and equally important, because he sensed
a winner. "Daley has sense enough to go with classy politicians, even if they're men he doesn't feel at ease with,"
said one student of machines. "That makes him different

from most machine people who shun anyone they don't feel at ease with." But with Bobby Kennedy it was a little different. They sensed in him a puritan; he was not above prosecuting dishonest local *Democratic* officials and in that sense, he was as dangerous as a Republican. (In Illinois, the Cook County machine cares more about who wins county attorney races than who wins the U.S. Senate race. The power of investigation is a very important negative power.)

In New York he had seemed to side increasingly, though sometimes ineffectually, with the reformers in their regular fights with the organization. He preferred to be photographed with the reformers and work in private with the apparatus people. In 1964, meeting with the varying bosses of New York State before deciding to run for the Senate, a photographer happened by the hotel suite and took a number of pictures. He was asked to throw them away. The machine people sensed that in future conflicts *this* Kennedy would side more and more with their enemies, and they did not like his style and his direction. The machines were dependent upon the old-style control of poor Negro areas. As it was, their own black leaders there (Toms) were being jeopardized by the new angry militants whom the poverty programs were supposed to help, and with whom Kennedy was so publicly identified. The apparatus people sensed that if Kennedy were elected, it would speed them that much more quickly to obsolescence. He was only forty-two and his people were often younger; they were all in their fifties and sixties.

(When Frank O'Connor was going to run against Rockefeller in New York, the Kennedys had opposed him. He was the best of the old breed, they noted, and they wanted the best of the new breed. If the young reformers did not understand what they meant, the worst of the old breed certainly did.) Kennedy was just very different, and he identified himself with all the new and threatening trends, even long hair. A story put out by Dick Daley's people tells of Kennedy's having gone, in 1967—when he was considering the race—to see the Mayor. He had said, my father is not well, and my brother is dead, and I now regard you as an old friend of the family. May I turn to you for advice? The Mayor said yes, that was fine. So Kennedy asked for advice, and Daley gave him some: "Get your hair cut." The story is perhaps apocryphal, but symbolic nevertheless. If the existing officials of the Democratic party lack a powerful sense of social change, they do have a sense of survival. Robert Kennedy, like Gene McCarthy, threatened that survival. Hubert Humphrey did not.

This had been a year of great surprises, though many of them highly predictable, and perhaps the greatest surprise was the resurrection of Hubert Humphrey. One was surprised by how easily it was done, and how readily the party faithful moved toward a man who had never proven himself in any sort of national election; a man who was closely tied to a deeply unpopular administration, and who was avoiding any primary fights, indeed a man who stood a very good chance of winning a nomination but losing an election (normally a patented Republican strategy). In early 1968 no one had seemed a frailer politician than Humphrey. Had one wanted to do a study of what the war in Vietnam had done to a generation of older American liberals, Humphrey would have been exhibit A. The war was destroying him with his liberal constituency, and as the war progressed, or failed to progress, his own style seemed increasingly out of date. He was a politician of the old school; hot and heavy oratory, never understate when you can overstate, party loyalty above all else (his Democratic arm around the Democratic arm of Lester Maddox)—they were all required qualities in the old politics, but dubious assets in this age. Even the old-style colleagues of Humphrey were now disappearing; Paul Douglas and Mennen Williams were out, Nelson Rockefeller, George Romney and Chuck Percy were in. (Romney and Percy were milestones in American politics. We had formerly trusted sons of very wealthy families in politics so long as they were not conservative—inherited wealth is intolerable in a conservative, for the rich do not need to steal. But now we had gone to trusting businessmen, even self-made businessmen, so long as they didn't look like businessmen.) Humphrey was markedly, relentlessly, of the old school.

In the age of cool he was out; in a time of understatement he overstated; in a time when television made brief speeches mandatory, he still spoke with the cadence and length of a radio orator. At a time when the intellectual theorists of his own party were increasingly dubious and pessimistic about the course of American life, Humphrey was incorrigibly ebullient, talking of the politics of joy and happiness. The more he talked, the more it grated. (Intellectuals consider optimism permissible if the times are clearly bad and frightening to an entire nation, i.e., a depression or a world war. Then the optimist who can inject new hope is desirable. But when the challenge seems hidden to much of the nation, as it did in 1968, optimism is unfashionable. The intellectuals demand someone who can convey to the rest of the nation that this is a dark time, and then hold up a glimmer of hope. Humphrey's optimism had been born during the New Deal days and both it and his style of projecting it had never changed. However, the country had changed a great deal.) Was the new style that of underplaying idealism? Humphrey shouted out. His ear was desperately bad and out of tune. He went on television and talked about himself in the third person, and it sounded like a relic of Fourth of July bombast. There was a quality of true sadness in all this; the liberals had loved Hubert back in the fifties. He was proof that liberalism did not necessarily exist only in the dark alien cities of the nation, but that it could flourish and win in the good clean air of the Midwest. They had not minded his good Midwestern enthusiasms and excesses, for they had been liberal excesses and enthusiasms. But now these excesses had been turned to a dubious cause; he had spoken in Saigon to American State Department officers about their *wonderful* mission there, God save the piaster, and now it was all ending badly because of the war. Joe Rauh of the ADA, an old friend of Humphrey's, would listen to all Humphrey's defenses of the war, and would nod and say yes, Hubert, yes. But don't you realize what everyone else in America realizes—that if you weren't vice-president you would be leading the dissent on it. Indeed a meeting had been arranged in December between Humphrey and the leaders of the ADA. Once his close friends, they were now his pickets. Feeling had run so high before he arrived that Arthur Schlesinger took the liberals aside and said, Look, I know we feel strongly, but he's a good man and he is the vice-president and our old friend. We've got to be polite and show restraint. Everyone agreed. Then Humphrey arrived and immediately began by saying that he had just talked with Adam Malik of Indonesia, and Malik had said that it was the U.S. intervention in Vietnam which had saved the Indonesian domino, and Schlesinger had interrupted: "Oh bullshit Hubert!"

Humphrey at the start of the year had been a badly crippled politician, a symbol of Lyndon Johnson's ability to take much and give little. (The Reverend Jesse Jackson, one of Martin Luther King's militant leaders in the North, would say in sadness of Humphrey, "Hubert Humphrey is a grape of hope that has been turned into a raisin of despair by the sunshine of Lyndon Johnson.") There was a touch of the clown in the tone with which Humphrey talked about the President. He could go on television and say: "I think I know who are men of peace, and the man of peace that I see in this country—but peace with justice and peace with freedom—is President Lyndon Johnson." It was one of the final victories of Lyndon Johnson that he had made Hubert Humphrey sound like Richard Nixon. But then suddenly Lyndon Johnson had withdrawn from the race and Humphrey had been reborn. Now all those great resources of the presidency which Lyndon Johnson had been unable to use for himself because of the war, could be used for Hubert Humphrey. He suddenly had the advantages of the presidency without the disadvantages. He could barely believe it. He had been out of the country when Johnson had withdrawn and when he came back the first question he asked his staff was whether Bobby had a lock on it. Kennedy did not, and day after day it was Kennedy who was further from the lock and Humphrey who was closer to it. For a moment the war had simply evaporated, the issue had disappeared. To an older generation of liberals he was the good Hubert again, the old Hubert. (It was a generational thing; among important younger members of the party his support was noticeably weaker. The only important young man on his way up who was backing Humphrey was Adlai Stevenson III—a tie bound in part out of family loyalty to his father, and also in part out of family dislike or uneasiness with the Kennedys.) It was back to 1948, all of this had never happened.

Humphrey suddenly started getting a very good press, particularly out of Washington. Washington is a company town and Humphrey was the good company liberal; indeed

he was the only company-certified candidate in either race.
Humphrey had been gathering due bills in Washington for
as long as he had been gathering them among the party
workers, and now he was calling them in. For the last year
or two he had managed to give the impression to those in
Washington, in the inner circle, that he was loyal, but
agonized and loyal. He might, knowing that a certain influential columnist was also agonized and loyal, stop by
for breakfast with him where they would share their agony,
and Humphrey's confidence would be protected. But his
deeper darker side would be properly viewed so that the
right men in Washington knew how agonized Humphrey
was, even if the rest of the country did not. Now running,
he got sympathetic columns from those liberals who liked
the war: Hubert really believes in the war, and understands
it, and from those liberal columnists who did not: Hubert
doesn't believe in the war, but has been imprisoned by
Johnson, just wait til he's on his own. Indeed if many of
the senior Washington commentators were upset by the
war, they seemed even more upset by what McCarthy and
Kennedy were doing with it. Perhaps it would all end badly,
for the Paris peace talks were a dubious proposition under
Lyndon Johnson: one did not hire the architect to tear down
his own prize building. Perhaps if they dragged on, the old
war would reappear and the new Hubert instead of the
old would be unveiled at Chicago. But for the moment the
Kennedy people were angry; they recognized all the good
and hard work Humphrey had done in the party vineyard,
but they were bitter about the good press he was getting
in liberal quarters (particularly *The New York Times* editorial page; if one were a former *Times* reporter one heard
about that regularly). They felt that this was giving a re-
spectability to an old outdated system which was trying to
protect itself; an alliance of Southern Democrats, big city

machines and big labor. An alliance which annoyed the
Kennedys primarily because it existed, and secondly because it wasn't going for them.

But Humphrey the party man was reaping the party
reward. He was like Richard Nixon in more than just
speech, perhaps speech was an outgrowth of association and
habit. He had been the good party loyalist, speaking at every
dinner, eating all those cold green peas, praising all those
overweight sheriffs, shaking hands with all those aldermen,
remembering their wives' names, showing up in Kansas
in the cold winter when the plane connections were terrible
and he had a cold, appearing at dinky fund raisings; always
ebullient and finding *virtue* in every Democrat there. If
there was any doubt in 1968 about how well Humphrey had
served the country (and there was a great deal of it), there
was no doubt at all about how well he had served the party.
And, of course, many of the faithful understood the party
better than the nation; a good many of them failed to make
any distinction at all.

For the party faithful Hubert was sound and safe and loyal,
and loyalty was the most important. The structure of the
party is not based on imagination or creativity or social
conscience, it is based on loyalty (the honest politician,
the joke goes, is the one who, when bought, stays bought).
It is based on working your way up one notch, not threatening the man above you, for you might be threatened from
below. Thus while Kennedy was out working the primaries,
Humphrey and his people were very quietly going around
and picking up the delegates, cashing in the due bills. Kennedy, campaigning on the road, was in serious trouble.
His delegate counts were not good, the delegates were pro-
Humphrey though Humphrey's hold was a very tenuous one.
Part of the problem was that as Kennedy plunged more

into the campaign and saw more and more of America, of the dispossessed and the under-privileged, the more he was moved by it and the more he identified with it. Accordingly, he identified less and less with the party apparatus and the professionals. He now began to see them as the kind of people who were responsible for the existing system, who were indeed blocking the needed changes, and he was not at ease with them. If they saw him as a threat, they were right, because he saw them as a stumbling block. In city after city he would meet with them. He was not good at the small talk, not good at the little jokes which were a staple of the profession; he could not do the little social things easily, press the flesh. Their stock in trade was small talk and his was not, and when they left they often thought him a cold one indeed.

During the campaign a curious phenomenon developed. At night when there might have been time to go to dinner with a delegate, or a politician or two, he rarely did. He went out with a few friends, occasionally an assistant, often journalist friends—not because they might write something nice about him, though that helped—but because he seemed almost bored by politics and wanted to talk about something else. One of his great favorites was Jack Newfield, a young radical writer for *The Village Voice*. Once, invited to Hickory Hill for a great party where all the old friends—Katzenbach, General Taylor, MacNamara—were also socializing, Newfield had balked: "You don't expect me to go in there and drink and talk with all those war criminals do you?" Kennedy would still meet with delegates and they would talk, but he would withdraw from them; and they sensed this.

All of this became clear one night in Omaha when Kennedy went before a Jefferson-Jackson Day dinner. It was a Friday, and Kennedy had enjoyed an excellent day; he had visited a dozen towns between Lincoln and Omaha, and his crowds had been good and his receptions warm. He had seemed to get stronger as the day went on, enjoying himself, relaxed. Then came the dinner. It was awkward to start with because Humphrey was to be the main speaker, and thus Kennedy seemed an interloper. Kennedy was to speak first and then leave. When he first walked into the hall (journalistic applausemeter: Kennedy polite applause; Humphrey warm applause), he already looked different, tense, his hands knotted. The band played the national anthem, the soloist sang, Bobby sang, and no one else sang. It was the kind of thing he loved. His speech was to be brief, but the prepared text was a good one. It was short, sharp, one of his best: "Too much and for too long we have confused our achievements with wealth, and measured our greatness with the statistics of the Gross National Product. But the Gross National Product counts air pollution and cigarette advertising and ambulances to clear our highways of carnage. It counts Whitman's rifle and Speck's knife and television programs that glorify violence—the better to sell goods to our children." Yet when he spoke he was terrible. He rushed through the speech, lost the balance and the cadence of it, dropped his lines, garbled his thoughts. He seemed in a hurry to leave; indeed the moment he finished he did.

Later, talking with a reporter about it, he was highly critical of his own performance. He had not turned them on, he said, and he had really blown the whole thing. A cold evening. Just cold. Then he added: "They're just not my kind of crowd." It was a curious thing for a candidate to say about other politicians.

A brief respite in Nebraska. His mother, campaigning on the west coast, had replied to criticism of Kennedy wealth by saying, "it's our money and we're free to spend it any way we please." Teddy Kennedy, asked about this quote, had partially saved the day by saying, "That's why we didn't make mother finance chairman." Now the candidate was being asked by a wire-service reporter about the quotes. He read Rose Kennedy's remarks and Teddy's reply and paled noticeably. No comment, he said. Not even an off-the-record comment? asked the reporter. Okay, said the candidate, "That's why we *did* make her finance chairman."

The day of the debacle with the Omaha party officials, he was relaxed again. It was a warm sunny day in the suburban areas of Omaha and the crowds were bigger than expected, more receptive. He spoke well and answered questions at length, in no rush to go anywhere on this lovely day. Was he worried about the population explosion? "I think every individual should work out his own arrangement. I've worked out my own arrangement, but obviously it won't work for everybody else." Would he lower the voting age? "Yes, to six." Then at the back of the crowd there was a disturbance. A heckler was being hauled off by the police. But he had been a curiously muted heckler, a mumbler really; no one had heard him, and the police were carting him off to protect him from Kennedy partisans. The candidate became interested. "Don't take him away," he shouted, "he has as much right to speak as I have." The police started to release the heckler, but the heckler refused. He was a proud heckler and he would not be freed by the word of a Kennedy. "Let him go," said Bobby. But he clung to the police. "Okay," said Kennedy, "if that's the way you want it. But I promise that if I'm elected President of the United States, one of the first things I'm going to do is get you out of jail."

There was, he thought, something comic about him,

a Kennedy, in Nebraska. He would tell audiences, "When
I first talked to my advisers about whether I should make
this race or not, they said I should. I asked why. They said
that if I did, I could come to Nebraska. To run in the Nebraska primary." Later that week at a rally, when a piece
of paper fluttered off the lectern and into the crowd, he said,
"Give me that back quickly. That's my farm program. I need
it." He sensed he was running well, and it was picking up—
the results were astonishing. Nebraska, the state they had
feared the most, had given him 53 percent of the vote
against two opponents. He ran well everywhere, with the
Negroes, with blue collar and stunningly well among the
angry farmers. (One Kennedy aide believed that the farmers went for Kennedy and not McCarthy because somehow McCarthy was identified with the Democratic party
farm establishment, a Midwestern colleague of Humphrey
and Orville Freeman. Kennedy, on the other hand, was
clearly an anti-establishment figure. This was borne out, at
about the same time, by a poll taken jointly in South Dakota
by three local newspapers. The poll, which seemed astonishing at the time, showed Kennedy beating Johnson and Mc-
Carthy, in that order, 52-to-24-to-17 among farmers and
ranchers; 51-36-11 among inhabitants of towns up to 2,500
people, and running only 34-34-17 among city inhabitants.

Election night in Omaha, the camp was pleased and
relaxed. Pierre Salinger was announcing that McCarthy was
dead as a candidate, and Tuck was only mildly annoyed
when he heard a network television man announcing ". . .
and again it was the classic Kennedy coalition: Negroes,
blue collar." "Negroes!" shouted Tuck, "one goddamn percent of the state is Negro." The truth was, and it did not
strike them immediately, that they had done well once again
in a conservative state. Now on to Oregon.

V

Oregon, the Kennedys would decide in retrospect, was a giant suburb. In disdain, Pat Moynihan, one of their very talented intellectuals (indeed, one of their few intellectuals who actually was an intellectual) would say that Oregon didn't even have crab grass. That was Oregon. Everything that could go wrong for the Kennedys went wrong in Oregon. McCarthy, on the other hand, would be at his best there; his advantages minimized, his assets maximized. The result would be that a Kennedy would be defeated for the first time in an election.

The Kennedys had looked forward to Oregon early in the campaign. It had seemed sweeter and more natural than the seemingly hostile road stops along the way, Indiana and Nebraska. Oregon and California had seemed, in contrast, God's country: liberal, more sophisticated. His staff was sure that Kennedy's liberalism would work well in both places, the staff members after all had been drawn to Kennedy because he was liberal, modern and urbane. They did not, at the beginning, take Gene McCarthy seriously. He was viewed as someone who flowered at a time when he was the only game in town. Now with the real man in the race, McCarthy would wither. But it was not so easy. During the campaign two patterns in white communities had developed: Kennedy was getting the blue-collar people, but McCarthy was running very well among the middle- and upper-class whites. Many of those who were for Kennedy were borderline backlashers who thought the choice in American politics narrowed to George Wallace or Bob Kennedy. They sensed that Kennedy was a tough little Irishman, someone they could understand. One Kennedy aide noted that both Kennedy and McCarthy were Irish Catholics, but they were not the same kind, particularly to Jews. Robert Kennedy was the tough little Irish kid who had punched you in the nose when you were little, while Gene McCarthy was the nice gracious English teacher who said, Yes, Mrs. Goldberg, your son writes very good essays. The Jews felt and sensed this. So did the poor whites; they liked his toughness and combativeness. They felt they could even understand the thing he was doing with the blacks, that was just something politicians had to do. McCarthy had somewhat petulantly remarked, after the first two primaries, that Kennedy could take pleasure in the fact that the least educated members of the society had voted for him.

If the Kennedy trend was true, so was the McCarthy trend. He was running well in the suburbs among both Independents and Republicans. Indeed he and Nelson Rockefeller had a strikingly similar constituency among white Americans. (Rockefeller was much stronger with blacks. He was the governor of a state with a sizeable Negro population, he had run several national races and he possessed a good physical ghetto-style. McCarthy came from a state with a minimal Negro population and he was too fiercely proud a man to make the kind of gestures to Negroes that might have won him their allegiance.) That constituency was middle class and moving up. It was white and it was above blue-collar. Questioned by pollsters about which party it favored, more and more it liked to answer that it didn't vote by party; it reacted to the man. McCarthy appealed to people who were worried about the war, and a little uneasy about the blacks, not exactly against them, but worried about them. To them he was quietly reassuring: he was intelligent; he had done the right thing—he had entered the presidential race and by doing so, he had been above politics whereas when Kennedy had entered it, he had been playing politics. To McCarthy's constituency the war was the crucial issue; otherwise they thought American life was all right. The race issue was something else. They had been for voting rights for Negroes, for integration, for the March on Washington, but they were worried and uneasy now. In the old days they had turned on their television sets and seen the white Alabama cops—slack-jawed—beating up those nice clean-cut Negro students, and they had known what they felt, and that what they felt was right. Now it was more difficult; the riots, the anger, black people calling them racists—who me? Someone shot Martin Luther King and that was bad, but then there was all that rioting and that was worse, and baffling. McCarthy was reassuring to them; he did not seem to represent the divisions. But one looked at Robert Kennedy and he looked a bit discordant—maybe, just maybe, he encouraged them a little, stirred them up.

The quiet man. That was McCarthy. One heard a lot about the quiet man. The sociologists of American politics, knowing that the new battleground would be in the suburbs, had taken their questionnaires and tape recorders and had gone there, in the last few years, to find out who these people were and what they wanted. At first they had been perplexed. It was an odd thing for there were no easily identifiable characteristics for the new candidate. Perhaps they had been looking for the wrong thing, indeed it might be precisely the *absence* of certain qualities which was reassuring to these people, particularly because thtey lived in such a charged up time. That was when the sociologists came up with the idea of the quiet man. The country, uneasy about the new passions being stirred up, the growing divisions, wanted someone to give it quiet confidence. Lyndon Johnson was not the quiet man, not with that bull horn, nor Hubert Humphrey, nor Robert Kennedy. But Gene McCarthy, walking down that street alone, throwing away his best lines, telling everyone how all the experts said his race was impossible because he didn't raise his voice (they didn't raise their voices either), scoffing at Washington—one sensed that if elected President he might just abolish the U.S. Government—was the quiet man. In many ways he sensed the mood of America better than almost any other candidate. He was an easy candidate to underestimate, and almost everyone had done it; first the President, then the press, then the pollsters, then the people around him, and finally the Kennedys. McCarthy's approach was not as haphazard as it seemed, there was a certain subtle calculation to it. He ran his own style of campaign very well, and now here he was in Oregon and Oregon was tailor-made for him. If he hadn't existed, Oregon would have invented Gene McCarthy. It liked underdogs up against famous rich candidates, and it distrusted Eastern favorites who wouldn't debate with poor but honest loners from the Midwest.

Oregon lacked all the Kennedy ingredients. The ghetto, Tuck complained, consisted of "just one block where the Reed professors could bring their kids to show them what *one* looked like." The Negro population barely existed; the Catholic population was very small. (There was usually a Catholic vote for Kennedy though the Kennedy people did not like to talk about it.) Oregon was beautiful, affluent, complacent, white, and far from the raw nerve of the rest of America. It was also far removed from the mood of the candidate: the challenge that America must be turned around, that the country was in serious trouble. Seeing Oregon one again remembered Barry Goldwater in 1964, remembered talking with him and suddenly realizing that in his hometown the person who drank or committed a crime was just the oddball. He was the offbeat person from an otherwise decent family who, in Goldwater's words, "simply couldn't hack it." There was no connection between crime and restlessness and social injustice. It was simply a very different life. All the great social problems had settled in the great cities of the Northeast and Midwest. There was the migration of frustrated illiterate Negroes from the South, but that problem was thousands of miles from Oregon. "Oh I'm not saying we don't have our troubles like everyone else," one Portland resident told a visiting reporter, "but in ten minutes' time I can be off fishing and forget about them." Oregon generated few of the ugly problems of modern America, and it neither understood nor wanted to understand them. It did not necessarily like what was going on in the rest of America, but it breathed better air and lived a better life. So Robert Kennedy entered Oregon without Negroes and Mexicans and Poles. He had the peace issue but that was a problem too. As the Kennedys would learn again in California, McCarthy had taken away the peace issue and with it the most dedicated, most activist, peace people. The people who desperately wanted Robert Kennedy to make the race six months earlier were now fighting him just as desperately. When peace people became committed they stayed committed. Only two things might have changed them: one was fear of Lyndon Johnson which might have made Kennedy a mandatory candidate, and the other was an even deeper commitment to the ghetto, and that was missing in Oregon.

Now the Kennedys had to deal with this new America

and it was particularly difficult for them because they had always based their races on shaking people up, challenging them, challenging complacency (a Kennedy runs because you need him in these particular times) and in Oregon they felt frustrated. They found the issues elusive; they could not get a handle on Oregon and what bothered its people. Larry O'Brien would recall visiting Oregon in 1960 and sensing the mood and the worries then; but now it was 1968. It was all different; it was all more affluent and subtle. The people who had been blue collar in 1960 were now making $9,000 a year and living in the new suburbs with one and a half cars and two and three-quarters children. "How do you get a handle on a state like this?" he would ask. Indeed about three weeks before the primary, the Kennedy people had a long strategy session with Edith Green, the Oregon congresswoman who was their campaign manager. They discussed exactly these problems; the affluence, the complacency, the undercurrent of resistance to the hard-driving Kennedy style. Someone had turned and asked her: "Edith, how do we do it? How can we shake them up?" She looked up stupefied. "You can't shake them up," she answered.

Everything went better for McCarthy in Oregon. His television money went further and there was more of it. On the heels of defeats in Indiana and Nebraska, there was no inclination to save for California; if he was beaten in Oregon, he was beaten in California as well. So they spent heavily. One minute of prime time in Oregon cost only $350 whereas in Los Angeles it was about $2,000. One radio minute of prime commuting time in Portland was about $18 whereas it would be $65 in Los Angeles. McCarthy had been used to a disorganized staff, but in Oregon he had his best organization: good people had been available early, and he had a good overall structure. As in New Hampshire—unlike Indiana and Nebraska—he again had, because of the war, the benefit of some of the most intense and dedicated activists in the state. The Kennedy campaign was just the opposite. The Kennedys were paying heavily for their late entry. They had been disorganized in general and in order to get off to a running start they had spent far too much time in Indiana, their first domino, and now there was too little time, and they were disorganized. Normally in a national campaign there should be time to organize slowly, to test out people, to try out ideas, to try out speeches without all the full focus of national publicity. Jack Kennedy had had this chance in 1960, and so had Gene McCarthy in 1968, but Robert Kennedy never had that time. In 1968 when he coughed, ten tape recorders picked it up.

Barrett Prettyman, a Washington lawyer, was Kennedy's first campaign coordinator, but that had worked out badly and at a somewhat belated date Bill vanden Heuvel, a wealthy and social young lawyer from New York, was shipped in. This became a point of considerable dispute within the Kennedy camp, for the politicians and some of the eggheads considered vanden Heuvel a social friend of the Kennedys and were dubious about him from the start. This touched on a fairly sensitive area for the Kennedys: Jack Kennedy who had enjoyed clubby people, whose wife disliked politicians and did not want them in her house, had almost completely separated his political and social worlds. Kenny O'Donnell would do the tough political work, but people like Lem Billings or Red Fay would be invited to the White House dinners—people whom Jack Kennedy, as one Kennedy pro put it, "wouldn't have trusted to run a dog-catcher race." There was a certain amount of feeling that this should never happen again. An assistant commented,

"When we came back this year some of us were very determined that this time we would be equals and friends, not employees, and there would be no lords and serfs. We talked about it at the beginning, and now, in retrospect, I think we looked pretty silly because Bob Kennedy just wasn't that way. He wouldn't separate his lives. But the other half of it was that his social friends would come in on politics."

There was always considerable doubt about vanden Heuvel among the pros; perhaps because he considered himself a politician—having managed one campaign for Congress and having had the misfortune to run once himself, against John Lindsay. When things went wrong in Oregon, as they did, the professionals blamed vanden Heuvel. In his defense he claimed that he had been warning the candidate for several weeks that they had very serious problems. But in the eyes of the professionals, Oregon just had not been put together properly: the scheduling wasn't good, the feel just wasn't right. While the Kennedy people thought vanden Heuvel hadn't done enough, some Oregon critics felt that he and his organization had pushed much too hard, made too many phone calls, been too eastern, too pushy. Perhaps if you are going to lose, you are simply going to lose and that's it. Nevertheless the pros were angry about the Oregon organization. "You can walk into an area and tell whether or not it's been organized, whether the advance man was any good, and Oregon was a problem," said one of the aides. "We should have done better than we did. There were too many people at certain levels in the campaign who had titles and slots but weren't really completing their assignments, weren't being pushed very hard."

The lack of organization had hurt them but they had probably been hurt even more seriously by their failure to debate. It was one of the ironies of the Kennedy camp that at the same time they both underestimated McCarthy (in what he was doing, how well he understood the media, and the type of appeal he was making) and overestimated his intellectual gifts. Because of this, they failed to debate in Oregon. It was a costly mistake, for Oregon has its own special style of politics. It is somewhat maverick, somewhat intellectually oriented; and for a variety of reasons it wanted the debate. It believed in debates. The Dewey-Stassen debates had been held there, and the failure to debate was a reminder again and again that it was McCarthy who had entered New Hampshire. The primary is a very big thing in Oregon; it is, said one Kennedy man, "the third largest industry in the state." By failing to debate they were irritating the Oregonians, leaving themselves open to the charges that they had simply muscled people aside with their money and organization, two distinctly non-Oregon attributes. McCarthy played skillfully on the lack of a debate. One of his television clips showed an old photograph of the two men together with the commentary, "This is probably the only time you'll see them together on television."

Within the Kennedy camp, the division over whether or not to debate McCarthy roughly paralleled that over whether or not to enter the race in the first place. The traditionalists argued against it; the young people, again particularly the Robert Kennedy people, argued for it. Walinsky, the most strong minded (Adamant Adam he was called), argued that you had to take high risks; that they had a quality candidate and therefore they should expose the candidate and take the chances. The others had seen what the debates had done to Richard Nixon in 1960. (At the studio in Chicago, Bob Kennedy had looked over at Nixon's picture on the monitor right before the first debate and had been appalled by his color and appearance. Nixon saw him looking and asked if he looked all right or whether he should change anything. "Dick, you look great!" said Kennedy.) They saw a relatively unknown Jack Kennedy destroy the front-running Nixon and they read this lesson from it: the well-known and supposedly front-running Kennedy must not give the unknown McCarthy so much exposure. We have the name this time and they don't; we are in and they are out. Walinsky and the others argued, in turn, that Kennedy had beaten Nixon because he was a higher quality candidate; that, if anything, Kennedy had been too conservative and cautious in the third and fourth debates; that the idea of denying exposure to McCarthy in the year 1968 was an exercise in mythology, the kind of thing the Kennedys normally let their opponents do. Because a fierce two-man race had been going on across the nation for almost two months, the exposure was there, McCarthy was on the news shows every night. McCarthy's very presence in the race had guaranteed his exposure. What they were doing, Walinsky argued, was helping McCarthy maintain his liberal constituency, since the failure to debate fed the idea that McCarthy was intellectually superior and that Bobby was a tough little prosecutor cashing in on the family name and wealth. Finally, Walinsky felt that McCarthy was overrated intellectually; that most of his speeches were of low quality, and most important, because Robert Kennedy bore exposure well, the very same qualities which drew so many bright people to him on a personal level would become apparent to a much larger audience through the debates. If he could impress people like Moynihan, Charles Evers, Harrington, and George McGovern, then he should also be able to impress the average white middle-class voter of Oregon. There was some extremely sound reasoning, but the essence of it was: to gain something you must risk something.

As for the traditionalists, they were somewhat older; they had sampled power. They were with a family which had never lost an election, and the long winning streak had made them conservative, protective of what they had, less willing to risk it. Had they little at stake, and no long winning streak, they might have been more willing to risk it. As it was, they held to the view that McCarthy should try and catch them. (In California Walinsky, who had been highly critical of some of the conservative tone of the campaign in Indiana and Nebraska, felt that Kennedy had been liberated by the defeat in Oregon; that he was a fresher, more relaxed man, more himself. He had been defeated and the aura of never having lost, and therefore of being conservative, was gone. He could now simply go out and campaign and be himself.) There was yet another problem here in the failure to debate, almost a subconscious one. These older men were still Jack Kennedy's people, and they had admired his intellect and Robert's organizational talent. While they realized that Robert had grown, they still didn't entirely believe it themselves; they automatically underrated him just a little. It was still hard not to think of him as the Robert Kennedy of 1960. Perhaps if he went on a debate he would be asked questions which he simply wouldn't be able to answer. Even someone like Dutton— who served as a swing man between the two factions; his ties going back to the older group, his social and political instincts often placing him with the newer one—was opposed to a debate near the end of the primary because he sensed that Kennedy was going to be defeated and he did not want the defeat to come right *after* the debate: That might be a serious mistake, for that would make it a lingering defeat. A myth would grow that McCarthy had beaten Kennedy only after the confrontation, and something like that might cost them California too.

Now the pace was wearing the candidate down. He looked tired and drawn. As if in response to his own fatigue, and the negative reports he was getting, he drove himself harder and harder, a longer schedule, smaller towns. His DC-4 landed on tiny airstrips which could barely accommodate it; at La Grande and Baker, he and his press party were de-planed by fork-lift, at Ontario, by a stepladder. He delighted in using such visits in his openings: "Ever since I was a little boy there were two things I wanted to do: Be a ventrilo-quist and see La Grande. . . ." The pace was exhausting and one night, as the plane lumbered back to Portland, the re-porters began chanting: "Hey hey, R.F.K., how many re-porters did you kill today?" Sometimes the very energy of the candidate seemed to offend the Oregonians; it was all too pushy. Even the innocent things backfired. About a week before the primary Kennedy visited a high school in a Portland suburb. About 4,000 students and parents had gathered to hear him, and they were offended by the manner of the press party: reporters shoving their way to telephones, photographers—cameras first—pushing everyone aside to get the best places. They decided that the press's manners were Kennedy manners and the next day, in the school's mock balloting, Humphrey upset Kennedy.

But there were lighter moments. Kennedy had his dog, Freckles, aboard now, and Tuck was in charge of the dog. (McCarthy, hitting harder and harder at Kennedy and his refusal to debate, was critical of the dog and the presence of John Glenn—the apple-pie front—saying, "He's afraid to debate me. He thinks he can beat me with an astronaut and a dog. . . .") Once Freckles got free on an airstrip and Tuck had to retrieve the dog. The reporters laughed and consoled Tuck. It's a terrible thing, Tuck, that a brilliant political in-

185

tellectual like you is in charge of a *dog*. Don't the Kennedys have any sense of merit? "It may look like a dog to you," said Tuck, "but it's an ambassadorship to me." Hearing this, Kennedy was pleased, and from then on whenever Tuck made a slip, he'd say, "You just lost Madrid, Tuck."

There were good days too, and the day before the primary, tired and sensing defeat, Kennedy went into southern Oregon. This was great outdoors land, hunting territory, and he had been told by all his advisers that the only issue here was guns and he was in trouble because of his strong stand on gun control. (McCarthy was playing this one pretty cool.) As Kennedy arrived in Roseburg he saw the signs everywhere: "Protect Your Right to Keep and Bear Arms." He looked around and asked if anyone from the crowd would like to come up and explain why he opposed gun legislation. After a few moments hesitation, up came a man named Bud Schoon, the owner of a floor-covering business and a director of the Association To Preserve Our Right To Keep And Bear Arms, Inc.

"Is there anything in this bill which says you can't have firearms?" Kennedy asked him.

No, Schoon answered. But then he added, "We think it's a backdoor bill for registration of guns and it will let the Secretary of the Treasury keep a registry of all firearms sale."

Then Kennedy took back the microphone, and with emotion showing in his voice—angered by the fact that there was so much deception on such a basic thing (there had been John Birch literature all over Oregon on the gun bill)—he said, "If we're going to talk about this legislation, can't we do it honestly, and not say it does something that it doesn't do? All this legislation does is keep guns from

criminals and the mentally ill and those too young. With all
the violence and murder and killings in the United States
I think you will agree that we must keep firearms from those
who have no business with guns or rifles." But the crowd
was not impressed; it was frightened about losing its guns.
One man in a cowboy hat booed and shouted, "They'll get
them anyway. Someone else yelled "Nazi Germany started
with the registration of guns."

"Well I don't think the registration of cars and the
registration of drug prescriptions destroyed democracy,"
the candidate said, "and I don't think the registration of
guns will either." He left shaking his head. It was a part
of America where the deepest concern was guns, and a fear
of what was happening in the rest of the country, a belief
that the authorities would take away their guns but permit
the rest of America, the bad America, which raped and stole,
to keep theirs. Easterners should not be allowed to take
away Westerners' guns. Kennedy was depressed by the day
and he could sense the defeat coming. The last few days
had been a disaster. The Saturday before the primary, the
day when you really turn out the crowds so that on Sunday
everyone in the state can see and read how you turned it on,
had been badly botched. A Saturday morning rally had
been scheduled late Friday night, at 11 P.M. It had been
organized so late that no crowd could be drummed up, and
worse, they had no permit for it so it had to be held outside
the city limits. The next stop was next to a carnival and he
was drowned out by the noise. His face took on that cold
icy look and two other meetings were scratched and he
went back to the hotel. He was going to be beaten and he
knew it. Humphrey would be the big winner in Oregon. He
also knew that this would hurt him in California; the people
within the party who opposed him would now have a club
to use against him.

The night of the election, as the returns came in, everyone sat around despondently. In the center of the room Edith Green kept watching the early returns and saying over and over again that perhaps it was the lunch-box vote (the non-working class which votes at midday at its leisure) coming in. No one answered her; they all knew they had been beaten. They drafted his concession speech. They were privately bitter about McCarthy's sharp anti-Kennedy attacks and his strange reluctance to attack Humphrey ("He just likes Hubert better than Kennedy," said one McCarthy aide), but decided to avoid rancor; they still might win in California and they still wanted McCarthy's troops. The concession speech was a generous statement; it praised the scenic beauty of Oregon ("one of the most beautiful places in the United States"), congratulated McCarthy on his victory and said that both candidates could take pleasure in the size of the anti-administration vote. Now it was on to California, but he had made a slip there earlier, the kind of slip that more traditional politicians do not make; he had told the Commonwealth Club that unless he won all the primaries he would not be a very viable candidate. Now he would have to campaign in the embers of that statement.

On the plane to California he and Tuck discussed the plan to redistribute the ethnic balance of America so that Oregon could have a ghetto. What can you do about a place like that? Kennedy asked. Airlift in a ghetto, Tuck said. Can you really do it? How many people? asked Kennedy. Tuck did some quick mental arithmetic. Two hundred thousand, he said; with 200,000 the vote will be turned around. He quoted an imaginary headline which gave Kennedy 53 percent of the Oregon vote. "You could airlift in 20,000 a day. But will they *like* it there?" asks Kennedy. "I mean, it's *Oregon,* and all those roses." "We could have a pre-fab ghetto," says Tuck, "have the whole thing brought in. Get to an exterminator and get him to save the rats. Soul food. Give Oregon a little class."

VI

He flew to Los Angeles from Oregon with the taste of ashes still in his mouth. Before he could spend too much time talking about defeat, analyzing it and being analyzed (the press writing their Kennedy-in-defeat stories: Kennedys take defeat well), he was back in Los Angeles, into a motorcade, and a tumultuous one. All the people who had disappeared in Oregon surfaced again; the faces were different, the jumpers were back, there were Negroes again. The motorcade drove through town and as it went, a fat blonde woman ran alongside shouting, "piss on Oregon, piss on Oregon." The candidate looked around him and said he felt like renaming Los Angeles Resurrection City.

California is radically different from other states. It is without traditional organization, rather it is the symbol of the new rootless, restless America; it tells more about what this country is going to be in the future than what it has been in the past. Its suburbs are bigger, and yes, more suburban, than other people's suburbs; its kooks are kookier than other states' kooks, and its political extremists more numerous, more extreme. Berkeley exploded four years before Columbia. California is gaudier, more neurotic, more innovative than the rest of the country. The ties that bind the older America, and fashioned its political order, the small neighborhoods, the sense of community; all passed on generation to generation, are changing slowly in the rest of the country, but barely exist in California. The people who have broken with all that, the people who were too restless for the quieter America, for whom the small towns never worked, are here, breaking with their families. Californians have broken with their social communities, their ethnic groups (by the time the Poles arrive here, they will no longer be Poles because they don't live among other Poles). It is a strange new society; its politics are media politics; its organizational structure is drowned out by the endless waves of new migration into the state, diluted by the countless new people who move in every month, and who are by and large not poor and not dependent on political organizations for jobs, welfare, and housing. California has a tap dancer-actor for a Senator, another actor for its Governor. California's known, identified political boss, Jesse Unruh, was the first important organization man to urge Robert Kennedy to run and to challenge the sitting President. It is the place where the organization is more fluid and less separated from the political and social turbulence than elsewhere in the country, and where the war was an intense political issue earlier than in most sections of the nation. California has wide-open fluid politics, the least structured in the country. Of California politics it has been said that if you took the 1,000 top Democratic party officials, put them on a barge and sank the barge, all you would lose is 1,000 votes. California is different. It is new politics and Kennedy was glad to be there.

There is a quality of release to California; one senses that at first newcomers either react against it, or join it. The youth of Indiana do not, for instance, live together as freely and as easily as the youth of California, nor do their somewhat older colleagues advertise themselves sexually in the, say, Terre Haute *Free Press* the way they do in the L.A. *Free Press*. The good youth of Indiana might not like

Robert Kennedy but they would be unlikely to view him as
a political opiate trying to trick them back into staying in
the system (a device of Lyndon Johnson), a system which
they feel has failed completely. If they question the system
at all, the good youth of Indiana question it very cautiously.
The liberals in Indiana, those who worried about the war
and were early doves, might have regretted that Kennedy
did not enter the race earlier, might have gone with Mc-
Carthy. Once Kennedy entered the race, they might have
forgiven him, or perhaps being of a strong moral sense, they
might have remained loyal to McCarthy. Whichever, they
would not, as many of the peace people in California did,
turn on Robert Kennedy with all the vengeance of betrayed
lovers. He had wronged them; he had failed to enter, then
he had entered and challenged their pure hero. With the
peace people in California, it was a blood war; it was emotional, for it is probably true of the new media-based politics
that the relationship between candidate and constituency is
much more emotional and neurotic. This would hurt Kennedy in California; and if it were true about the parents,
then it was even more true among the alienated and embittered kids.

Kennedy had sampled some of the intensity and neu-
rosis of California's politics early in the campaign. He had
been campaigning in Indiana and had flown out to California for a day and a half—a hectic emotional time. It had
started in San Diego when he had arrived; a huge crowd of
blacks and whites was at the airport, and among them, a
group of young radicals, bitter and hostile. One of them,
hearing the rest of the crowd cheer, turned to Pete Hamill,
a free-lance writer and a friend of Kennedy's and said, "He's
a fink like the rest of them."

Why? asked Hamill.

"He's not talking about revolution. He just wants to

put Band-Aids on the problems. He doesn't want to destroy the System."

What's the system, Hamill asked.

"Finks like you," the kid said. Paper revolutionaries, Hamill thought.

At the airport members of the newly formed Peace and Freedom Party were handing out mimeographed sheets of paper quoting from *MacBird. MacBird*, the play written by Barbara Garson, accuses Lyndon Johnson of murdering John Kennedy with the aid of Robert Kennedy. It is considered a fashionable play in radical and even some liberal circles, though if Mrs. Garson had been a right-winger instead of a left-winger, and had written the exact same words, it probably would have been considered a less respectable play. The lines from the play went:

> *We must expose this subtle bobcat's claws*
> *He even now collects the straying sheep*
> *And nudges them so gently toward the fold.*
> *O sheep, awake and flee this fenced corral*
> *He's just like all the rest. They're all alike.*

But it would get worse that night, at a rally at the University of San Francisco auditorium. The audience, though composed of different parts, was dominated by the Peace and Freedom kids. They were well-organized, angry, bitter, and they hated someone like Kennedy more than Johnson or Rusk, because to them Kennedy was more dangerous, he was the chocolate coating which might lull the others back to the system. When he entered they were screaming and chanting, Victory for the Vietcong; Free Huey Newton (a Black Panther currently in prison charged with killing a policeman and thus a local radical hero); Victory for the Vietcong. A kid rushed up and spit in his face, screaming "Fascist Pig." The face went cold. Kennedy put away his prepared text, it was the only thing to do, and tried to answer questions. Did you work for Joe Kennedy, someone shouted, getting the name wrong in his excitement, and Kennedy, released from the ugly shouting, laughed. Joe Kennedy, Yes, I worked for Joe Kennedy; he's my father.

Why are you running, someone shouted, and Kennedy traced his involvement in government, the Cuban Missile crisis, the Bay of Pigs. He thought he could make a contribution, he said, trying to save the peace. He wanted to keep America from being involved in other Vietnams.

Victory for the Vietcong, a kid yelled.

Victory for the Vietcong? Kennedy said, somewhat surprised, No, I don't agree with that.

Victory for the Vietcong, the kid repeated. (Later Kennedy told a reporter: those people, the ones who yell Victory for the Vietcong, I can't help people like that, someone who hates this country. Someone who comes up to me, and says, look, this and this and this are wrong, we've got to change it—I can help them. I can understand that, and I can understand some of the bitterness. I can understand the alienation and the eighteen year old black kid who comes to me and says this country means nothing to me, I'm outside it; prove it to me, prove that it's worth it. I can understand that. What has this country offered to a kid like that? Someone like that can be helped. But not the ones who hate it and want to destroy it. How can you help them? It's psychological with so many of them. I can't be their psychiatrist.)

Another kid asked a belligerent question, a question filled with hate spilling over so that in the end one forgot what the question was about and remembered only the hatred and the edge and the bitterness. Kennedy, a little tired, answered, "What we need in this country is to cut down the belligerence. If we let this hatred and emotion control our lives, we're lost."

"It's our lives," one of the kids yelled.

He continued to talk and it got worse; they shouted and booed and yelled for the Vietcong. It was a nightmare evening; he handled it well. Later, when the Kennedy people left, some of the Peace and Freedom kids threw pebbles and apple cores at the motorcade. Bright, upper-middle-class kids, children of affluence, they believed in the doctrines of the New Left, that if a society is wrong you can do anything you want to redress it, and if someone says something you don't like, you can drown him out and deprive him of his speech. It was an ugly hour, for one sensed that it would get worse, that this was not going to be the last such evening in American life. Later Kennedy would talk with a reporter about it, and talk about the cycle of extremism and violence; that violence and extremism on one side beget extremism on the other. Each somehow makes the other feel that it is permissible and justifiable to do whatever you like.

That night on the plane a group of reporters were talking about the evening, how unpleasant it had been, so much hatred.

"I thought he handled it well," Mankiewicz said.

"But it was so goddamn demeaning," said a reporter.

"So is politics," said another reporter.

A few minutes later someone mentioned the evening to Kennedy. "That was pretty nice back there," the candidate said.

"For a fascist pig you did all right," the reporter answered.

"Yes," he said, "as one fascist pig to another."

Now he was back in California, and all along he had counted on this state to save him. There had been times when it had seemed as if he would be able to take 60 percent in California, though that had been while Johnson was still in the race. Now hopes for sixty were gone, but perhaps in the fifties, the mid-fifties. He had a good base, the Mexicans and the Negroes, but he had to work on the liberals; he was in serious trouble there. Some reports were that he was around 35 percent in middle class liberal districts.

Not among the Mexicans and the Negroes, however. The new complexities, the subtleties of the new politics, were far from their minds. Their issues were survival issues, they were involved in the kind of politics that went back to the early days of the New Deal. Robert Kennedy symbolized to them that America might care. His relationship with the Mexicans was unique; other politicians had courted the Negroes, but no other major political figure had made the cause of the grape pickers his own. That was a special act, for the grape owners are very powerful in the Democratic party. Robert Kennedy, baited a little by his young staff, had finally gone out there, had been moved, and had returned to go to Mass with Cesar Chavez. Could there have been a more symbolic moment? It was the kind of political symbolism which had passed from most of America in our new affluence, the dramatization of a relationship with an ethnic group. Going to a synagogue with Arthur Goldberg would not get back the Jews. It was a momentous occasion; within hours after it had happened, every Mexican American in the area knew of it—it was history. Kennedy had visited the strikers in 1966, had visited the fields and then had held hearings on the strikes. The local sheriff had testified that they were making preventive arrests because they were afraid of violence on the part of the pickets or on the part of the local people who did not like the pickets. The sheriff was very benign about this, pointing out also that he took photographs of all the pickets, and finally Kennedy had looked at him, all the coldness and the controlled anger there, and said: "I just want to ask you one thing. Have you ever read the Constitution of the United States?" The Mexicans had not forgotten. Now in 1968 they would say again and again that he had visited them in *1966;* a great man come to honor their little cause, and now wherever he went, the crowds were enormous. His speeches were terribly simple. Decency is the heart of the matter, he said to them. The death and maiming of young men in the swamps of Asia is indecent. For a man to work with his hands in the valley of California with no hope of sending his son to college, that is also indecent. I think we can do better in America. It was simple enough, but the question had always been whether the Mexicans would vote. Mexicans are bad voters. But they did turn out. In Mexican districts that morning, in house after house, workers came around saying very simply: "Cesar says this is the day to vote for Robert Kennedy." It was the biggest turnout in their history. They voted roughly 15-to-1 over McCarthy, and turned the towns, where anti-Mexican feeling went to McCarthy, into Kennedy camps.

The Negroes would do the same. Kennedy had the Negroes, there was no doubt—it was one of the few remaining love affairs in American politics. In part it was the product of the John Kennedy years. At the beginning of the campaign a poll showed that while only 39 percent of the general population believed that Robert Kennedy "has the same outstanding qualities of his brother," 94 percent of the black people felt that way, an astonishing and quite revealing statistic. It was of course helpful that in an inordinate number of American homes the photographs on the wall were of Jesus Christ, the Pope, Martin Luther King and John Kennedy—but it was also Robert Kennedy himself.

He was drawn to them, felt their cause was the most important thing in America. He did not think one had to

go through formal channels to talk with the anointed leaders, but rather he made himself available to a vast variety
of black spokesmen. He had listened, was not bored, was
not condescending, and they knew this, and were touched
by him. He would campaign in the ghettos, always going
beyond the allotted time, teasing with the youngsters, asking
them what they studied in history, whether they liked school.
Who's your favorite president? he would ask. You, you you,
they'd shout. No, no, that's not what I mean. He'd grin, he
was touched by them. He said to Jimmy Breslin one day
in Watts, "These are the best-looking people in the country
until they're twelve. You look at the faces. They're alive and
have such expressions. What is it? These kids growing up
face so many challenges right where they live that it shows
in their faces. A character. Then when they get to about
twelve, the challenges become too much for them. They get
overwhelmed. Then the faces change. They become these
masks. But until they're twelve they're marvelous. Much
better-looking children than these kids you'd see on Fifth
Avenue with their maids walking them."

The affection was there. Every time the candidate entered a ghetto it would begin again, black hands reaching
for white hands, a rare enough sight in the America of the
late sixties, and he would be very gentle, occasionally ad-
monishing an extra body guard to be more gentle, "Easy
Jimmy, your hands are white and theirs are black." But the
question always was, Would they reciprocate, would they
really go out and vote? There had been a smear campaign
at the end. Drew Pearson, who wrote favorably about Humphrey, had written a column saying that Kennedy had au-
thorized the bugging of Martin Luther King's telephone.
That King's telephone had been tapped was not exactly news.
Everyone in the country, it seemed, knew the FBI had
bugged King's phone. The FBI had the tapes and would
play them for reporters and for Southern congressmen. It

was one of the finer smears in America since there was no way of combatting it; it was the old Communist throttler at his best, saving Democracy for future generations. The column had been picked up by the McCarthy people, and there were radio spots, in a heavy Negro voice, saying, "I used to be for Robert Kennedy, but then I learned about how he bugged my brother Martin Luther King's phone." For a while Kennedy was a little nervous, but then Charles Evers, who was in California speaking for Kennedy, went around Watts sampling barbershop opinion and reported back that it was nothing to worry about. Most Negroes, he said, felt they did not need Drew Pearson to tell them how to vote. One man told Evers, "It's like someone comes to you and tells you your wife is cheating but you love her so much anyway you just don't care."

The mythology of black politics is that Negroes too are bad voters. But there were people in the Kennedy camp who felt that just the reverse was true, that they are very good voters, simply more sophisticated than white people realize. Often they don't care; the choice of two white politicians normally doesn't move them very much and they see marginal differences. Given two candidates whom they measure in degrees of hostility, they will not vote in opposition to the slightly more desirable man. They just will not vote for him either. Thus in Los Angeles they have traditionally voted about 15 percent below the county turnout for whites, with the exception of the 1936 Roosevelt campaign, and the 1950 Helen Gahagan Douglas Senate race (she had been badly smeared on the race question). In 1968 the turnout would prove to be staggering; they would not only vote up to the white level, but in many sections went 5 and 10 percent above it. It is very easy to keep the pressure on in California to get out the vote. There are lists of voters at every polling booth and every hour the list is posted, with those who have voted scratched out. Thus a poll watcher with phone numbers can tell exactly who has voted and who hasn't and can contact those who haven't.

The California people working for Kennedy could not believe the enthusiasm or number of Negroes working for him. In 1956 Dutton, working for Pat Brown and needing precinct workers, had called a number of domestic agencies and hired workers at ten dollars a head; for this election there were about 5,000 volunteers. Later, after the vote, after the assassination, Jesse Unruh would understand what it all meant. He would turn to a friend and say that that was the Negro vote for this year. "We can't get them out again. They'll never come back like that."

But there was a strategy battle over where to make the effort among the whites. There was so little time, so little organization. They were already annoyed with Unruh; they liked him, but they decided his machine was typical of California, he was a boss without a real organization. "Jesse was a real poor boy. Came out of the dust bowl. He was very bright and very ambitious; in fact he reminded us a lot of a young Lyndon Johnson," one Kennedy staff member said. "But we had a hell of a time convincing him to broaden the delegation out. His idea of it was his immediate family, a few of their friends, his staff people and a few of their friends. That's not exactly the way to win in California. We liked him a lot. There's something good there. But sometimes I think we'd have been a lot better off without him, just going in there by ourselves." Now, late in the campaign, they were regretting their early confidence and dependence on him.

In Indiana and Nebraska they had realized they didn't have the local organization and as such they had no illusions; they had gone in and done the whole thing themselves, made the tough decisions, put their own people in from top to bottom. But in both Oregon, where they had what they thought was Edith Green's organization, and now in California, where they had the Unruh organization, they had picked up more illusions than anything else. In retrospect, an Edith Green organization just does not exist, or if it does, it is a highly nontransferable apparatus (except for the enemies), and they felt afterward that they would have been better off going in on their own and creating their own organization. Now in California it was worse, because there was more illusion and less organization than anywhere else. Unruh, whom they considered a good man ("one of the most humane professional politicians in the country," one Kennedy man called him), had nevertheless been feuding with the liberals, and they picked up all those animosities. In addition, he simply did not understand the breadth and intensity of a Kennedy campaign. "Jesse was always trying to keep everyone out but his own people, without realizing it he was really narrowing our base. His theory was a small operation, and our theory always was that if five people could do the job, and twenty-five showed up, you found places for the twenty-five." The California situation, which had been very good at the start, slipped badly, and by May the Kennedys had been forced to send Steve Smith and John Seigenthaler in full time, and had even detached Mankiewicz from the traveling party to work full time in Los Angeles, his original home.

There remained the growing dispute over where to make the effort among the whites; among the liberals, who had turned to McCarthy, in the suburbs or among the white backlashers. Unruh and his people wanted to go for the backlashers and the suburbs; it was an area where they were more at ease and, according to one Kennedy man, where they "had fewer enemies; so they were pulled that way." But the outsiders, the Kennedy people, wanted to make the effort among the liberals because by all the laws of American politics they felt the liberals should be for Kennedy, and they were uneasy about what would happen if he failed to run well among the liberals in California. It might harden and become part of the permanent political and journalistic ethos of Robert Kennedy: liberals don't like Kennedy and won't vote for him. Perhaps they would never turn it around. The liberal suspicion had haunted him all during this campaign, and it probably was the one thing that got under his skin. It was a product of many things. The liberals, after all, had not changed very much over the last sixteen years, since that first exhilarating Stevenson campaign, and Robert Kennedy had changed a great deal; they found that hard to accept. He had carried on his education in public and his mistakes were a matter of record. He had been the tough lightening rod of his brother's years, handling all the thankless jobs. He liked power, and he looked like he liked power, and many of the liberals, particularly the Stevensonians, drew back from power; there was something inherently evil in power. For the liberal intellectuals, many of them Jews, it was almost an ethnic thing—he looked too Irish-Catholic for them; they believed him more like his father than his brother; and they remained uneasy with him. Their defection hurt him the most. He had gone through it all once before, wearing a yarmulke all over New York City, sensing the strength of their distrust, but finally winning their votes if not their affection. Now in the campaign the Jews were retaining all the old suspicions, and this hurt him. Again and again with friends (at times, half of his advisers seemed to be Jewish) he would ask why it was happening and they would try to explain. But I thought we had established a relationship, and then they did not come across, he said. Some of the McCarthy support he could understand, he said, but now some of these people in New York and California, people who had asked him to make the race, were for Humphrey. *Humphrey*. Someone said not to worry, that if he got the nomination they would all come home. It's not the same thing, he said; if they vote for me against Richard Nixon, what does that mean? What kind of consolation prize is that?

Now in California, his advisers suggested that the major effort be to court the liberals. The Kennedy people thought the Unruh people looked down on the liberals and, more important, underestimated them as a force in California politics. There was a group of people which the Kennedys grouped as intellectual-liberals-academic-professional-people. They were roughly one half Jewish, said a Kennedy aide, and the rest might just as well be; they had the same voter profile. They equaled about 8 percent of the California population, 4 percent Jewish, 4 percent non-Jewish, but since they were almost all Democrats, they equaled about 10 percent of the total Democratic party. But since they voted with a special fervor, they represented roughly 15 percent of the voting Democrats, and since they were respected and influential, they could carry satellites with them, making a total of 20 percent. But in early May they were for McCarthy in roughly a 2-to-1 ratio and so a major effort was initiated to swing it around the other way. A collection of very distinguished liberals was imported to talk to small groups, coffee klatches, synagogues—always looking for groups which were either anti-Kennedy or fence-sitting. In they came, Pat Moynihan, Robert Coles, Arthur Schlesinger, Michael Harrington, Edwin Reischauer, Roger Hilsman, Roswell Gilpatric, Cesar Chavez (for white liberals). On one campus, Moynihan was speaking about the

Negroes, and up came the question, What about wire tapping. Moynihan, too busy with the blacks all those years,
didn't really know about the wire tapping. But he happened
to look up and there was a sign which said "Alexander Bickel
will speak here at 2 P.M." and he said, well when Bob Kennedy was appointed Attorney General, Alex Bickel had
called it the worst appointment in the history of the republic, but when Kennedy left office he wrote in the *New Republic* that Kennedy had the best record on civil liberties of
anyone in years, and now he's speaking here today for
Kennedy and if you have any questions you can ask him.

In a sense the strategy probably worked. Some of the
Kennedy people thought it was a waste of manpower, and
that the guests didn't reach enough people, but the general
feeling was that they had made ripples beyond expectation
for Kennedy. McCarthy still carried the liberal areas, but
by a much narrower margin. The problem, of course, was
California's rootlessness. The California experts remained
dubious about the idea of the imported speakers. Yes, sure,
they spoke to a group of fifty people, and those fifty people
had fifty wives, and fifty friends to whom they could say,
"Well, you know, I had a pretty interesting talk with that
Pat Moynihan, and he told me some things about Kennedy
I didn't know and I want to think about this election a little
longer." But finally, even those many converts, if they were
all converted, would be too few. The Unruh regulars, of
course, wanted a more traditional campaign, and had more
confidence in the efficiency of their organization than the
outsiders; but they were all bewildered by the same question: how do you reach the people?

The people had come to California and lost their roots,
their dependence on one another, their knowledge of and
ties with their neighbors. They no longer lived in the neat
little neighborhoods in which they had grown up. California

was a long way from Thornton Wilder's *Our Town,* another country. (One wondered what Wilder would do with the new America of California; would he sound more like Harold Pinter?) Now their new relationships came from the media—it existed, it was dependable, it was there every night, and had certain known, identified, friendly characteristics. They knew and felt at ease with the talk shows—Merv, Johnny, Joey—and inevitably California politics became media politics; it was the only way of reaching into those great disorganized scattered neighborhoods. So Kennedy now turned, for guidance on how to run a media campaign in California, to Dutton, the expert on California politics who had helped run those surprisingly successful early Pat Brown races. Dutton, not a close friend at the start, had grown closer and closer to Kennedy as the campaign developed. He had always been one of the brightest men that the Kennedys had brought to Washington in 1961, bright, talented, honest but modest. He lacked a capacity for self-glorification and dramatization and he was not nearly as widely known as he should have been. Dutton fashioned a television campaign which everyone in the Kennedy camp agreed was the most brilliant ever done in California—until afterward, when they realized what McCarthy had done, and realized that he, a rank outsider, had done it better.

There are three major television markets in California: the San Francisco area, the Los Angeles area, and the San Diego area. Traditionally a candidate would arrive in California, spend a day in Los Angeles, then the next day on to San Francisco, and then the next day on to San Diego. But Dutton had changed that; jet travel was so simple these days that they would begin in San Diego in the morning, fly to another market in the afternoon, and finish in the third market area in the evening. That way they would touch all three major markets in one day, and the local television stations would all rush out and get the scene: candidate arriving, jet coming to a halt, candidate shaking hands, jostling of the airport crowd, into town, five words from his speech; it was free television time in all three areas each day. They were all pleased with this. The candidate told people often Fred Dutton had the best political judgment of anyone he knew, and they were very pleased until they realized what McCarthy had done.

McCarthy could not draw crowds the way Kennedy could. Where Kennedy would draw 15,000, he would draw 1,500, and he knew this, and the press knew this, and nothing would irritate him more than to read the stories the next day where the press would judge him for his crowd gap. The crowds bored him anyway; he did not like the grabbing and the thrashing; and so rather than be judged badly on something he didn't like in the first place, wearing himself down, burning up his time and energy, he skipped crowd stops as much as he could and went instead on the radio shows and the televisions talk shows. There are hundreds, perhaps thousands, of them in California, and there is a great secret to getting on them—show up at the studio. The proprietors, of course, are delighted, and by and large it is the sweetest kind of questioning in the world. Good morning Senator, could you please tell us what a hell of a good guy you are and what your fine record is. Then, fifteen minutes later, Thank you Senator for taking the time to come by and explain to us what a terrific guy you are. And this was McCarthy at his best, witty, sometimes gentle, being a little nasty about Robert Kennedy. Suddenly the Kennedy camp realized what had happened. There would be two minutes on television each night of Robert Kennedy being mauled, losing his shoes, and then there would be fifteen *free*—that was painful—minutes of Gene McCarthy talking leisurely and seriously about the issues. That Gene McCarthy, the people would say, is a serious man; and the quiet man had turned a liability into an asset. Kennedy could draw crowds, it was one of his special strengths, and he was tied to doing the crowd thing. McCarthy was not able to do the things of the past, such as draw crowds, and thus was freer to take advantage of the new things. Now the Kennedy people realized that McCarthy had run, perhaps not by intention, a better television campaign in California.

In a somewhat modified form, this had bothered the Kennedys earlier in the campaign. The TV men covering him would always shoot him with the crowds, good stuff though rarely of substance, and the film clips would come in to the great networks. On that particular day McCarthy would do little because there was little in the way of crowds, but in order to have *something,* he and the TV reporters covering him might do small-spot interviews so that networks, who would not want to run Kennedy without McCarthy, would have something to balance the Kennedy coverage. So again they would portray a mauled Kennedy and a serious thoughtful McCarthy. A few days later the Kennedy people would want to show a Serious Kennedy and, in the morning, they would summon a TV man and give him a small exclusive, serious interview; then they would all go out campaigning and the crowds would maul Kennedy and the TV men would shoot that too. Both cans of films would come in to the networks and since one can was action, it was also *news,* and it would be used and the interview would be thrown away. In desperation one of Kennedy's aides finally told him that if he wanted to be serious and thoughtful he would have to stay in his hotel room all day and be serious and thoughtful there.

But now the campaign was almost over, and he was driving himself relentlessly. Just these few more days and he could ease off, reduce the twenty hour day to a sixteen hour day, a fifteen stop day to a four stop one. He rested only for the great debate with McCarthy; the debate was to be on a Saturday night and on Friday he told an aide: "I'll have my biggest crowd of the year out here tomorrow."

"No, no," said the aide, "you have the day off except for the debate. We canceled everything off."

"No, it's my largest crowd of the year," he insisted. "All my advisers are flying in from all over the country to tell me what to say. It'll be a hell of a crowd." He was in a good mood.

The debate, like most highly promoted things in American political life, such as conventions, contained less than met the eye. It was not a debate, it was a love-in; they had no great dispute. They complemented each other: McCarthy would fire Dean Rusk; Kennedy would not deal in personalities. McCarthy wanted only the exposure that went with challenging Kennedy face to face; Kennedy wanted only to soften the ruthless image which had built up against him. It was a mutually pedestrian performance, and as far as convincing people went, it probably had a marginal effect; most people would watch it and see what they wanted to see and hear what they wanted to hear. *The New York Times* editorial page gave it to McCarthy; I gave it to Kennedy. It seemed to me that the great issue of the campaign, at this point in California, was not Vietnam or ghettos, but Bobby himself. He succeeded in softening the issues against himself; he did not look ruthless and he seemed McCarthy's intellectual equal that night though even the announcer seemed both men's intellectual equal that night. But now it was over and there was precious little time left. McCarthy was blitzing now, coming on hard with a strong television campaign. There are only two ways of doing your television programming: either you save up your television money and blitz at the end, or you spread it out evenly. McCarthy, who was less well known, decided to blitz hard at the end, pound away with the name right before the election. It was the right strategy for him, the Kennedy people acknowledged, whereas with Kennedy the problem was different; he was already well known, so they spread it out more evenly to ease the ruthless issue.

The mood in the Kennedy camp was becoming a little more optimistic and more relaxed. Abba Schwartz, who had handled immigration in the state department, came out and helped work with the Chinese and had explained to some of the Kennedy people how to vote the Chinese. Tuck had answered, yes, that was fine, but the only problem was that two hours after you voted them you had to vote them again.

They were convinced now that they would come out of the state running hard, so all through the California campaign they hammered away at Humphrey, the enemy. It was good politics; implicitly it said that McCarthy was not a serious figure, and this was helping to ease some of the Eastern liberal feeling against Kennedy. For McCarthy was slightly trapped; he had to run against Kennedy to stay in and he was doing this, sharply and caustically, but the impression was growing among some of McCarthy's foremost supporters that he was too hard on Kennedy and too soft on Humphrey. Clean Gene, among some of the kids and some of the intellectuals, was becoming tarnished for the first time.

For some reason Oregon no longer seemed so final; Kennedy's advisers sensed they were going to come out of California with a real chance. They had already evolved a fairly sophisticated post-California strategy; a national grass-roots television campaign would be mounted, which would be similar in some ways to the one Rockefeller finally used, except much less emphasis would be on newspaper advertising and more on television. They would have five-minute spots five nights a week, right before the 11 o'clock news: *This is Robert Kennedy and I want to talk to the people of the nation just as I did to the people in the states with primaries.* Then finally one long thirty-minute program, virtually a speech by the candidate, spliced in with documentary shots of the public life of Robert Kennedy. Then an intense travel schedule from California to New York where the New York primary was to be held June 18, and where the Kennedy people were in serious trouble fighting a well-organized peace campaign. (As in California, the best people had gone over to McCarthy, and they had the best slates; he was still fighting the late entry.) Then from New York all over the country, a schedule arranged by Sorensen; twenty-six states where the delegates were still flexible. They would stop by in Chicago. "A good meeting with Daley. We'll be very respectful, very polite. Here, Mister Mayor, is what we can do, where we run strong, and here's Humphrey's strength and McCarthy's strength. All very polite. Then we'll go into the ghetto and get one hell of a response." Then a quick flying trip overseas to show that a major American political figure can still be acclaimed: *Robert Kennedy Wildly Cheered in Paris, Rome, Warsaw.* All of this, of course, designed for crowds, for publicity, for impact, and mostly to touch the polls and thus the delegates.

They felt that the delegates could still be wooed. Humphrey was far ahead in delegate strength, but Kennedy did not believe that it was a particularly strong hold; indeed Kennedy and the people around him sensed that Humphrey's position would go not up but down as the convention approached, and this, his strength, would erode. They believed that much of Humphrey's resurrection was tied directly to the euphoria of the Paris peace talks and Johnson's magnanimous gesture. That had taken place on March 31; it would last for six or seven weeks, but then, as June moved along and July arrived, the euphoria would end, the old malaise about the war and about the administration would return. By early July it would be the new Hubert and the old war and the old malaise, for Humphrey was tied directly to things which were outside his control and which looked insoluble. (Although the Kennedy people felt the Humphrey delegate counts were inflated, they deliberately refused to challenge the figures. There were two reasons. The first was that they thought Humphrey's grip was soft and they did not want to alert the Vice-President's people to this until after the primaries when it would be too late. The second reason was that they were sure that after the primaries there would be erosion from Humphrey's total, and they were anxious to create a reverse bandwagon psychology for the Vice-President.) In addition, Kennedy thought McCarthy's hold on his young people was bound to slip. There were already signs that it was slipping; the Oregon campaign, with its attacks upon Kennedy rather than Humphrey, had given rise to some disillusionment.

So he pushed harder and harder. The Monday before the California primary he put in the final, most bone-crushing day of all. He covered 1,200 miles of the state, touched every ethnic group, and made a triumphant visit to Watts. Teasing with them, he said, Yes, you come out to see me. Are you just going to wave to Mr. Kennedy and then tomorrow when I'm gone forget about me, or are you going to vote? I think you'll probably forget about me. The exhaustion showed; in San Diego where he spoke to a rally—

divided into two sections because there were so many people; 2,500 in the first seating, 2,500 in the second—he collapsed momentarily between speeches. But it was a strong day. The response of the crowds encouraged him, and at one point while discussing why he was running, he said, "My first responsibility is to the United States, not to the Democratic party. It is a responsibility to the country itself. Now, feeling as strongly as I do, I can do nothing other than what I am doing."

Election day. A good day. Enormous Negro and Mexican turnouts. The results were very good; the day was looking better and better. Early in the evening the results came in from South Dakota, and they were impressive; indeed they may have spelled the beginning of the end for Humphrey. South Dakota, where Kennedy had spent so little time, is Humphrey's backyard—a rural state and the vice-president's birthplace—and now it was giving Kennedy 50 percent, McCarthy 20 percent, and a Johnson slate, which was pledged to Humphrey, only 30 percent. It was astounding news, a staggering victory, and Kennedy knew this would have a powerful effect on Daley. Humphrey could not even run well in his own region, where he is best known. It was one of the least-noticed political events of the year, but a persuasive piece of evidence, and Kennedy immediately and joyously recognized its significance. Earlier in the evening he had talked with Dun Gifford, a young lawyer on Teddy's staff who was helping to handle delegate counts. He had asked him about the delegate counts and Gifford said they'd be assembled for him tomorrow, "and you're going to like them." Curiously, they had gotten better since Oregon; the defeat there had taken the edge off some of the hostility toward the candidate. It was a remarkable thing, Oregon had made him more attractive. "Don't try and kid me with delegate counts," Kennedy said. "I used to do them myself." Now the air was expectant and the early results were good; they showed Kennedy winning a major victory. One of the networks said it would be 54 percent, a smashing victory. Not sixty, but with South Dakota it was enough to remove most of the stigma of Oregon. His spirits were buoyant. Earlier in the evening Pat Paulsen, the new television comic, had referred to Humphrey as Herbert Humphrey ("I will debate all of the candidates for President in a place of their choosing. I will even debate Herbert Humphrey in a smoke-filled room"), and that caught Kennedy's fancy. It somehow seemed to fit Humphrey and now, grinning, he said, "I'm going to chase Herbert's ass all over the country. Every-where he goes I'll go too." Then he descended to acknowl-edge his victory, to talk about the violence and the divisive-ness, and to let a nation discover in his death what it had never understood or believed about him during his life.

ABOUT THE AUTHOR

Born in New York City thirty-four years ago, DAVID
HALBERSTAM graduated from Harvard in 1955. For
five years he worked for newspapers in Mississippi
and Tennessee before joining *The New York Times*
in 1960. As a foreign correspondent for that paper,
he served in the Congo, Vietnam and Poland, and
his dispatches from Southeast Asia won him the
Pulitzer Prize in 1964.

Mr. Halberstam is the author of *The Making of
a Quagmire,* an account of our commitment in Vietnam, and of two novels, *The Noblest Roman* and
One Very Hot Day. For the last eighteen months he
has been a contributing editor of *Harper's Magazine,* covering the American political scene.